MW00997875

STUDY GUIDE *for* KINN'S THE MEDICAL ASSISTANT AN APPLIED SCIENCE LEARNING APPROACH

Eleventh Edition

Alexandra Patricia Young-Adams, BBA, RMA, CMA (AAMA), MA
Adjunct Instructor
Everest College, Arlington Midcities Campus
Arlington, Texas
Professional Writer
Grand Prairie, Texas

Deborah B. Proctor, EdD, RN
Professor and Medical Assistant Program Director
Butler County Community College
Butler, Pennsylvania

SAUNDERS
ELSEVIER

SAUNDERS
ELSEVIER

3251 Riverport Lane
St. Louis, Missouri 63043

STUDY GUIDE FOR KINN'S THE MEDICAL ASSISTANT
AN APPLIED LEARNING APPROACH

ISBN: 978-1-4160-5443-6

Copyright © 2011, 2007, 2003, 1999, 1993, 1988, 1981, 1974, 1967, 1960, 1956 by Saunders, an imprint of Elsevier Inc.

All rights reserved. No part of this publication may be reproduced or transmitted in any form or by any means, electronic or mechanical, including photocopy, recording, or any information storage and retrieval system, without permission in writing from the publisher.

Notices

Knowledge and best practice in this field are constantly changing. As new research and experience broaden our understanding, changes in research methods, professional practices, or medical treatment may become necessary.

Practitioners and researchers must always rely on their own experience and knowledge in evaluating and using any information, methods, compounds, or experiments described herein. In using such information or methods they should be mindful of their own safety and the safety of others, including parties for whom they have a professional responsibility.

With respect to any drug or pharmaceutical products identified, readers are advised to check the most current information provided (i) on procedures featured or (ii) by the manufacturer of each product to be administered, to verify the recommended dose or formula, the method and duration of administration, and contraindications. It is the responsibility of practitioners, relying on their own experience and knowledge of their patients, to make diagnoses, to determine dosages and the best treatment for each individual patient, and to take all appropriate safety precautions.

To the fullest extent of the law, neither the Publisher nor the authors, contributors, or editors, assume any liability for any injury and/or damage to persons or property as a matter of products liability, negligence or otherwise, or from any use or operation of any methods, products, instructions, or ideas contained in the material herein.

Executive Editor: Susan Cole
Associate Developmental Editors: Jennifer Presley and Jamie Augustine
Publishing Services Manager: Julie Eddy
Project Manager: Rich Barber

Printed in the United States

Last digit is the print number: 9 8 7 6 5 4 3 2 1

Working together to grow
libraries in developing countries

www.elsevier.com | www.bookaid.org | www.sabre.org

ELSEVIER BOOK AID International Sabre Foundation

To the Student

This study guide was created to help you to achieve the objectives of each chapter in *Kinn's: The Medical Assistant: An Applied Learning Approach* and to establish a solid base of knowledge in medical assisting. Completing the exercises in each chapter in this guide will help reinforce the material studied in the textbook and learned in class.

Study Hints for All Students

Ask Questions!

There are no stupid questions. If you do not know something or are not sure about it, you need to find out. Other people may be wondering the same thing but may be too shy to ask. The answer could mean life or death to your patient. That is certainly more important than feeling embarrassed about asking a question.

Chapter Objectives

At the beginning of each chapter in the textbook are learning objectives that you should have mastered by the time you have finished studying that chapter. Write these objectives in your notebook, leaving a blank space after each. Fill in the answers as you find them while reading the chapter. Review to make sure your answers are correct and complete. Use these answers when you study for tests. You should also do this for separate course objectives that your instructor has listed in your class syllabus.

Vocabulary

At the beginning of each chapter in the textbook are vocabulary terms that you will encounter as you read the chapter. These terms are in bold type the first time they appear in the chapter.

Summary of Learning Objectives

Use the Summary of Learning Objectives at the end of each chapter in the textbook to help you review for exams.

Reading Hints

As you read each chapter in the textbook, look at the subject headings to learn what each section is about. Read first for the general meaning and then reread parts you did not understand. It may help to read those parts aloud. Carefully read the information given in each table and study each figure and its legend.

Concepts

While studying, put difficult concepts into your own words to determine whether you understand them. Check this understanding with another student or the instructor. Write these concepts in your notebook.

Class Notes

When taking lecture notes in class, leave a large margin on the left side of each notebook page and write only on right-hand pages, leaving all left-hand pages blank. Look over your lecture notes soon after each class, while your memory is fresh. Fill in missing words, complete sentences and ideas, and underline key phrases, definitions, and concepts. At the top of each page, write the topic of that page. In the left margin, write the key word for that part of your notes. On the opposite left-hand page, write a summary or outline that combines material from the textbook and the lecture. These can be your study notes for review.

Study Groups

Form a study group with some other students so that you can help one another. Practice speaking and reading aloud. Ask questions about material you find unclear. Work together to find answers.

References for Improving Study Skills

Good study skills are essential for achieving your goals in medical assisting. Time management, efficient use of study time, and a consistent approach to studying are all beneficial. Various methods can be used for reading a textbook and taking class notes. Some methods that have proven helpful can be found in *Saunders Health Professional's Planner*.

Copyright © 2011, 2007, 2003 by Saunders, an imprint of Elsevier Inc. All rights reserved.

Additional Study Hints for English as a Second Language (ESL) Students

Vocabulary

If you find a nontechnical word you do not know (e.g., drowsy), try to guess its meaning from the sentence (e.g., With electrolyte imbalance, the patient may feel fatigued and drowsy.). If you are not sure of the meaning or if it seems particularly important, look it up in the dictionary.

Vocabulary Notebook

Keep a small alphabetized notebook or address book in your pocket or purse. Write down new nontechnical words you read or hear, along with their meanings and pronunciations. Write each word under its initial letter so that you can find it easily, as in a dictionary. For words you do not know or for words that have a different meaning in medical assisting, write down how each word is used and how it is pronounced. Look up the meanings of these words in a dictionary or ask your instructor or first-language buddy (see the following section). Then write the different meanings or uses that you have found in your book, including the medical assisting meaning. Continue to add new words as you discover them.

First-Language Buddy

English as a second language (ESL) students should find a first-language buddy—another student who is a native speaker of English and who is willing to answer questions about word meanings, pronunciations, and culture. Maybe, in turn, your buddy would like to learn about your language and culture; this could be useful for his or her medical assisting career.

Copyright © 2011, 2007, 2003 by Saunders, an imprint of Elsevier Inc. All rights reserved.

Contents

Copyright © 2011, 2007, 2003 by Saunders, an imprint of Elsevier Inc. All rights reserved.

Copyright © 2011, 2007, 2003 by Saunders, an imprint of Elsevier Inc. All rights reserved.

Copyright © 2011, 2007, 2003 by Saunders, an imprint of Elsevier Inc. All rights reserved.

1 Becoming a Successful Student

VOCABULARY REVIEW

Match the following terms and definitions.

1. ________ The constant practice of considering all aspects of a situation when deciding what to believe or what to do
2. ________ Actions that identify the medical assistant as a member of a healthcare profession, including dependability, respectful patient care, initiative, positive attitude, and teamwork
3. ________ The way an individual looks at information and sees it as real
4. ________ The manner in which an individual perceives and processes information to learn new material
5. ________ The way an individual internalizes new information and makes it his or her own
6. ________ The process of considering new information and internalizing it to create new ways of examining information
7. ________ Sensitivity to the individual needs and reactions of patients

A. Learning style

B. Reflection

C. Professional behaviors

D. Processing

E. Empathy

F. Perceiving

G. Critical thinking

SKILLS AND CONCEPTS

Time Management

Answer the following questions.

1. List five time management skills.

   a. ____________________

   b. ____________________

   c. ____________________

   d. ____________________

   e. ____________________

   Which of these do you think will require the most effort on your road to becoming a medical assistant? How can you better prepare yourself for the challenges ahead?

   ____

   ____

2. Describe five strategies for breaking the cycle of procrastination.

   a. ____________________

   b. ____________________

   c. ____________________

   d. ____________________

   e. ____________________

Copyright © 2011, 2007, 2003 by Saunders, an imprint of Elsevier Inc. All rights reserved.

3. What barriers cause you to procrastinate? How can you prepare yourself to avoid procrastination?

____

____

____

____

Problem Solving and Conflict Management

True and False: Indicate which statements are true (T) and which are false (F).

1. _______ The best way to deal with conflict situations is through open, honest, assertive communication.
2. _______ The first step in conflict resolution is examination of the pros and cons.
3. _______ Conflicts should be resolved immediately.
4. _______ Sometimes you will not be able to solve problems, or a conflict may not be important enough for you to act to change the situation.
5. _______ It is best if you attempt to solve the conflict in a private place at a prescheduled time.
6. _______ You need to understand the problem and gather as much information about the situation as possible before you decide to act.
7. _______ As a future member of the healthcare team, you will frequently face problems and conflict.

Assertive Behaviors

True and False: Indicate which statements are true (T) and which are false (F).

1. _______ We are born either assertive or passive, and there is nothing we can do to change those behaviors.
2. _______ Assertive communication will get you what you want.
3. _______ A person who responds to conflict passively really is not bothered by the situation.
4. _______ Nonassertive individuals ultimately may respond with anger or an emotional outburst if pushed too far.
5. _______ Aggressive individuals ignore the needs of others.

Briefly answer the following questions.

6. Describe four different nonassertive behaviors.

   a. ____

   b. ____

   c. ____

   d. ____

7. Describe four different aggressive behaviors.

   a. ____

   b. ____

   c. ____

   d. ____

 Copyright © 2011, 2007, 2003 by Saunders, an imprint of Elsevier Inc. All rights reserved.

8. Explain the process of developing and delivering an assertive message.

STUDY SKILLS

1. Examine your own note-taking ability. Review the note-taking strategies in Chapter 1 and record the ideas you plan to incorporate into your academic goals for this term.

CASE STUDIES

Read the case studies and answer the questions.

1. Dr. Weaver is running late seeing patients this afternoon. Sara Kline has been waiting in the examination room for Dr. Weaver for 30 minutes. She peeks her head out of the examination room doorway and demands to know what is taking so long. How should you, the medical assistant, approach this patient? How do you calm her down and explain the physician's situation without compromising other patients' confidentiality? What are some things you can do for the patient to make the wait not seem so long?

2. Victoria Graham, a 68-year-old woman with diabetic retinopathy, arrives today for diabetes disease management education. How might the medical assistant approach Ms. Graham's learning style? What are some possible barriers and how can the medical assistant help Ms. Graham overcome them?

3. You have been working with another student to prepare for your next exam. The student asks to borrow your notes but has yet to return them so you can study for the exam. You are usually a nonassertive person, but you know that you have to get your notes back or you will not do well on the test. How can you formulate an assertive message? Summarize the steps to take and exactly what "I" message you will deliver.

Copyright © 2011, 2007, 2003 by Saunders, an imprint of Elsevier Inc. All rights reserved.

WORKPLACE APPLICATIONS

1. You are the office manager for a busy family practice office. Over the past week, you have noticed that one of your employees has been 15 minutes late every day. Should you approach this employee? If so, how would you manage the situation? What are the main points you would want to stress to this employee? Are there any consequences? What follow-up, if any, should be done?

2. Physicians' offices are extremely busy and must deal with many daily demands. How should one prepare for proper time management? Why is it necessary to prioritize tasks? What are some ideas the medical assistant can use to get the most out of the day and stay organized?

3. Connie is the manager of a busy family practice office. The insurance clerk has complained that the receptionist takes too many smoking breaks and accepts too many personal calls while at work. What type of information should Connie obtain before approaching the receptionist? How should this situation be handled? Where? Who should be present?

4. After being on vacation for a week, Laura returns to the office to find her desk piled high with the following tasks. Laura decides to get organized and make a list of the items that need attention. Prioritize the tasks from "most important and urgent" to "needs to be done later today" and "may be done later this week." Explain your answers.

   a. Make staff schedule for next week

   b. Pull patients' charts for the laboratory results the office received this morning for the physician's review

   c. Call and order immunization vaccines (the staff has informed you they are on the last vial)

   d. Call and confirm the patient appointments for tomorrow

   e. Order general stock supplies (e.g., bandages, gauze, needles, and sharps containers)

   f. Review the insurance reimbursements the practice received for last month and address any claims that have not been paid

   g. File charts

   h. Edit the physician's schedule for a meeting scheduled next month

 Copyright © 2011, 2007, 2003 by Saunders, an imprint of Elsevier Inc. All rights reserved.

2 The Healthcare Industry

VOCABULARY REVIEW

Fill in the blanks with the correct vocabulary terms from this chapter.

1. A nurse sees several patients in a hospital emergency department and determines which patient is the most ill and should be seen by the physician first. The process the nurse is using is called ________________.
2. An administrative assistant in a large clinic must write a letter to another state to determine whether a physician whom the clinic wants to hire has ever had his license revoked. This action is part of a process called ________________.
3. A patient arrives at a physician's office and sees the physician. This event is called a(n) ________________.
4. Accrediting agencies look for ________________ or ________________ to determine whether a healthcare facility is following required policies and regulations.
5. A physician who has been ________________ has been charged with a crime but has not yet been tried in a court of law.
6. A person who is unable to pay for medical expenses is often called ________________, and most hospitals will provide such patients with emergency care.
7. A group of healthcare practitioners involved in reviewing the charts of patients with a certain disease to determine the medical necessity of procedures might be serving in a(n) ________________ organization.
8. When families look for an assisted living facility for a relative, they often consider the ________________ that will add to the comfort and convenience of the patient.
9. Physicians who conduct a great amount of research are often ________________ in medical journals and articles within their field of study.
10. A new hospital contacts The Joint Commission (formerly JCAHO) to begin the ________________ process, which verifies that the facility meets or exceeds standards.
11. Dr. Robertson uses mostly herbs and natural supplements in his practice of medicine. Although he could be any type of physician, he probably practices ________________.
12. Dr. Wray combines conventional medicine with manipulative techniques when treating his patients. This type of medicine is called ________________.
13. Dr. Stern treats patients by locating slight misalignments of the vertebrae and corrects them using manipulative techniques. He practices ________________ medicine.
14. Dr. Margolis practices ________________, which is a medical discipline in which treatments and medications are used to counteract the signs and symptoms of disease. Most of the physicians in the United States practice this type of medicine.
15. Susan works for Dr. Burns and has forwarded information about his medical license, medical training, and experience to Mercy Hospital. He is applying for ________________ at the hospital.

Copyright © 2011, 2007, 2003 by Saunders, an imprint of Elsevier Inc. All rights reserved.

SKILLS AND CONCEPTS

Part I: Pioneers in Medicine

Fill in the blanks.

1. The surgical research technician who contributed to the success of the Blalock-Taussig procedure was ________________.
2. ________________ presented rules of health to the Jews around 1205 BC, making him the first advocate of preventive medicine and the first public health officer.
3. ________________, known as the father of medicine, was the most famous of the ancient Greek physicians, best remembered for an oath that has been taken by many physicians for more than 2,000 years.
4. ________________ was a Greek physician who migrated to Rome in AD 162 and became known as the "Prince of Physicians."
5. ________________ was a Belgian anatomist who is known as the "Father of Modern Anatomy."
6. In 1628 ________________ announced his discovery that the heart acts as a muscular pump, forcing and propelling the blood throughout the body.
7. ________________ was the first to observe bacteria and protozoa through a lens.
8. English scientist, ________________, is known as the "Founder of Scientific Surgery."
9. ________________ observed that those who had contracted cowpox never contracted smallpox.
10. ________________ directed that in his wards, the students were to wash and disinfect their hands before examining women in labor and delivering infants.
11. ________________ saved the dairy industry of France from disaster in the nineteenth century by developing a process now called *pasteurization*.
12. ________________ reasoned that microorganisms must be the cause of infection and should be kept out of wounds.
13. ________________ was the first to use ether as an anesthetic agent.
14. Marie and Pierre ________________ discovered radium in 1898, and they were awarded the 1902 Nobel Prize in Physics for their work on radioactivity.
15. ________________, the founder of nursing, is known as "The Lady With the Lamp."
16. In 1881 ________________ organized a committee in Washington that became the American Red Cross.
17. ________________ became the American leader of the birth control movement.
18. ________________ wrote about death and dying.
19. Salk and ________________ almost eradicated polio, which was once a killer and crippler of thousands in the United States.
20. David ________________, MD, considered by many to be one of the most brilliant minds today, is helping to piece together the puzzle of the human immunodeficiency virus (HIV).
21. During his terms as the Surgeon General of the United States, ________________ became a proponent of tobacco awareness, insisting that tobacco advertisements must be made less attractive to the youth of today.

Copyright © 2011, 2007, 2003 by Saunders, an imprint of Elsevier Inc. All rights reserved.

Part II: Word Find

Using the answers from the previous section, find the names of past and present leaders in the healthcare industry.

S	K	H	U	N	T	E	R	Q	T	W	L
E	E	O	S	S	G	R	E	N	N	E	J
M	O	L	O	H	M	E	I	B	C	V	M
M	H	I	P	P	O	C	R	A	T	E	S
E	N	S	C	Y	S	X	U	R	C	S	A
L	E	T	K	E	E	P	C	T	E	A	N
W	W	E	H	V	S	D	K	O	G	L	G
E	U	R	I	R	T	C	V	N	X	I	E
I	E	J	G	A	L	E	N	O	Z	U	R
S	E	E	K	H	W	B	P	B	X	S	K
S	L	O	N	G	V	S	A	B	I	N	M
E	L	A	G	N	I	T	H	G	I	N	Y
P	A	S	T	E	U	R	Z	F	M	G	E
F	Y	Z	S	A	M	O	H	T	X	M	O
K	U	B	L	E	R	R	O	S	S	C	T
O	B	T	S	K	O	O	P	L	D	N	C

Part III: National Healthcare Organizations

Spell out the following acronyms.

1. WHO

____

2. DHHS

____

3. USAMRIID

____

4. CDC

____

5. NIH

____

6. CLIA

____

7. OSHA

____

Part IV: Healthcare Professionals

Use the appropriate terms to complete the sentences.

1. Dr. Hazlehurst bears responsibility for her practice 7 days a week. This practice is called a(n) _______________.
2. A(n) _______________ is formed when two or more physicians elect to associate in the practice of medicine without incorporating.
3. Dr. Sorrow and Dr. Wester sold their practice to a large artificial entity with legal and business status, and now they work for a(n) _______________.

Copyright © 2011, 2007, 2003 by Saunders, an imprint of Elsevier Inc. All rights reserved.

4. A(n) ______________ is trained to locate subluxations of the spine and repair them, using x-ray examinations and adjustments.

5. ______________ physicians, or DOs, complete requirements similar to those for MDs to graduate and practice medicine.

6. Duncan wants to become a(n) ______________, who treats and prevents problems related to the teeth and gums and the tissue surrounding them.

7. The professional who is trained and licensed to examine the eyes, test visual acuity, and treat defects of vision by prescribing correctional lenses is called a(n) ______________.

8. A(n) ______________ is educated in the care of the feet, including surgical treatment.

9. ______________ and medical laboratory technicians perform diagnostic testing on blood, body fluids, and other types of specimens to assist the physician in obtaining a diagnosis.

10. ______________ provide direct patient care services under the supervision of licensed physicians and are trained to diagnose and treat patients as directed by the physician.

11. ______________ are registered nurses who provide anesthetics to patients during procedures performed by surgeons, physicians, dentists, or other qualified healthcare professionals.

12. ______________ assist patients in regaining their mobility and improving their strength and range of motion, which may have been impaired by an accident or injury or as a result of disease.

Part V: Healthcare Facilities

Fill in the blanks.

1. Roger's hands were injured in an accident, and he must undergo rehabilitation. He is obtaining treatment at a(n) ______________ health center so that he can prepare to return to work.

2. Susan's son, Brandon, had his tonsils removed at the ______________ unit of their local hospital and went home later that evening.

3. ______________ facilities have become very popular because they give the residents a sense of independence while still providing supervision and various amenities.

4. ______________ centers provide patients an alternative to hospital emergency departments.

5. ______________ diagnose and treat people who have sleep disorders.

Part VI: Matching Patients with Physicians

Match the following patients with the physician who should treat them. The specialties are based on the divisions of medicine recognized by the American Board of Medical Specialties. Write the corresponding letter for the physician on the blank next to the patient's name.

1. _______	Mr. West has complained of problems with excessive gas and bloating after meals. He also has some pain in his lower abdominal area.	a. Dr. Stayer
		b. Dr. Quincy
2. _______	Ms. Jindra has suffered from severe acne most of her adult life. She hopes to find a treatment that will give her more confidence in her appearance.	c. Dr. Haskins

 Copyright © 2011, 2007, 2003 by Saunders, an imprint of Elsevier Inc. All rights reserved.

3. _______ The results of Ms. Robles' amniocentesis are abnormal, and her obstetrician suspects that she may be carrying a child who will be born with a birth defect.

4. _______ Ms. O'Neal is pregnant with her first child.

5. _______ Ms. Sklaar had gastric bypass surgery 2 years ago and now wants to undergo abdominoplasty to remove excess skin.

6. _______ Mr. Taylor experiences pain in his left eye when he is exposed to bright sunlight. He is concerned, because his mother and grandmother both lost their eyesight in their later years.

7. _______ Jack Monroe is the lead singer for a popular rock band. He experienced laryngitis during a world tour and needs to see a physician quickly to help him get back on the road.

8. _______ Sarah is 1 year old and needs several immunizations.

9. _______ Jimmie suffers from asthma related to reactions that occur when he is around grass, shrubs, and some animals.

10. _______ Mrs. Downey had a stroke and needs surgery to remove a small clot that has lodged in her brain.

11. _______ Andrea is having a hysterectomy and will be given a general anesthetic. While in the hospital, she meets the physician who will administer the anesthetic during surgery.

12. _______ Mrs. Ballard had an ovarian cyst, which was removed after a visit to the emergency department. She received a bill later from the physician who evaluated the cyst for malignancies.

13. _______ Mrs. Harris had several polyps in her gastrointestinal tract. She was referred for surgery by her family physician.

14. _______ Mrs. Richardson has had migraine headaches for about 6 months. Her family physician thinks she should see a specialist.

15. _______ Bobbie broke his arm and was taken to the emergency department. X-ray films were taken, and they were read by a physician.

16. _______ Mr. Oldman periodically suffers from kidney stones and may need surgery.

17. _______ Rhonda was taken to the emergency department after a car accident.

18. _______ Mr. Anton contacted a physician for removal of a minor cyst on his back.

19. _______ The entire Blair family sees one physician.

20. _______ Mr. Saxton will have surgery tonight to treat a punctured lung.

d. Dr. Marrs
e. Dr. Cantrell
f. Dr. DuBois
g. Dr. Gleaton
h. Dr. Kirkham
i. Dr. Jones
j. Dr. Faught
k. Dr. Martin
l. Dr. Rowinski
m. Dr. Antonetti
n. Dr. Jackson
o. Dr. Tips
p. Dr. Roberts
q. Dr. Skylar
r. Dr. Burns
s. Dr. True
t. Dr. Williams

Part VII: Short Essay Questions

Answer the following questions using complete sentences.

1. Why was the education offered by Johns Hopkins University Medical School so effective in training physicians?

____

____

____

Copyright © 2011, 2007, 2003 by Saunders, an imprint of Elsevier Inc. All rights reserved.

2. Explain the differences between the two medical symbols discussed in the chapter and what each icon represents.

____

____

____

3. Why is the history of medicine important to us today?

____

____

____

4. Which ancient cultures contributed to the medical terminology we use today?

____

____

____

5. Which medical pioneer do you feel contributed the most to medicine?

____

____

____

6. Explain the role of the hospitalist.

____

____

____

Part VIII: Healthcare Occupations

Match the following descriptions with the appropriate healthcare occupation.

1. _______ Provides services such as injury prevention, assessment, and rehabilitation
2. _______ Is qualified to implement exercise programs designed to reverse or minimize debilitation and enhance the functional capacity of medically stable patients
3. _______ Practices medicine under the direction and responsible supervision of a medical doctor or doctor of osteopathy
4. _______ Performs diagnostic examinations and therapeutic interventions of the heart and/or blood vessels, both invasive and noninvasive
5. _______ Assists licensed pharmacists by performing duties that do not require the expertise of a pharmacist
6. _______ Assists in developing and implementing the anesthesia care plan
7. _______ Helps improve patient mobility, relieve pain, and prevent or limit permanent physical disabilities

a. Audiologist
b. Cardiovascular technologist
c. Therapeutic recreation specialist
d. Physical therapist
e. Pharmacy technician
f. Dietetic technician
g. Anesthesiology assistant
h. Specialist in blood bank technology
i. Diagnostic medical sonographer

Copyright © 2011, 2007, 2003 by Saunders, an imprint of Elsevier Inc. All rights reserved.

8. ______	Helps patients use their leisure in ways that enhance health, functional abilities, independence, and quality of life	j. Kinesiotherapist
9. ______	Identifies patients who have hearing, balance, and related ear problems	k. Occupational therapist
10. ______	Integrates and applies the principles from the science of food, nutrition, biochemistry, food management, and behavior to achieve and maintain health	l. Orthoptist
11. ______	Evaluates, treats, and manages patients of all ages with respiratory illnesses and other cardiopulmonary disorders	m. Physician assistant
12. ______	Evaluates disorders of vision, eye movement, and eye alignment	n. Surgical technologist
13. ______	Performs routine and standardized tests in blood center and transfusion services	o. Respiratory therapist
14. ______	Uses equipment that produces sound waves, resulting in images of internal structures	p. Athletic trainer
15. ______	Uses the nuclear properties of radioactive and stable nuclides to make diagnostic evaluations of the anatomic or physiologic conditions of the body	q. Medical technologist
16. ______	Prepares the operating room by selecting and opening sterile supplies	r. Emergency medical technician
17. ______	Uses purposeful activity and interventions to achieve functional outcomes to maximize the independence and maintenance of health	s. Health information specialist
18. ______	Performs tests to detect and diagnose various diseases and works closely with pathologists	t. Nuclear medicine technologist
19. ______	Provides medical care to patients who have suffered an injury or illness outside the hospital setting	
20. ______	Formulates strategic, functional, and user requirements related to the processing of health data	

CASE STUDY

Read the case study and answer the questions that follow.

Rebecca is a new employee at the Blackburn Clinic. She recently graduated from an accredited medical assisting school and completed her externship in a family practice clinic. She enjoys the variety of patients who come to the office, and she respects the physicians for their dedication to the art and science of medicine. The physicians with whom Rebecca works are strong proponents of continuing education, and they want Rebecca to attend no less than two seminars each year. Research the history of family practices and answer these questions:

1. What types of patients are seen in family practice clinics?

____

____

____

2. What educational background does the physician need to become a family practitioner?

____

____

____

Copyright © 2011, 2007, 2003 by Saunders, an imprint of Elsevier Inc. All rights reserved.

3. What are some of the more common illnesses that present in a family clinic?

___

___

___

4. What are the goals of the American Association of Family Practitioners?

___

___

___

Workplace Applications

Read the following information and complete the exercises.

1. Visit a local hospital and introduce yourself to five medical professionals. Make an appointment to interview them and find out their job duties and their professional backgrounds. Write a thank-you note to each person after the interview.

2. Interview an office manager at a family practice. Ask about the positive and negative aspects of working with a variety of patients each day.

Internet Activities

1. Choose one of the early medical pioneers discussed in this chapter and research him or her using the Internet. After conducting the research, write a report and present the person to the class. Be creative with the presentation, using PowerPoint or some type of audiovisual equipment.

2. Research the history of a particular illness. Prepare a short report on that illness and present it to the class.

Copyright © 2011, 2007, 2003 by Saunders, an imprint of Elsevier Inc. All rights reserved.

3 The Medical Assisting Profession

VOCABULARY REVIEW

Fill in the blanks with the correct vocabulary terms from this chapter.

1. Sandra should consider both the ________________ and the ________________ as she considers the various positions offered to her on graduation from her medical assisting training.
2. Robert is anxious to learn ________________, because he would like to draw blood and possibly work in a local hospital laboratory.
3. The Wray Clinic recently began to offer ________________ ________________ to the employees, which gives them a part of the profits the clinic earns over the year.
4. It is important for graduates of medical assisting programs to gain ________________ as soon as possible after graduation and to maintain it throughout their medical assisting career.
5. It is clear to Paula that there are many ________________ to working as a medical assistant that make the profession worthwhile in ways other than compensation.
6. Alberta is interested in administrative medical assisting, because she is unsure whether she would enjoy performing ________________ procedures.
7. Some high schools offer classes that allow students to explore the ________________ ________________ ________________.
8. Both the American Association of Medical Assistants and the American Medical Technologists offer ________________ ________________ ________________ for medical assistants.
9. ________________ helps a team of medical assistants cover for one another in the event of illness or absence.
10. Medical assistants are the most ________________ allied health professionals.
11. Some for-profit organizations offer ________________ ________________ after an employee has worked there for a specific period.
12. Bethany is looking forward to her ________________ in a family practice clinic next month.

SKILLS AND CONCEPTS

Part I: The Medical Assisting Profession

1. Name the two major areas of medical assisting practice.

____

____

Copyright © 2011, 2007, 2003 by Saunders, an imprint of Elsevier Inc. All rights reserved.

2. List five administrative duties a medical assistant might perform.

3. List five clinical duties a medical assistant might perform.

4. Provide an example of cross-training.

5. Explain why hiring a medical assistant without any formal training often is more expensive.

6. Explain in your own words the history of medical assisting as a profession.

Part II: Professional Appearance

Determine which of the following normally would be part of the medical assistant's professional appearance. Place a check mark in the box marked "yes" or "no" to indicate whether that item would be acceptable in today's medical facilities.

	Yes	No	
1.	❑	❑	Hoop earrings
2.	❑	❑	Clear nail polish
3.	❑	❑	White uniforms
4.	❑	❑	Red nail polish
5.	❑	❑	One ear piercing
6.	❑	❑	Scrub tops
7.	❑	❑	Facial piercings
8.	❑	❑	Tennis or running shoes
9.	❑	❑	Excessive jewelry
10.	❑	❑	Tongue rings
11.	❑	❑	Lab coats
12.	❑	❑	Heavy eye makeup
13.	❑	❑	Street clothes with a lab coat
14.	❑	❑	Jeans

Copyright © 2011, 2007, 2003 by Saunders, an imprint of Elsevier Inc. All rights reserved.

Part III: Externships and Internships

Explain briefly the solution you would choose for the following situations that might occur during an externship or internship. Discuss and compare answers during class.

1. Anna notices that her supervisor at the externship frequently arrives late and leaves work early. The physician asks Anna casually one day if the supervisor is helpful and cordial to her. What should Anna say about the supervisor?

____

____

____

2. One of Dr. Hammersly's patients, Brock Anderson, is extremely attractive, and Suzanne, the extern at the clinic, would like to get to know him better. When working with Brock's chart, Suzanne notices his home telephone number. She considers writing it down and contacting Brock after her externship is completed. Would this be acceptable behavior?

____

____

____

3. On a very stressful day, Georgia assists a drug representative in placing drug samples in the storage area. She has battled a headache for most of the day. One of the drugs left behind is a mild painkiller called Ultram. Georgia has taken Ultram before for her headaches and doesn't think the physician will mind if she takes one at work. Would this be appropriate?

____

____

____

4. Natasha was one of the most industrious medical assistant students in her class, always working hard and going the extra mile. When she begins her externship, she notices that the other assistants in the office are allowing her to do a large part of the work while they gossip and explore the Internet during working hours. How should Natasha handle this when her supervisor asks her how the externship is going?

____

____

____

5. Randy graduated from the same school Angela currently is attending for medical assisting training. The two meet during Angela's externship at the office where Randy works, and they quickly become friends. Randy would like to ask Angela, a single parent, to a company picnic the following weekend, after Angela finishes her externship. Would this be acceptable behavior?

____

____

____

6. Dr. Morton confides in Catrina, an extern, that he plans to fire Ashley, the medical assistant who books appointments for the clinic. He offers Catrina the job, which pays slightly more than she expected to make just out of school. The office is located very close to Catrina's apartment. Later in the week, Ashley and Catrina go to lunch together, and Ashley mentions that she is about to buy a new car. Should Catrina steer her away from such a major purchase, knowing that she is about to be fired?

____

____

____

Copyright © 2011, 2007, 2003 by Saunders, an imprint of Elsevier Inc. All rights reserved.

7. Bailee, an extern, is shocked to see one of the other medical assistants, Kristen, take $20 from the petty cash drawer and put it in her purse. When the physician asks about the petty cash balance, Kristen mentions that she gave a Girl Scout troop a $20 donation. What should Bailee do?

____

____

____

8. Dr. Schilling storms into the clinic and calls a meeting. Taylor, an extern who has been at the clinic for 1 week, attends the meeting with the two other medical assistants in the office. When the physician insists that one of the three of them took a vial of Demerol from the drug cabinet, the two medical assistants look at Taylor. If Taylor is not guilty, how should she handle this situation professionally?

____

____

____

Part IV: Professional Organizations

Fill in the blanks with the correct word choice.

1. Gail uses the CMA credential after her name, which stands for ______________ ______________ ______________.

2. The CMA examination is offered by which organization? ______________

3 Patty uses the RMA credential after her name, which stands for ______________ ______________ ______________.

4. The RMA examination is offered by which organization? ______________

5. Two agencies that accredit medical assisting programs are the ______________ and the ______________.

6. Explain the purpose of CEUs.

____

7. Do both the AAMA and the AMT either require CEUs or offer them as an option for recertification?

____

8. Explain the mission of the AAMA.

____

____

____

9. Explain the mission of the AMT.

____

____

____

Copyright © 2011, 2007, 2003 by Saunders, an imprint of Elsevier Inc. All rights reserved.

Part V: Short Essay Questions

Answer the following questions using complete sentences.

1. List several personal attributes a student should display during his or her externship.

2. Explain why continuing education is critical to the success of the medical assistant.

3. What are some of the subjects that will be included in most medical assistant training programs?

CASE STUDY

Read the case study and answer the questions that follow.

Maryanne entered a medical assisting training program in June, and by mid-July she was struggling to do homework, take care of her infant son, and work part-time. She loves her classes but feels overwhelmed by the amount of work school requires. At times she thinks about quitting school, but she also realizes that a job as a medical assistant will be more rewarding than her current part-time job. Maryanne wants a position that she can be proud to hold. One of her instructors suggested that she make plans for the situations that could prompt her to give up her schooling.

1. How can Maryanne make plans for situations that might go wrong throughout her time in school?

2. What types of situations could present problems for her?

3. How can Maryanne budget her time effectively so that she is able to meet all her responsibilities?

Workplace Applications

Write a reasonable dress code policy for a fictional medical office. Include regulations for both male and female employees. Be specific about jewelry (e.g., nose rings, piercings, and so on), fingernail length, clean shoes, and all other aspects of an acceptable dress code.

Copyright © 2011, 2007, 2003 by Saunders, an imprint of Elsevier Inc. All rights reserved.

Internet Activities

1. Research the requirements for taking both the CMA and RMA examinations. Request or download an application to become a member of the American Association of Medical Assistants and the American Medical Technologists. Obtain a money order for the application fee and send the fees with your application. Answer the following questions:

   What CMA examination date is closest to your graduation? ________________

   What is the fee for the CMA examination? ________________

   How much are the initial dues for joining the AAMA based on your state of residence? ________________

   How much are annual dues for the AAMA based on your state of residence? ________________

   What local chapter is closest to you? When and where are the meetings held?

   ____

   ____

   What RMA examination date is closest to your graduation? ________________

   What is the fee for the RMA examination? ________________

   How much are the initial dues for joining the AMT? ________________

   How much are annual dues for the AMT? ________________

   What local chapter is closest to you? When and where are the meetings held?

   ____

   ____

2. Research the medical assistant's scope of practice and write a report on this subject. Present the report to the class.

3. Research the requirements of other certifications that you might be interested in obtaining. Which would you like to work toward, if any? Secure applications for those additional certifications.

Copyright © 2011, 2007, 2003 by Saunders, an imprint of Elsevier Inc. All rights reserved.

4 Professional Behavior in the Workplace

VOCABULARY REVIEW

Fill in the blanks with the correct vocabulary terms from this chapter.

1. Dr. Babinski struggles with ________________, often putting off doing tasks that should be completed.
2. Anna has worked as a medical assistant for almost 30 years, and her professionalism and compassion are above ________________.
3. Susan Bessler is a CMA who has supervised externships for almost 10 years; she expects students to display ________________ when performing their duties at her clinic.
4. ________________ is one of the most important attributes that medical assistants should display as they go about their duties.
5. James has learned that he must use ________________ when dealing with the patients in the clinic, being careful not to reveal any confidential information to an unauthorized third party.
6. Roberta ________________ the notes from the last staff meeting to all employees.
7. A few of the ________________ that the professional medical assistant should show include loyalty, initiative, and courtesy.
8. Because Julia has been dishonest about her reasons for missing work, her ________________ has been called into question.
9. Kristen has a pleasant ________________ when working with patients.
10. Medical assistants receive pay that is usually ________________ with their experience and training.
11. Jessica holds drawings for small gifts at her staff meetings, which helps to raise employee ________________.
12. Gene evokes a professional ________________ when talking with patients that encourages them to place their trust in him.
13. Medical assistants must take ________________ when they are performing both externship and job duties.
14. ________________ is a cause for immediate dismissal from employment.
15. The phrase "office politics" has a negative ________________.

SKILLS AND CONCEPTS

Part I: Short Answer Questions

Briefly answer the following questions.

1. List the eight characteristics of the professional medical assistant.

   a. ________________________________

   b. ________________________________

   c. ________________________________

   d. ________________________________

   e. ________________________________

Copyright © 2011, 2007, 2003 by Saunders, an imprint of Elsevier Inc. All rights reserved.

f. __________

g. __________

h. __________

2. List five obstructions to professionalism.

a. __________

b. __________

c. __________

d. __________

e. __________

3. Define teamwork in your own words.

Part II: Practicing Professional Behavior

Answer the following questions.

1. Karen has developed a friendship with Angela, who has a wonderful personality but does not always do her share in the family practice clinic where they work together. Dr. Rabinowitz tells Karen that Angela is going to be terminated on Friday, and she asks Karen to take over some of Angela's duties until a replacement is found. How can Karen demonstrate loyalty to her employer in this situation? To her friend, Angela?

2. Martin Smith is a patient who always disrupts the clinic. He constantly complains about everything from the moment he enters until the moment he leaves. Karen is at the desk when he arrives to check out and pay his bill. When she tells him that he has a previous balance from a claim that his insurance did not pay, he argues that Karen filed the claim incorrectly. Karen is not in charge of filing insurance claims and did not handle any part of the claim in question. How can she be courteous to this patient?

3. Karen works in the office laboratory. She is often asked questions about insurance and billing that she must refer to other personnel. How should Karen efficiently request information or assistance for the patient from other office personnel?

Copyright © 2011, 2007, 2003 by Saunders, an imprint of Elsevier Inc. All rights reserved.

4. Karen and her fiancé ended their relationship last week. How can she deal with personal stressors while she is in the workplace?

____

____

____

____

5. A patient needs to be scheduled for an outpatient endoscopic examination. When Karen gives the instruction sheet to the patient, she suspects from his reaction that the patient is unable to read. How can Karen professionally handle this situation without causing embarrassment to the patient?

____

____

____

____

6. Which of the characteristics of professionalism is your greatest strength? Explain why.

____

____

____

____

7. Which of the five obstructions to professionalism will be most difficult for you to overcome? Explain why.

____

____

____

____

8. Explain the difference between drug abuse and drug addiction.

____

____

____

____

9. List the four criteria of substance abuse.

   a. ____

   b. ____

   c. ____

   d. ____

Copyright © 2011, 2007, 2003 by Saunders, an imprint of Elsevier Inc. All rights reserved.

10. List the seven criteria that determine abuse if three are met within a 12-month period.

a. ______________________________

b. ______________________________

c. ______________________________

d. ______________________________

e. ______________________________

f. ______________________________

g. ______________________________

CASE STUDY

Read the case study and answer the questions that follow.

Aaron is a new medical assistant in Dr. Royce's family practice. He was an exceptional student, and he consistently performed well on his externship, receiving commendations from the externship office manager as well as a written recommendation from the physician. One month after he started his job, Bethany asked him to make a bank deposit for her, usually a duty that she performs daily. Bethany told him she was leaving the bank deposit in Aaron's bottom left drawer at his desk. When Aaron looked for the deposit at the end of the day, it was not anywhere in his desk; he looked in every drawer and even took the drawers out to make sure it had not fallen behind them. All the employees looked for the deposit, which was not found. No one was able to reach Bethany on the phone. The next morning when Aaron opened his left bottom desk drawer, the deposit bag was there, but it was empty. Bethany had already reported to the physician that the deposit had not been made. The physician calls Aaron to his office to discuss the situation.

1. What do you think happened?

____

____

____

2. How can you deal with employees who are determined to cause problems for others in the clinic?

____

____

____

3. How can situations such as this be proven effectively when one is unsure about exactly what happened?

____

____

____

WORKPLACE APPLICATIONS

Professionalism is a word used often with regard to medical personnel. What does professionalism mean? Write a report on the meaning of professionalism, highlighting a person you believe is the epitome of professionalism in the medical field. This person could be an instructor, a physician, or some other healthcare worker whom you have come to know. Be specific about the ways professionalism is apparent in this individual's actions and speech.

Copyright © 2011, 2007, 2003 by Saunders, an imprint of Elsevier Inc. All rights reserved.

INTERNET ACTIVITIES

1. Find four articles on medical professionalism. What seems to be the primary issues in attempting to maintain professionalism in medical facilities?

2. What are some ways medical professionalism is taught in medical schools? Do these methods apply to medical assistants?

Copyright © 2011, 2007, 2003 by Saunders, an imprint of Elsevier Inc. All rights reserved.

5 Interpersonal Skills and Human Behavior

VOCABULARY REVIEW

Fill in the blanks with the correct vocabulary terms from this chapter.

1. Jill commented that the new office policies are confusing and ________________.
2. Giving a patient an injection against his or her will could be considered ________________.
3. Shane's remark was insulting and ________________.
4. Whitney ________________ denied leaving the narcotics cabinet unlocked.
5. With the increasing number of lawsuits, medical personnel can conclude that our society is quite ________________.
6. Angry employees who are being terminated might turn ________________ in a short time.
7. The notion that large individuals are lazy is an example of a(n) ________________.
8. Sayed uses positive ________________ while training a new employee.
9. Rahima demonstrates ________________ when she attempts to get her way in every situation.
10. Paula has learned that she uses ________________ ________________ when she feels threatened by her supervisor.
11. Karen felt intense ________________ when her grandmother died.
12. ________________ helps Angela make sure she understands exactly what a patient meant.
13. Roberto eventually was terminated for using ________________ with several of the patients in the clinic.
14. Bobbie attended a seminar last week and learned about ________________, which included the study of the spatial separation that individuals naturally maintain.
15. Sue Ann definitely felt out of her ________________ ________________ when she was asked to be a guest speaker at a regional AAMA meeting.
16. Mrs. Robinson is able to ________________ her words quite distinctly.
17. Dr. Kirkham warned that no employee should speak to the ________________ about any of his celebrity patients.
18. Rodman has a(n) ________________ ________________ at work, because he speaks so little English.
19. It is important to consider the patient's ________________ of the staff, clinic, and physician.
20. Dr. Rockwell took Julia off phone duty because the high ________________ of her voice was disconcerting to many patients.

Copyright © 2011, 2007, 2003 by Saunders, an imprint of Elsevier Inc. All rights reserved.

SKILLS AND CONCEPTS

Part I: Open-Ended and Closed-Ended Questions

Label the following questions or statements as either open ended (O) or closed ended (C).

1. _______ Are you taking blood pressure medication?
2. _______ Are you allergic to aspirin?
3. _______ Would you tell me about your past surgeries?
4. _______ Do you have asthma?
5. _______ What types of attempts have you made to stop smoking?
6. _______ Explain what you feel when your migraines begin.
7. _______ Do you have hospitalization insurance?
8. _______ Do you want a morning or afternoon appointment?
9. _______ How are you feeling today?
10. _______ What type of trouble do you have when swallowing pills?

Part II: Defense Mechanisms

Match the following defense mechanisms with the appropriate statements.

1. _______ "Everyone forgets to clock in from lunch once in a while. Why am I being singled out and written up?"
2. _______ "I refuse to believe that I'm HIV positive. I've only had sex with two people in the past 5 years."
3. _______ "I would do a better job at work, but I can't do everything in 1 day like I'm expected to."
4. _______ "I know that the office manager is angry with me because I've been late, and I should talk to her, but I just can't deal with that stress right now."
5. _______ "Why are you attacking me about not filling out the narcotics log? You certainly aren't the perfect medical assistant!"
6. _______ "I know my blood sugar is high, and I have tried to avoid sugar, but at least I'm doing my exercises twice a week."
7. _______ "Dr. Roberts only yells at me because he's stressed about his patient load."
8. _______ "It doesn't matter what I do to please my family. They hate me anyway, and there's nothing I can do about it."
9. _______ "I have enough on my mind and don't need my co-workers complaining that I'm not doing my share of the work!"
10. _______ "I can't bear to go to Memorial Park for our office picnic, because that's where my ex-husband told me he wanted a divorce."
11. _______ "Sure she looks good, if you like people from the 60s!"

a. Verbal aggression
b. Projection
c. Sarcasm
d. Compensation
e. Physical avoidance
f. Regression
g. Apathy
h. Rationalization
i. Displacement
j. Repression
k. Denial

Part III: Barriers to Communication

Determine which of the five barriers to communication applies in each example given.

1. Cylinda has lived in the South all her life, and when Bruce came to work at the office, his brusque attitude made her feel defensive. She was so offended by his manner of speaking that she began to avoid him in the hallways and during breaks. He constantly spoke of how much more he'd been paid in New York and stressed the efficiency of the clinic where he formerly worked. Cylinda considers him a typical Northerner, and her dislike of him is based largely on the fact that he is different from her and most of the people she knows.

____

Copyright © 2011, 2007, 2003 by Saunders, an imprint of Elsevier Inc. All rights reserved.

2. Aretha dreads the days that Rahima Bathkar comes to the office. She is a pleasant patient, but Aretha cannot understand her well and feels as if she is not providing Rahima with the care she deserves. She is always worried that she is missing some information the physician needs to know to diagnose and treat the patient properly. Aretha takes extra time with Rahima, but she is concerned, because there is no one to interpret for Rahima when she cannot find the right word in her broken English.

___

3. Allan and Rebecca Poe are an elderly couple who visit the clinic twice a month for Rebecca's diabetes. Rebecca is blind in one eye and cannot read easily. Allan has vision problems as well, so the staff must read to them any documents they are required to sign to ensure that they understand the information.

___

4. Tommy Lightman approached the office manager because he was concerned about the manner in which Sarah spoke to him in the office. He expressed that Sarah was quite short with him last Tuesday and seemed very distracted as she talked with him in the examination room before the physician came in to treat him. He also said that the physician seemed to spend less time with him that day than usual. Tommy was concerned that he was not wanted in the clinic and wanted to have his records sent to another physician. The office manager checks the appointment book and realizes that Tommy was in the office last Tuesday at 11 o'clock, which was the exact time that another patient was being transported to the hospital because of heart failure.

___

5. Teresa has a difficult time dealing with Orlando Guiterrez. He comes for appointments twice a month and is trying desperately to lose weight. He currently weighs 435 pounds. He is a pleasant person, but Teresa has been raised to believe that those who are overweight are lazy individuals. She tries to avoid caring for him when he visits the clinic.

___

Part IV: Dealing with Barriers to Communication

Reread the scenarios in the previous section and explain how each situation could be professionally handled by the medical assistant using good communications skills.

1. How can Cylinda develop a positive working relationship with Bruce?

___

___

___

2. What can Aretha do to improve communication with Rahima?

___

___

___

3. How can the medical assistant make Rebecca Poe feel more comfortable with her disability in the physician's office?

___

___

___

4. What can Sarah and the office manager do to change Tommy's perception about the incident that happened during his last office visit?

___

___

___

Copyright © 2011, 2007, 2003 by Saunders, an imprint of Elsevier Inc. All rights reserved.

5. What does Teresa need to do personally to deal with patients she doesn't care for who visit the clinic?

Part V: Communication During Difficult Times

Read the following descriptions and suggest effective ways to communicate with the patient. Identify whether the patient is probably experiencing anger, shock, grief, or a combination of these emotions.

1. Joanna Taylor has just been brought to the physician's office after learning that her 16-year-old son was killed in a car accident. She is not responding to questions.

2. Lafonda Williams has come to the physician's office because of injuries she sustained when her estranged husband assaulted her.

3. Jackson Holland is seeing the physician today for antidepressants because of work-related stress, as well as difficulty dealing with the death of his elderly mother.

4. James Ackard comes to the physician's office for treatment of a work-related injury.

Part VI: Death and Dying

List the stages of grief in proper order.

1.
2.
3.
4.
5.

Copyright © 2011, 2007, 2003 by Saunders, an imprint of Elsevier Inc. All rights reserved.

Part VII: Resolving Conflict

1. List three ways to resolve conflict.

   a. ___

   b. ___

   c. ___

2. How would the medical assistant professionally resolve a conflict with a co-worker?

   ___

   ___

   ___

3. How would the medical assistant professionally resolve a conflict with a supervisor?

   ___

   ___

   ___

Part VIII: Boundaries

1. Define self-boundaries.

   ___

   ___

   ___

2. List the four steps of setting boundaries at work.

   a. ___

   b. ___

   c. ___

   d. ___

Part IX: Communicating with People of Other Cultures

1. If a non–English-speaking patient comes to the office without an interpreter, what should the medical assistant do?

   ___

   ___

   ___

2. How can the medical assistant put a patient at ease who seems nervous about an office visit or a procedure?

   ___

   ___

   ___

3. Why should the medical assistant avoid the phrase "I know how you feel"?

   ___

   ___

   ___

Copyright © 2011, 2007, 2003 by Saunders, an imprint of Elsevier Inc. All rights reserved.

Part X: Maslow's Hierarchy of Needs

Draw and label the Hierarchy of Needs as shown in Figure 5-7 in the text.

Part XI: The Process of Communication

Draw and label the transactional communication model as shown in Figure 5-4 in the text.

CASE STUDY

Read the case study and answer the questions that follow.

Janet has tried for months to reach Mr. Robinson, a cancer patient who comes to the clinic every 3 weeks. He does not have any family in the area, and he feels that no one is interested in him or the problems he faces. He is estranged from both of his daughters, whom he has told to stay out of his life. They have not seen or spoken to him in more than 10 years. Each visit, Mr. Robinson complains about how worthless his family is and how they have all deserted him in his time of need. However, Janet knows from reviewing the chart that Mr. Robinson was insistent that his daughters stay out of his life.

1. How involved should Janet get in this patient's life?

___

___

___

2. How can she deal with Mr. Robinson's attitude during his office visits?

___

___

___

Copyright © 2011, 2007, 2003 by Saunders, an imprint of Elsevier Inc. All rights reserved.

3. Does Janet or the physician have the right to contact the daughters and discuss Mr. Robinson's condition with them?

WORKPLACE APPLICATIONS

Solicit 10 volunteers to come to the classroom and role-play patients and co-workers. Develop several personalities by writing a synopsis of the chief complaints and general personality traits. Allow each student to experience each "patient" or "co-worker" and react to them using professional interpersonal behavior and good human relations skills. Discuss the activity in class and talk about what this role-play activity can teach medical assisting students.

INTERNET ACTIVITIES

Use the Internet to answer the following questions.

1. How many different career fields do human relations and interpersonal skills affect?

2. What is organizational behavior?

3. How are human relations and interpersonal skills practiced in classrooms?

Write a classroom policy that stresses positive interpersonal skills and human relations. Share this policy with the class.

Copyright © 2011, 2007, 2003 by Saunders, an imprint of Elsevier Inc. All rights reserved.

6 Medicine and Ethics

VOCABULARY REVIEW

Fill in the blanks with the correct vocabulary terms from this chapter.

1. Melissa believes that one of her roles as a medical assistant is to be a patient ________________, supporting both the patient and family members during illnesses.
2. Ben has conflicting views about ________________ and is unsure as to whether he would want the option to die with dignity if he had an incurable, debilitating disease.
3. Jill understands that the ________________ of her actions while she is at work could affect whether a patient complies with the physician's instructions.
4. ________________ allows the medical assistant to consider his or her personal feelings about various ethical issues before being faced with those decisions while working with actual patients.
5. ________________ or handicapped patients need special understanding and patience from those who are employed in medical facilities.
6. Bianca is an infertile patient who is participating in ________________ ________________ to research a new drug that may help her to conceive a child.
7. The members of the Council on Ethical and Judicial Affairs issue ________________ about medical situations, similar to the way that the Supreme Court justices consider matters that are brought before the court.
8. ________________ is a devotion to the truth.
9. Kristy considers being friendly toward the patients in the clinic as her ________________ and a vital part of her job performance.
10. When a person has breached an ethical standard, ________________ may be necessary to atone for the action.

SKILLS AND CONCEPTS

Part I: Making Ethical Decisions

List the five steps of ethical decision making.

1. ____
2. ____
3. ____
4. ____
5. ____

Copyright © 2011, 2007, 2003 by Saunders, an imprint of Elsevier Inc. All rights reserved.

For the following scenarios, determine the type of ethical problem presented, the agent or agents, the course of action, and the outcome. Although these situations may present more than one ethical problem, choose only one possibility for each exercise.

Two sisters have arrived at a medical facility to discuss with the attending physician the course of action they should take regarding their dying father. Mr. Roberts, the patient, is no longer responsive. Cassandra wants to continue all possible medical treatment to keep her father alive. Janet insists that her father would not want his life prolonged by artificial means. Mr. Roberts did not give either sister a power of attorney, and he did not leave a written record of his wishes on this issue.

1. Type of ethical problem

____

2. Agent or agents

____

3. Course of action (Suggest one.)

____

4. Outcome (Suggest one.)

____

5. How can the medical assistant refrain from inflicting his or her own opinions on patients?

____

____

____

Dr. Patrick is the chief of staff at a regional medical center. His specialty is oncology, and the hospital is considering the construction of a cancer center as part of a multimillion-dollar project. One of Dr. Patrick's partners, Dr. Adams, is vehemently opposed to the project because of the cost to the local taxpayers who support the hospital. Dr. Adams has threatened to leave the practice unless Dr. Patrick votes against the project. Dr. Patrick wants the center to be built, but he also realizes that if Dr. Adams leaves, the practice will suffer a drastic loss of income.

1. Type of ethical problem

____

2. Agent or agents

____

3. Course of action (Suggest one.)

____

4. Outcome (Suggest one.)

____

5. How would you handle an ethical decision that has an equal number of pros and cons?

____

____

____

Copyright © 2011, 2007, 2003 by Saunders, an imprint of Elsevier Inc. All rights reserved.

Part II: Types of Ethical Problems

Identify the type of ethical problem that each diagram represents.

1.

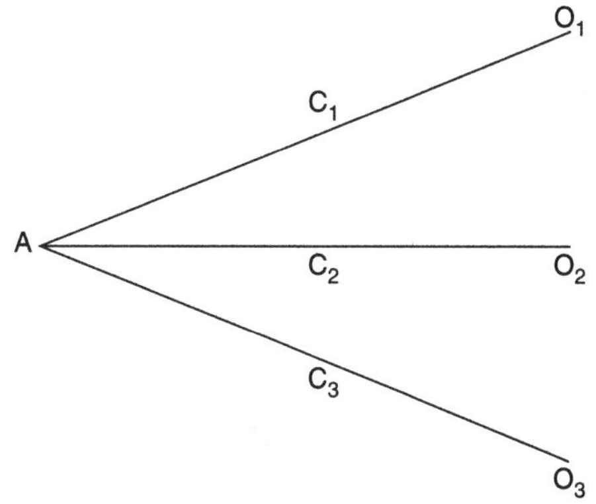

2.

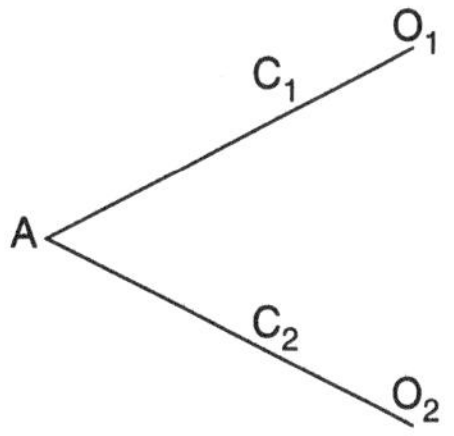

3.

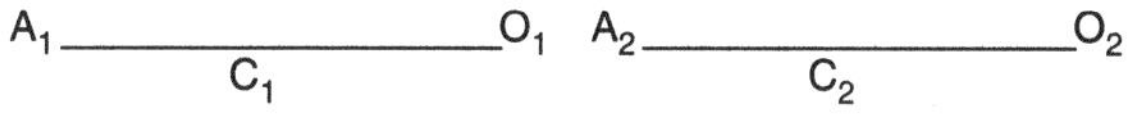

4.

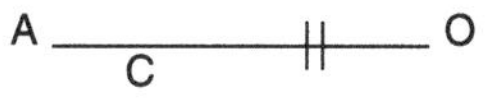

Part III: Opinions on Medicoethical Issues

Write your personal opinion regarding the following medicoethical issues. After writing your opinion, consider differing opinions by writing a brief opposing argument.

1. Abortion

____

____

____

2. Abortion: opposing opinion

____

____

____

Copyright © 2011, 2007, 2003 by Saunders, an imprint of Elsevier Inc. All rights reserved.

3. Stem cell research

4. Stem cell research: opposing opinion

5. Human cloning

6. Human cloning: opposing opinion

7. Genetic counseling

8. Genetic counseling: opposing opinion

9. Physician-assisted suicide

10. Physician-assisted suicide: opposing opinion

 Copyright © 2011, 2007, 2003 by Saunders, an imprint of Elsevier Inc. All rights reserved.

Part IV: Ethics and the Medical Assistant

1. Describe the behavior of an ethical medical assistant in your own words.

Part V: Rights and Duties

Identify the following as a right, a duty, or neither.

1. Healthcare services for all Americans

   right duty neither

2. Owning a gun when licensed

   right duty neither

3. Providing care to an elderly parent

   right duty neither

4. Nondiscrimination

   right duty neither

5. Life

   right duty neither

6. Are there times when a right or duty in the preceding list is invalid or could be argued to be so? Explain your answer.

Part VI: Confidentiality

1. List several physical places within the physician's office where confidentiality could be breached.

2. What are the usual consequences of breach of patient confidentiality?

3. Explain why confidentiality is critical in the medical environment.

Copyright © 2011, 2007, 2003 by Saunders, an imprint of Elsevier Inc. All rights reserved.

CASE STUDIES

Read the case studies and answer the questions that follow.

1. Robert is a patient who has tested positive for the human immunodeficiency virus (HIV). His employer invites the local blood bank to come to the workplace every 6 months and conduct a blood drive. Robert has declined to donate in the past because of his HIV status, but he often feels pressured by co-workers to give blood. None of them is aware that he is HIV positive. How do blood banks handle this situation today? Does Robert have alternatives that will resolve the situation? Explain your answer.

2. Cameron works for Dr. Christian, and she works hard to earn the trust of the patients. Mrs. Rainer confides to Cameron that she has been smoking, against Dr. Christian's advice, and she asks Cameron not to tell the physician. How should Cameron handle this situation? What should she tell the patient?

WORKPLACE APPLICATIONS

Stepping into the medical environment, where confidentiality is so important, may be a difficult adjustment for some new medical assistants. In any medical facility, you must think before speaking. At times, discussion of patients and their conditions will not be appropriate. How can you change your way of thinking and be constantly aware of the constraints that patient confidentiality places on discussion of patient information?

INTERNET ACTIVITIES

1. Peruse the Web site for the Health Insurance Portability and Accountability Act (HIPAA) and download the quick fact sheets. Study this information to gain a basic knowledge of HIPAA guidelines before studying the law in more detail in Chapter 16.
2. Discuss ethics in the classroom. How do medical assisting students perform ethically while completing their education? Research this issue on the Internet and talk about it in class.
3. Read the preamble and the nine principles of medical ethics posted on the American Medical Association's Web site. Discuss each principle. What changes would you make to these principles? Are they applicable to the situations that arise in the medical world today?

Copyright © 2011, 2007, 2003 by Saunders, an imprint of Elsevier Inc. All rights reserved.

7 Medicine and Law

VOCABULARY REVIEW

Fill in the blanks with the correct vocabulary terms from this chapter.

1. Dr. Parker insists that a medical assistant be present during all of his patient examinations in order to avoid any ________________ of wrongdoing or abuse.
2. Many physician offices require patients to sign a(n) ________________ agreement, which means disagreements may be settled by a qualified third party.
3. If a person contributes to a patient's poor condition, he or she may be charged with ________________.
4. Dr. Samantha Beddingfield was called to court to discuss her knowledge of malpractice cases as a(n) ________________.
5. When a patient offers his or her arm to have blood drawn, he or she has ________________ consent.
6. A doctor of ________________ studies the law.
7. Dr. Cartwright failed to follow the care of a hospital patient to whom he was assigned and may be guilty of ________________ and/or ________________.
8. Civil cases must be proved by a(n) ________________ of the ________________.
9. Criminal cases must be proved by ________________ ________________.
10. Roger Askew is bringing a case against a physician in the death of his wife during surgery, making him the ________________ in the case.
11. Something put into one's own words is ________________.
12. A court must have ________________ over a case before it can hear the arguments and make a judgment.
13. If Alisha writes down comments that are untrue and inflammatory about another person, she might be accused of ________________.
14. City court is often called ________________ court.
15. City regulations are often called city ________________.
16. If either side in a lawsuit is unhappy with the results, in most cases the decision can be ________________.
17. Vince suffered the loss of use of his arm after surgery, loss of wages by being rendered unable to work, and loss of his ability to earn a living. These losses are called ________________ in court.
18. The constitutional guarantee that legal proceedings will be fair is called ________________.
19. Judge Roberts has 12 cases on the ________________ for the day.
20. The person who stands accused of a crime in court is called the ________________.
21. The person who stands accused in a civil trial is called the ________________.
22. Alyssa may be held ________________ for damaging her boyfriend's car.
23. An intentional attempt to injure another person is called ________________.

Copyright © 2011, 2007, 2003 by Saunders, an imprint of Elsevier Inc. All rights reserved.

24. The unlawful use of force or violence against another person is called ________________.

25. A(n) ________________ is a major crime, such as rape or murder.

26. Consent that is detailed and usually in writing is called ________________ consent.

27. Judge Conlin uses previous cases as models to determine his decisions on current cases. The previous cases are called ________________.

28. Barbara Harris was served a(n) ________________, which required her to appear in court.

29. The document requiring that records be produced in court is called a(n) ________________ ________________.

30. The final decision of the judge or jury is called the ________________.

SKILLS AND CONCEPTS

Part I: Classifications of Law

1. The three basic categories of criminal law discussed in this chapter are:

   a. ________________________________

   b. ________________________________

   c. ________________________________

2. The three basic categories of civil law discussed in this chapter are:

   a. ________________________________

   b. ________________________________

   c. ________________________________

3. A law that is minor in nature and usually a breach of municipal regulations is called a(n) ________________.

4. Civil law involves cases that are brought to court by ________________.

5. Criminal law involves a crime against the ________________ or ________________.

6. Medical professional liability falls under what category of civil law? ________________

Part II: Anatomy of a Medical Professional Liability Lawsuit

1. List the four elements of a valid, legal contract.

   a. ________________________________

   b. ________________________________

   c. ________________________________

   d. ________________________________

2. List the three steps in the creation of the physician-patient relationship.

   a. ________________________________

   b. ________________________________

   c. ________________________________

Copyright © 2011, 2007, 2003 by Saunders, an imprint of Elsevier Inc. All rights reserved.

3. What must a letter of withdrawal of care state?

a. ____________________

b. ____________________

c. ____________________

4. How should a letter of withdrawal be mailed? ____________

5. Does the letter of withdrawal have to explain to the patient the reason the physician chose to withdraw from care of the patient? Explain your answer.

____

____

____

6. Explain what is meant by having jurisdiction over a case.

____

____

____

7. What is the ultimate appellate court in the United States?

____

8. Explain the difference between a deposition and an interrogatory.

____

____

____

9. List three of the five ways to determine whether a subpoena is valid.

a. ____________________

b. ____________________

c. ____________________

10. Briefly explain how a person called to testify in court should dress.

____

____

____

11. What is a defendant in a civil trial often called? ____________

Copyright © 2011, 2007, 2003 by Saunders, an imprint of Elsevier Inc. All rights reserved.

Part III: Medical Professional Liability and Negligence

Find the words in the list in the following puzzle.

Y	S	R	Z	S	T	F	P	E	M	Z	S	T	D	B	P	X	K	F	Q	W	U	T	F
M	R	K	O	F	U	N	H	C	H	A	F	C	B	M	N	G	J	K	M	M	T	E	U
Y	R	O	T	U	B	I	R	T	N	O	C	T	F	E	W	X	L	A	B	J	D	Y	O
M	R	U	T	T	P	A	A	Q	M	S	N	B	I	L	E	V	U	Y	K	I	W	Y	S
S	D	E	L	A	N	O	I	S	S	E	F	O	R	P	G	S	G	J	L	U	G	S	R
B	E	C	N	A	S	A	E	F	L	A	M	O	I	Y	V	P	G	H	K	W	P	E	G
V	N	N	K	Y	B	N	J	M	A	B	X	H	H	T	R	E	P	X	E	I	Z	W	S
T	I	A	Q	F	Y	E	E	U	U	E	A	T	I	U	A	I	M	B	S	Q	H	O	U
B	C	S	A	P	H	G	N	P	W	H	A	K	D	D	O	G	S	E	P	H	F	R	B
T	I	A	I	H	I	L	E	O	M	Z	H	E	I	M	V	B	E	J	M	N	B	K	M
S	D	E	R	E	L	I	C	T	I	O	N	A	C	Z	M	F	G	L	J	E	F	F	Z
C	E	F	F	O	F	G	N	G	Q	T	C	N	V	F	Q	K	A	T	L	D	G	S	S
K	M	S	R	U	R	E	A	S	O	N	A	B	L	E	X	E	M	P	L	A	R	Y	S
B	W	I	C	I	D	N	S	W	Z	G	Q	G	D	V	E	D	A	T	L	I	R	N	N
K	X	M	V	E	Z	C	A	C	S	U	V	N	I	I	V	H	D	T	O	M	R	R	T
R	D	F	C	L	O	E	E	A	P	O	N	D	K	T	X	I	J	W	K	L	M	K	I
Q	K	E	K	H	U	D	F	W	D	W	G	S	K	I	I	Y	R	U	D	E	W	U	S
L	D	R	P	X	Z	F	N	P	A	Z	R	B	V	N	F	L	P	Y	P	X	V	M	I
L	Y	Y	S	O	J	S	O	P	L	D	G	Q	U	U	V	G	P	E	F	R	U	J	P
A	V	P	J	X	X	J	N	C	L	W	U	I	S	P	S	N	N	I	P	A	V	F	T
D	B	W	T	R	U	V	R	V	C	Z	Q	D	X	O	W	U	F	E	Q	S	T	W	Z

Act
Allegation
Compensatory
Contributory
Damages
Decedent
Dereliction
Duty
Exemplary
Expert
Litigation
Malfeasance
Misfeasance
Negligence
Nonfeasance
Professional
Prudent
Punitive
Reasonable

Copyright © 2011, 2007, 2003 by Saunders, an imprint of Elsevier Inc. All rights reserved.

Part IV: Fill in the Blanks

Fill in the blanks with the correct answers.

1. The formal action of a legislative body is called a(n) ________________.
2. The performance of an act that is wholly wrongful and unlawful is ________________.
3. The agency that regulates safety in the workplace is ________________.
4. A law enacted by the legislative branch of a government is called a(n) ________________.
5. Failure to perform an act that should have been performed is ________________.
6. A solemn declaration made by a witness under oath in response to interrogation by a lawyer is called ________________.
7. The pretense of curing disease is called ________________.
8. The improper performance of a legal act is ________________.
9. Something that is easily understood or recognized by the mind is called a(n) ________________.
10. An authoritative decree or direction usually set forth by a municipal regulation is called a(n) ________________.
11. The law that promotes accuracy in medical laboratories is ________________.

Part V: Inside the Courtroom

Circle T or F to indicate whether the statement is true or false.

1. T F Lying under oath constitutes perjury.
2. T F Arriving late to the courtroom is acceptable if the witness has a good excuse.
3. T F Attorneys usually discover new information when questioning their clients in the courtroom.
4. T F A sustained objection means that the judge disagrees with the objection and will allow the question to stand.
5. T F It is not necessary to use "ma'am" or "sir" in the courtroom when addressing the judge.
6. T F If a question is confusing to a witness, he or she should ask the attorney to restate or repeat the question.
7. T F Discovery is pretrial disclosure of pertinent facts or documents pertaining to a case.
8. T F Arbitration is a cost-saving alternative to trial.

Part VI: The Four Ds of Negligence and Damages

1. A patient was given the wrong medication. No adverse effects occurred. Which of the four Ds is missing? Why does this affect the possibility of a lawsuit?

____

____

____

2. A car accident occurs at an intersection outside a physician's office during normal business hours. Do the physician and staff have a duty to provide direct care for the injured? Why or why not?

____

____

____

Copyright © 2011, 2007, 2003 by Saunders, an imprint of Elsevier Inc. All rights reserved.

3. A patient is treated for low back pain caused by a fall at the local mall. The patient sues the physician, because the pain is unresolved. Which of the four Ds would be the most difficult for the patient's attorney to prove? Why?

____

____

____

4. A medical assistant mislabeled a vial of blood that was sent to an outside laboratory. Because of this mistake, a child was given the wrong diagnosis and later died. The child's family sued the medical assistant, the physician, and the hospital that owned the practice. The child's family was awarded $4 million. What type of damages is this?

____

____

____

5. A female patient was awarded punitive damages after a physician sexually molested her during her annual pelvic examination. What are punitive damages designed to do? Do you think punitive damages should be limited to a specific amount of money?

____

____

____

CASE STUDY

Read the case study and answer the questions that follow.

A 10-year-old girl was brought to a physician's office with a complaint of a headache after gymnastics practice in mid-August. The clinic was a freestanding, minor emergency center and not the child's regular physician's office. The girl and the adult who had brought her to the clinic, her aunt, both denied that she had been in any type of accident and stated that her only complaint was the headache and being tired and hot. The aunt mentioned that the girl also seemed a bit disoriented during the drive to the clinic. The girl didn't recall having been at gymnastics practice less than an hour earlier. The child told the physician that she had been a gymnast for 6 years and that she really liked her coach.

The outside temperature had reached 101° F that day. The physician examined the patient and suggested that she be taken home to rest and rehydrate. No prescriptions were written, and the girl left the clinic. Two hours later, she could not be roused from sleep; her aunt immediately took her to the emergency department (ED) at the closest hospital. The girl's mother met them at the hospital just in time to be told that the girl had slipped into a coma. The ED physician suspected that the girl had experienced heat stroke. The aunt was shocked and mentioned that she had taken the girl to a clinic earlier; she questioned why this diagnosis has not been considered at that time. The girl's mother immediately called the clinic and berated the physician for putting her child in a coma.

What went wrong in this case? Who is responsible for the child's condition? Is this a "good" malpractice case?

____

____

____

____

____

____

____

____

____

Copyright © 2011, 2007, 2003 by Saunders, an imprint of Elsevier Inc. All rights reserved.

WORKPLACE APPLICATIONS

Research the laws that apply to medical clinics in your state. If possible, interview an office manager about the laws that apply to local clinics and ask what challenges arise in trying to comply with them. Share what you learn with the class.

INTERNET ACTIVITIES

1. Use the Internet to find the place in your area where a small claims case would be filed. Obtain the paperwork necessary to file a claim. Create a fictional case and complete the paperwork as if you plan to file it in court.

2. Research mediators in your area using the Internet. Find the name and contact information for at least three. With your instructor's permission, contact a mediator and ask the individual to speak to the class.

3. Research medical malpractice attorneys in your area using the Internet. Find the name and contact information for at least three. With your instructor's permission, invite the attorney to speak to the class on how medical assistants can help prevent medical malpractice claims.

Copyright © 2011, 2007, 2003 by Saunders, an imprint of Elsevier Inc. All rights reserved.

8 Computer Concepts

VOCABULARY REVIEW

Fill in the blanks with the correct vocabulary terms from this chapter.

1. Jacob uses a(n) ________________ ________________ to write data onto a blank compact disk and stores the CD as a backup for the clinic's blank forms.
2. To assist with patient diagnosis, Dr. Matthews uses software that is equipped with a type of ________________ ________________.
3. The smallest unit of information inside the computer is called a(n) ________________.
4. Olivia installed new ________________ ________________ on the office computers that will allow patients to check in without the assistance of a receptionist.
5. Ethan has asked that all the computer users in the clinic clear the computer ________________ periodically so that Web sites stored there will be erased and the system will run faster.
6. The office manager asked Samantha to print a(n) ________________ ________________ of the minutes of the meeting for each person attending.
7. Daniel likes to change the ________________ in the different sections of the clinic's patients' newsletter to make it more readable and attractive.
8. A picture that represents a program or an object on the computer is called a(n) ________________.
9. Information entered into and used by the computer is called ________________.
10. Tyler is responsible for the operation of the clinic's ________________, which manages shared network resources.
11. Information that is processed by the computer and transmitted to a monitor or printer is called ________________.
12. Christian was able to easily connect a(n) ________________ to his home computer, which allows information to be transmitted over telephone lines and enables him to connect to the Internet.
13. Any type of storage of files used to prevent their loss in the event of hard drive failure is called ________________.
14. The ________________ tracks all patient information, including addresses, phone numbers, and details about insurance coverage.
15. Megan purchased a(n) ________________ ________________ to backup the patient database and archive computer files.
16. A personal ________________ assistant is a handheld computer that can perform many functions.
17. The initial part of a URL listing is called a(n) ________________ ________________.

Copyright © 2011, 2007, 2003 by Saunders, an imprint of Elsevier Inc. All rights reserved.

SKILLS AND CONCEPTS

Part I: Matching Exercises

Match the following terms with their definitions.

1. ______ Approximately 1 billion bytes
2. ______ Approximately 1 trillion bytes
3. ______ 8 bits
4. ______ Binary digits
5. ______ Approximately 1,024 bytes
6. ______ Approximately 1 million bytes

A. Terabyte
B. Bit
C. Megabyte
D. Byte
E. Kilobyte
F. Gigabyte

Part II: Input, Output, and Storage Devices

Label each of the following as an input, output, or storage device.

1. Mouse	Input	Output	Storage
2. Keyboard	Input	Output	Storage
3. Printer	Input	Output	Storage
4. Scanner	Input	Output	Storage
5. Speakers	Input	Output	Storage
6. CD-ROM	Input	Output	Storage
7. Zip drive	Input	Output	Storage
8. Touch screen	Input	Output	Storage
9. Floppy disk	Input	Output	Storage
10. Flash drive	Input	Output	Storage

Part III: Parts of the Computer

Provide the name of the computer part described below.

1. Central unit of the computer that contains the logic circuitry and carries out the instructions of the computer's programs

   ____

2. Main circuit board of the computer

   ____

3. Devices inserted into a computer that give it added capabilities

   ____

4. Device used to display computer-generated information

   ____

5. Magnetic disk inside the computer that can hold several hundred gigabytes of information and is used to store the application software that runs on the computer

   ____

6. Device used to take information from one CD-ROM and write it to another CD-ROM

   ____

Copyright © 2011, 2007, 2003 by Saunders, an imprint of Elsevier Inc. All rights reserved.

7. Device over which data can be transmitted via telephone lines or other media, such as coaxial cable

___

8. Allows music or MIDI files to be heard from the computer

___

9. Software installed on a computer to allow a hardware device to function

___

Part IV: The Computer as a Co-Worker

List seven ways computers assist workers in medical offices.

1. ___
2. ___
3. ___
4. ___
5. ___
6. ___
7. ___

Part V: Basic Computer Functions

Describe how the following functions are performed on the computer.

1. Open a document

___

___

2. Save a document

___

___

3. Rename a document

___

___

4. Cut and paste text

___

___

5. Copy text

___

___

6. Exit a program

___

___

Copyright © 2011, 2007, 2003 by Saunders, an imprint of Elsevier Inc. All rights reserved.

7. Turn the computer on

____

____

8. Turn the computer off

____

____

Part VI: Short Answer Questions

1. The three elements that differentiate microprocessors are:

   a. ____

   b. ____

   c. ____

2. Explain peripheral devices and give one example of a peripheral device.

____

____

3. What is the function of a browser?

____

____

4. Define computer networking.

____

____

5. Why is computer security so important in today's medical office?

____

____

Part VII: File Formats and Printer Types

Match the following terms with their definitions.

1. _______ Inexpensive printer that provides a moderate-quality hard copy
2. _______ File format that supports color and often is used for scanned images
3. _______ Bitmapped graphics compiled by a graphics image set in rows or columns of dots
4. _______ Printer output similar to that of a photocopier; capable of complex graphics
5. _______ File format in which characters are represented by their ASCII codes
6. _______ File type commonly used for photographs

a. .doc
b. .gif
c. Laser
d. .jpeg
e. .bmp
f. Dot matrix

Copyright © 2011, 2007, 2003 by Saunders, an imprint of Elsevier Inc. All rights reserved.

7. ________ File type that combines ASCII codes with special commands that distinguish variations

8. ________ File usually created by a word processor for various documents, including letters and forms

9. ________ Printer that uses a heating element that is energized during the printing process

10. ________ Type of printer that serves as a scanner, fax, and copier

g. .txt

h. Ink jet

i. .rtf

j. Multifunctional

CASE STUDY

Read the case study and answer the questions that follow.

Brooke Comis works for Dr. Tomms as a clinical medical assistant. She is a former office computer specialist who worked in the computer field for 12 years before she entered medical assisting school. She changed career fields because of the work prospects in technology and acted on her dream to enter the medical field. Unfortunately, she is the only person in the office who is knowledgeable about computers, the Internet, and networking. Whenever a computer is not functioning correctly or a problem occurs with the network, Dr. Tomms asks Brooke to fix it. When he decided to buy new computers, he expected Brooke to assemble all of them and set up a new network. Brooke gets more and more irate each time she is asked to perform these duties, because she is not compensated other than her normal hourly pay. She knows that if Dr. Tomms paid someone to do this work, it would cost him more than her monthly salary. Brooke is not certain how to handle this situation. What should she do first? How should she approach the physician? Should she refuse to perform computer work? What could happen if she refuses?

____

____

____

____

____

____

____

____

____

WORKPLACE APPLICATIONS

Assume that you have been selected to order a new computer system for the physician. The clinic's personnel include three physicians, six administrative personnel, and four clinical assistants, plus you, the office manager. Describe the minimum equipment needed. Consider printers, Internet access, scanners, and wireless needs. Investigate computers using the Internet and prepare a folder with photos and/or specifications that detail the equipment you have selected.

INTERNET ACTIVITIES

Use the Internet to locate a company that sells computers in your geographic area. Explore the site. Find a computer that you might consider purchasing, then answer the following questions.

1. How much RAM and ROM does the system have?

Copyright © 2011, 2007, 2003 by Saunders, an imprint of Elsevier Inc. All rights reserved.

2. What is the clock speed?

3. What is the baud rate of the modem?

4. What software, if any, comes with the system?

5. What is the total cost before taxes are applied?

 Copyright © 2011, 2007, 2003 by Saunders, an imprint of Elsevier Inc. All rights reserved.

9 Telephone Techniques

VOCABULARY REVIEW

Fill in the blanks with the correct vocabulary terms from this chapter.

1. Taylor Medical USA sells durable medical equipment and supplies to the public, so the company is considered to be a(n) ________________.
2. Julie is careful of her ________________, because she wants her voice to be clear and effective when she is speaking on the telephone.
3. Cassie's voice has a nice ________________, which is a change in pitch or loudness when speaking.
4. Dr. LeGrand wants to ________________ her relationships with patients of different cultures so that she can understand their needs.
5. The office manager cautions the medical assistants to avoid ________________, because most patients do not understand complicated medical terms.
6. The highness or lowness of sound is called its ________________.
7. Laura ________________ will be at work on time and will stay until the last patient leaves.
8. When speaking on the phone or in public, Dr. Conn knows that he should avoid ________________ speech to keep the listeners interested and enthusiastic about what he has to say.
9. The medical assistants at Wray Medical and Surgical Clinic are proficient at ________________.
10. Being placed on hold for an extended time becomes quite ________________.
11. The utterance of articulate, clear sounds is ________________.
12. It is pleasant to hear a person speak with ________________.
13. Dr. Beard ordered the laboratory tests ________________ so that the results would be reported to him immediately.
14. Mackenzie has learned to be ________________ when she speaks with patients on the phone so that she maintains a good relationship with them.
15. Dr. Lightfoot prefers that the receptionist ________________ all his calls so that he can concentrate on the patients in the office during their examinations.

Copyright © 2011, 2007, 2003 by Saunders, an imprint of Elsevier Inc. All rights reserved.

SKILLS AND CONCEPTS

Part I: Answering Incoming Calls and Taking Phone Messages

Read the following incoming calls. Then use the telephone message forms to take an accurate message for each caller. The calls in quotations are taken from voice mail. Determine who should receive the message; three questions to ask the patient when the call is returned; and what actions need to be taken for proper follow-through. Although you are not required to list questions that are clinical in nature, you may include clinical questions if you like.

Staff Members at Dr. Julie Beard's Office

Physician	Dr. Julie Beard
Office Manager	Julia Carpenter
Clinical Medical Assistant	Trina Martinez
Clinical Medical Assistant	Dean Howell
Scheduling Assistant	Stephanie Dickson
Receptionist	Ginny Holloway
Insurance Biller and Medical Records	Gloria Richardson

1. "Hello, this is Peter Young. I saw Dr. Beard on Monday about a rash on my forearms. This thing isn't getting any better, and the cream she prescribed for me isn't helping the itching, and it's very uncomfortable. Is there anything else we can do to help it? My number is 972-555-9873." The message was received at 8:30 AM on Thursday, February 3.

   Who should receive this message?

   ____

   Questions to ask the patient when returning this call:

   a. ____________________

   b. ____________________

   c. ____________________

   What action should be taken after speaking with the patient?

   ____

   ____

   ____

2. Gerald Morris calls Dr. Beard's office to ask whether his insurance has paid for his last office visit. He is an established patient and has worked as a city police officer for more than 10 years. After asking to place Mr. Morris on hold, you pull up his account on the computer. No insurance payment has been credited to his account, and a note indicates that his insurance was not in effect at the time of his office visit. Mr. Morris asks you to check with the insurance company and call him back, because he is concerned about resolving this issue. His phone number is 972-555-8824. This message was taken at 3:45 PM on September 4.

   Who should receive this message?

   ____

   Questions to ask the patient when returning this call:

   a. ____________________

   b. ____________________

   c. ____________________

Copyright © 2011, 2007, 2003 by Saunders, an imprint of Elsevier Inc. All rights reserved.

What action should be taken after speaking to the patient?

____

____

____

3. "Hello, this is Savannah Yarborough. I visited with your receptionist earlier today, and she indicated that one of the medical assistants has resigned and you will have a position available in a few weeks. I am very interested in interviewing and presenting myself as a candidate for the job. I am a certified medical assistant with 6 years' experience. Please give me a call at your convenience. My telephone number is 817-555-9902. I look forward to speaking with you and perhaps scheduling an interview." This message was taken at 1:30 PM on May 1.

   Who should receive this message?

   ____

   Questions to ask when returning this call:

   a. _______________

   b. _______________

   c. _______________

   What action should be taken after speaking to Ms. Yarborough?

   ____

   ____

   ____

4. Mr. Juan Ross called today at 10:15 AM to get his prescription for Ambien refilled. His pharmacy is Wolfe Drug, and the drugstore phone number is 214-555-4523. He is allergic to penicillin. Mr. Ross's phone number is 214-555-2377. Mr. Ross's message was received on July 23.

   Who should receive this message?

   ____

   Questions to ask the patient when returning his call:

   a. _______________

   b. _______________

   c. _______________

   What action should be taken after speaking to the patient?

   ____

   ____

   ____

5. Mr. Benjamin Adams called to speak to the office manager to express his dissatisfaction with the times he was offered for an appointment. His job is strict about attendance, and he cannot leave work until 4 PM. He has requested appointment times after 4 PM, but the scheduling assistant tells him that he cannot have an appointment any later than 4 PM. Mr. Adams is concerned that he will not be able to be at the clinic at that exact time, and he is frustrated that the clinic is not more responsive to his needs. He called at 2:15 PM on March 14. His phone number at work is 972-555-6343, and his cell phone number is 214-555-8080.

   Who should receive this message?

   ____

Copyright © 2011, 2007, 2003 by Saunders, an imprint of Elsevier Inc. All rights reserved.

Questions to ask the patient when returning the call:

a. ______________________________

b. ______________________________

c. ______________________________

What action should be taken after speaking to the patient?

____

____

____

6. "This is Ms. Garrett from Blue Cross/Blue Shield, and it's 10 AM on June 5. I am calling to discuss employee benefits for the coming year with the office manager. BCBS provides insurance coverage for your clinic employees. Would you please have the office manager return my call when she has a few moments to talk? My number is 800-555-0024, extension 415. Thank you!"

   Who should receive this message?

   ____

   Questions to ask when returning the call:

   a. ______________________________

   b. ______________________________

   c. ______________________________

   What action should be taken after speaking to Ms. Garrett?

   ____

   ____

   ____

7. "This is Sarah at Cline Meador Lab with a stat lab report. It's 9:35 AM on November 16. The patient's name is Laura Williamson, and her WBC count is 18,000. Please notify Dr. Beard immediately. The lab phone number is 800-555-3333, and my extension is 255. If she has any questions, please have her give me a call. Thanks."

   Who should receive this message?

   ____

   Questions to ask or information to verify when returning the call:

   a. ______________________________

   b. ______________________________

   c. ______________________________

   What action should be taken after speaking to Sarah?

   ____

   ____

   ____

Copyright © 2011, 2007, 2003 by Saunders, an imprint of Elsevier Inc. All rights reserved.

8. Judy Jordan has migraine headaches and occasionally takes hydrocodone to relieve the pain. Dr. Beard leaves the office for the weekend at noon on Friday, and office policy dictates that she is not to be paged except in emergencies. Patients with routine or lesser health issues are to be instructed either to make an appointment to come in and see the physician or to go to the emergency department. Ms. Jordan calls at 4:45 PM on Friday afternoon, March 9, after Dr. Beard has left the office. She requests that the staff authorize a refill for her pain medicine and insists on speaking to the office manager, who is in a meeting. Ms. Jordan's phone number is 214-555-9822.

   Who should receive this message?

   ____

   Questions to ask or information to verify when returning the call:

   a. ______________________________

   b. ______________________________

   c. ______________________________

   What action should be taken in this situation?

   ____

   ____

   ____

9. Gary Burritt is moving out of state, so he calls the office because he needs a copy of his medical records. Dr. Beard prefers to send medical records directly to the receiving physician. Mr. Burritt's phone number is 512-555-6679. Today's date is December 20, and this message was received at 11:45 AM.

   Who should receive this message?

   ____

   Questions to ask or information to verify when returning the call:

   a. ______________________________

   b. ______________________________

   c. ______________________________

   What action should be taken in this situation?

   ____

   ____

   ____

10. Allan Jenkins is calling from the cleaning service to let the office manager know what supplies he needs. He leaves a message stating that the office needs window cleaner, paper towels, liquid cleanser, and floor cleaner. He says that the office manager does not have to call him back, but the service will be cleaning again on Friday evening and will need the supplies at that time. This message was received on Wednesday, April 7 at 8:10 AM. The caller leaves his phone number, 903-555-2378, in case the office manager has questions.

    Who should receive this message?

    ____

    What action should be taken in this situation?

    ____

    ____

    ____

Copyright © 2011, 2007, 2003 by Saunders, an imprint of Elsevier Inc. All rights reserved.

11. "Hello. My name is Christina Cawtel, and I was referred to your office by Dr. Preston for evaluation of an ovarian cyst. Today is Wednesday, October 4, and it is 8 AM. I would like to make an appointment for early next week if possible. My phone number is 817-555-9325. Oh, and by the way, I need to know if you are a provider for Aetna, because my company just changed to their managed care plan. I probably need to have a mammogram, too, and I want to see if you will order it before I come in for the appointment. Thanks."

    Who should receive this message?

    ____

    Questions to ask or information to verify when returning the call:

    a. ______________________________

    b. ______________________________

    c. ______________________________

    What action should be taken in this situation?

    ____

    ____

    ____

12. "My name is Janeen Shaw and I am Dr. Beard's patient. It is just before 2 PM, and I am trying to reach you as soon as you open your office after lunch. I am having a hard time breathing, and I have stomach pains. I am hurting all over my upper body, on my chest, my arms, my neck, just everywhere. I'm sweating, and I'm very nauseated. I'm 45, and I'm almost never ill. I wanted to find out if I can come in for an appointment today. Please call me back as soon as possible. My phone number is 601-555-3423. Thank you. Please call as soon as you can. I really feel awful."

    Who should receive this message?

    ____

    Questions to ask or information to verify when returning the call:

    a. ______________________________

    b. ______________________________

    c. ______________________________

    What action should be taken in this situation?

    ____

    ____

    ____

Part II: Handling Difficult Calls

Briefly explain how the following callers and types of calls should be handled.

1. Angry callers

    ____

    ____

    ____

2. Sales calls

    ____

    ____

    ____

Copyright © 2011, 2007, 2003 by Saunders, an imprint of Elsevier Inc. All rights reserved.

3. Emergency calls

____

____

____

4. Unauthorized inquiry calls

____

____

____

5. Callers with complaints

____

____

____

Part III: Using a Telephone Directory

Using your local telephone directory or internet directory, find the following telephone numbers for your city or community.

1. Nonemergency number for the police department

____

2. General information number for the nearest airport

____

3. Local tax office

____

4. American Red Cross office

____

5. Acute care hospital

____

6. Mental health and mental retardation center

____

7. Meals on Wheels

____

8. American Cancer Society

____

Copyright © 2011, 2007, 2003 by Saunders, an imprint of Elsevier Inc. All rights reserved.

Part IV: Answering the Telephone

Use the local telephone directory or internet directory to find telephone numbers for the following medical specialty offices in your area. Call these offices to determine how they answer the telephone. Explain the purpose of your call to the staff member who answers the phone and record the phone greeting they use in the space provided below. Alternatively, write an original phone greeting for each of these medical specialty offices.

1. Ophthalmologist

   ____

2. Oncologist

   ____

3. General practitioner

   ____

4. Chiropractor

   ____

5. Cosmetic surgeon

   ____

6. Dermatologist

   ____

Part V: Short Answer Questions

Fill in the blank with the correct answer.

1. Selecting which calls will be forwarded to the physician immediately is a process called ______________.
2. A study by Harvard University claims that the physician's ______________ of voice has a direct link to medical professional liability claims.
3. The medical assistant should not eat, drink, or ______________ while answering the office telephone.
4. The mouthpiece of the telephone handset should be held ______________ inch(es) from the lips.
5. The medical assistant must maintain patient ______________ at all times, even when on the telephone.
6. Telephone calls should be answered by the ______________ ring.
7. Unsatisfactory progress reports from patients should be directed to the ______________.
8. ______________ calls help the physician communicate with family members in different parts of the country.
9. Medical offices should have a set of clearly written ______________ that can be read to the caller who requests the information.

Part VI: Time Zones

Determine the correct times.

1. When it is 3 PM in Dallas, Texas, it is ______________ in Los Angeles, California.
2. When it is 2 PM in Washington state, it is ______________ in New York City.
3. When it is 5 PM in Las Cruces, New Mexico, it is ______________ in Flint, Michigan.
4. When it is 4 PM in Augusta, Maine, it is ______________ in Columbia, South Carolina.
5. When it is 11 AM in Biloxi, Mississippi, it is ______________ in Chicago, Illinois.

Copyright © 2011, 2007, 2003 by Saunders, an imprint of Elsevier Inc. All rights reserved.

Part VII: Telephone Technique

1. List five questions that might be asked of a patient who calls with an emergency situation:

   a. ______

   b. ______

   c. ______

   d. ______

   e. ______

2. The phrase that often calms an angry patient is ______ ______ ______ ______.

3. Explain the procedure for transferring a phone call.

   ______

4. What should the medical assistant do if a caller refuses to identify himself or herself?

   ______

5. List the seven components of a proper telephone message.

   a. ______

   b. ______

   c. ______

   d. ______

   e. ______

   f. ______

   g. ______

CASE STUDY

Read the case study and answer the questions that follow.

Denise has been the receptionist for a moderately large clinic for the past 3 months. She replaced Dorothy, who retired. Denise has been overwhelmed by the number of calls to the clinic, and the office manager has spoken to her twice about missing calls. Denise insists that she is constantly on the phone answering and transferring calls. She is beginning to lose faith in herself, but as she considers why she is failing at her job, she realizes that two new physicians have joined the practice since Dorothy left, and numerous calls come to the clinic for those two physicians. Denise wants to suggest to the office manager that perhaps the time has come for a second receptionist, but she is unsure how to broach the subject. How can Denise begin her conversation with the office manager? What should she not do or say?

______

Copyright © 2011, 2007, 2003 by Saunders, an imprint of Elsevier Inc. All rights reserved.

WORKPLACE APPLICATIONS

Contact a clinic office manager and ask whether he or she would allow you to shadow the office receptionist for a day. Take note of the types of calls that come into the clinic and how they are handled. Discuss the results of the visit with the class.

INTERNET ACTIVITIES

1. Investigate telephone techniques and skills on the Internet and bring three tips to class. Share these with your classmates.

2. After researching information on the Internet, write a report that explains why the telephone is so important in making a good first impression.

3. Research the way telephones actually work. Prepare a brief report for the class.

4. Research the way Internet connections are made through phone systems. Prepare a brief report for the class.

Copyright © 2011, 2007, 2003 by Saunders, an imprint of Elsevier Inc. All rights reserved.

10 Scheduling Appointments

VOCABULARY REVIEW

Fill in the blank with the correct vocabulary term from this chapter.

1. Angela arranged for a short time ________________ between Dr. Patrick's speaking engagement and his first afternoon appointment so that he would have time for lunch.
2. Gayle gained ________________ in computers by taking Saturday classes on the newest software.
3. A(n) ________________ noise came from the autoclave when it was turned on this morning, so Pamela called service personnel to repair the machine.
4. Olivia realized that she needed to take a(n) ________________ medical terminology course before she could register for anatomy and physiology.
5. All the medical assistants in the facility know that a(n) ________________ ________________ must be noted in the medical record, as well as the appointment book.
6. Before using an appointment book, establish the ________________ by marking all times the physician is unavailable, so that patients will not be scheduled during those times.
7. A patient from a neighboring clinic caused a(n) ________________ in the hallway as he left, because he disagreed with a billing statement.
8. ________________ ________________ are those who have been seen as patients in the clinic more than once.
9. The ________________ among the staff at Dr. Wykowski's office has become strained since the office manager was terminated.
10. Cooperation and willingness to help other staff members is a(n) ________________ part of the success of a practice.
11. The payment of benefits to the physician for services rendered is called ________________.
12. A(n) ________________ is a predeveloped page layout used to make new pages with a similar design, pattern, or style.

Copyright © 2011, 2007, 2003 by Saunders, an imprint of Elsevier Inc. All rights reserved.

SKILLS AND CONCEPTS

Part I: Appointment Reminder Cards

Practice completing appointment reminder cards on the forms provided.

1. Gayle Jackson has an appointment for August 23, 20XX, at 3 PM with Dr. Lupez.

Blackburn Primary Care Associates, PC
1990 Turquiose Drive • Blackburn, WI 54937 • 608-459-8857

has an appointment on ______ provider ______

date ______ time ______

Please telephone one day in advance if you will be unable to keep the appointment

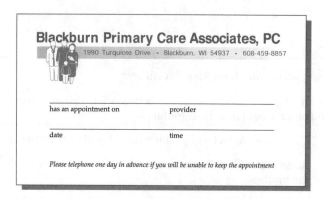

2. Debra Odom has an appointment for May 1, 20XX, at 9 AM with Dr. Hughes.

Blackburn Primary Care Associates, PC
1990 Turquiose Drive • Blackburn, WI 54937 • 608-459-8857

has an appointment on ______ provider ______

date ______ time ______

Please telephone one day in advance if you will be unable to keep the appointment

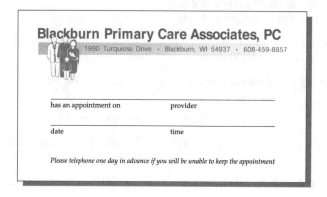

3. Katrina Shaw has an appointment for June 13, 20XX, at 11:45 AM with Dr. Hughes.

Blackburn Primary Care Associates, PC
1990 Turquiose Drive • Blackburn, WI 54937 • 608-459-8857

has an appointment on ______ provider ______

date ______ time ______

Please telephone one day in advance if you will be unable to keep the appointment

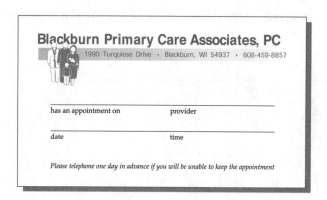

Copyright © 2011, 2007, 2003 by Saunders, an imprint of Elsevier Inc. All rights reserved.

4. Joni Perry has an appointment for September 12, 20XX, at 2:40 PM with Dr. Lawler.

Blackburn Primary Care Associates, PC
1990 Turquiose Drive • Blackburn, WI 54937 • 608-459-8857

____
has an appointment on provider

____
date time

Please telephone one day in advance if you will be unable to keep the appointment

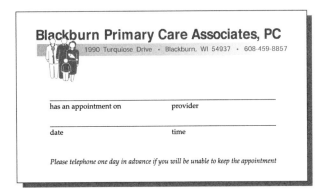

5. Savannah York has an appointment for December 15, 20XX, at 4:30 PM with Dr. Lupez.

Blackburn Primary Care Associates, PC
1990 Turquiose Drive • Blackburn, WI 54937 • 608-459-8857

____
has an appointment on provider

____
date time

Please telephone one day in advance if you will be unable to keep the appointment

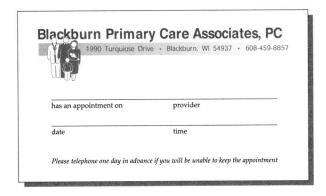

Part II: Guides for Scheduling

1. What three items must be considered when scheduling appointments?

   a. ____

   b. ____

   c. ____

2. Why is patient need an important consideration when planning the services the clinic will offer?

   ____

   ____

3. How can the medical assistant handle a physician who habitually spends more than the allotted time with patients?

   ____

   ____

4. List one advantage and one disadvantage to using an appointment book for scheduling.

   Advantage ____

   Disadvantage ____

5. List one advantage and one disadvantage to using a computer for scheduling.

   Advantage ____

   Disadvantage ____

Copyright © 2011, 2007, 2003 by Saunders, an imprint of Elsevier Inc. All rights reserved.

6. Explain why the time length of appointments is important.

____

____

7. Define a template and explain its use with regard to appointment scheduling.

____

____

8. What is a repeating appointment?

____

____

9. What is the difference between an emergency appointment and an urgent appointment?

____

____

10. Explain why an emergency call should never be placed on hold.

____

____

Part III: Advance Preparation and Establishing a Matrix

Prepare Appointment Page 1 (See Work Product 10-1 on p. 47 of the Procedures Checklists) according to the following directions.

1. The date is Monday, October 13, 20XX.
2. Dr. Lawler and Dr. Hughes have hospital rounds from 8 to 9 AM.
3. Dr. Lupez sees patients from 8 AM to noon and then has a medical conference.
4. Lunch is from noon until 2 PM.
5. Dr. Lawler has a 4 PM meeting at the hospital.
6. Dr. Hughes and Dr. Lawler both prefer a break from 3:15 to 3:30 PM to catch up on telephone calls and other duties.

Part IV: Scheduling Appointments

Prepare Appointment Page 2 (See Work Product 10-2 on p. 49 of the Procedures Checklists) according to the following directions. Appointments can be scheduled for subsequent days in these exercises.

1. The date is Tuesday, October 14, 20XX.
2. Lunch is from noon until 2 PM.
3. Dr. Lawler will be out Tuesday afternoon.
4. Dr. Hughes is out of town speaking at a conference.
5. Tracey and Keith Jones would like an appointment with Dr. Lawler right before lunch. Both are new patient physical examinations, and they would like to come to the office at the same time so that they can also discuss family planning.
6. John Edgar, Lydia Perry, and June Trayner are established patients who need follow-up appointments with Dr. Lupez.

 Copyright © 2011, 2007, 2003 by Saunders, an imprint of Elsevier Inc. All rights reserved.

7. Wayne Harris needs a new patient appointment with Dr. Lawler as early as possible.
8. Lucy Fraser needs an appointment with Dr. Lawler or Dr. Hughes and has to make the appointment after 3:30 PM, because she picks up her children from school.
9. Asa Nordholm, Carrie Jones, and Seicho Ando need follow-up appointments with Dr. Lawler.
10. Talia Perez called and is having trouble with her new blood pressure medication. The soonest she can get off work and come to the clinic is 2:15 PM.
11. Paula Nolen needs an allergy shot in the morning.
12. Amy Wainwright needs a well-woman examination and can come to the clinic any time before 3 PM.
13. Pam Billingsley wants to come to the clinic in the later afternoon for a return check about her migraine headaches.
14. Adam Angsley needs an appointment with Dr. Lawler in the afternoon.

Prepare Appointment Page 3 (See Work Product 10-3 on p. 51 of the Procedures Checklists) according to the following directions. Appointments can be scheduled for subsequent days in these exercises.

1. The date is Wednesday, October 15, 20XX.
2. All of the physicians are in the office today.
3. Lunch is from noon until 2 PM.
4. Dr. Lawler has three rechecks today, with Ella Jones, Fred Linstra, and Mary Higgins.
5. Winston Hill is an established patient coming in for an annual physical with Dr. Lawler. His neighbor can drive him to the clinic for a 2 PM appointment.
6. Elnar Rosen, an established patient, needs a physical with Dr. Hughes at around 10:15 AM.
7. A staff meeting is scheduled for 9 AM.
8. A representative from Allied Medical Supply is demonstrating a self-scheduling computer program at 4:30 PM for all staff members.
9. Bob Jones needs a morning appointment with Dr. Lupez.
10. Talia Perez is extremely nauseated and needs to return to the clinic today.
11. Robin Tower is a new patient who wants to see Dr. Lawler or Dr. Hughes.
12. Audrey Rhodes is a new patient who wants to see Dr. Lawler.
13. Victor Garner is a follow-up patient whom Dr. Lupez saw last week in the hospital. He is new to the clinic.
14. Charlie Robinson missed his appointment today at 11 AM with Dr. Hughes.
15. Peter Blake calls to see if he can be seen by one of the physicians at 11:15 AM.

Prepare Appointment Page 4 (See Work Product 10-4 on p. 53 of the Procedures Checklists) according to the following directions. Appointments can be scheduled for subsequent days in these exercises.

1. The date is Thursday, October 16, 20XX.
2. Dr. Hughes is not in the office, because his daughter is having a baby.
3. Lunch is from noon until 2 PM.
4. All patients must be seen in the morning because the clinic is closed on Thursday afternoons.
5. Cassie LeGrand is coming to the clinic as a new patient to see Dr. Lupez.

Copyright © 2011, 2007, 2003 by Saunders, an imprint of Elsevier Inc. All rights reserved.

6. Cassandra LeBrock is coming to the clinic as an established patient to see Dr. Lupez.

7. Raymond Smith wants to make an appointment at 1:45 pm with Dr. Lawler.

8. Benjamin Charles requests an appointment with Dr. Lupez at 3:45 PM.

Prepare Appointment Page 5 (See Work Product 10-5 on p. 55 of the Procedures Checklists) according to the following directions.

1. The date is Friday, October 17, 20XX.
2. Dr. Lupez is the only provider in the office today.
3. Lunch is from noon until 2 PM.
4. Cassie LeGrand returns today for laboratory work and to consult with Dr. Lupez for surgery.
5. Bruce Wells is scheduled for a follow-up appointment at 10:15 AM.
6. Ronald Trayhan calls to make an appointment with Dr. Lupez for 2:30 PM.
7. Dr. Hughes calls to ask Dr. Lupez to see one of his young patients, Barbara Scott, at 3 PM for a high fever.
8. Stanley Allred calls for an appointment to see Dr. Lupez at 3 PM.

Part V: Types of Scheduling

Briefly describe each type of scheduling, and list one advantage and one disadvantage of each.

1. Scheduled appointments

____

____

2. Open office hours

____

____

3. Flexible office hours

____

____

4. Wave scheduling

____

____

5. Modified wave scheduling

____

____

6. Double booking

____

____

Copyright © 2011, 2007, 2003 by Saunders, an imprint of Elsevier Inc. All rights reserved.

7. Grouping procedures

8. Advance booking

Part VI: Special Circumstances

1. How can the medical assistant deal with patients who are consistently late for appointments?

2. How does the medical assistant handle a patient who arrives at the clinic to see the physician but does not have an appointment?

Part VII: Verifying Appointments

1. Write a brief script that could be used to verify patient appointments and that does not violate patient privacy.

Part VIII: Scheduling Inpatient and Outpatient Admissions and Procedures

Complete the referral forms in Work Products 10-6 to 10-9 on pp. 57-64 of the Procedures Checklists for the following patients. Create fictional demographic information.

1. Cassie LeGrand is to report to Mercy Hospital for excision of a nasal polyp on Tuesday, October 24, 20XX. Dr. Lupez is her attending physician. Surgery is scheduled for Tuesday at 2 PM. She will need blood work that morning. The procedure is considered outpatient, and Cassie will go home later that day if she does well. ICD code: 471.0 (Work Product 10-6).

2. Bob Jones arrives at Presbyterian Hospital to have a magnetic resonance imaging (MRI) scan on his right knee on Friday, November 2, 20XX. He needs an early morning appointment. ICD code: 715.8 (Work Product 10-7).

3. Lucille Saxton is to be admitted to the hospital for surgery for a bowel obstruction. Her surgery date is June 14, 20XX, and she must be admitted a day in advance for laboratory work and a chest x-ray examination. ICD code: 560.9 (Work Product 10-8).

4. Pam Burton needs to be admitted for several tests because of recurrent irritable bowel syndrome. She will be in the hospital for at least 3 days and should check in on July 23, 20XX, in the afternoon so that she will have taken nothing by mouth (NPO) before the blood tests are performed and x-ray films are taken the following morning. ICD Code: 564.1 (Work Product 10-9).

Copyright © 2011, 2007, 2003 by Saunders, an imprint of Elsevier Inc. All rights reserved.

CASE STUDY

Read the case study and answer the questions that follow.

Janie Haynes consistently arrives at the clinic 15 to 45 minutes late. She always has a "good" excuse, but she could make her appointments on time if she had better time management skills. The office manager has mentioned to Paula, the receptionist, that Janie is to be scheduled at 4:45 PM and if she is late, she will not be seen by the physician. Paula books Janie's next three appointments at that time, and Janie actually arrives early. However, on the fourth appointment, Janie arrives at 5:50 PM, and Paula knows it is her responsibility to tell Janie she cannot see the physician. How does Paula handle this task? Is more than one option available?

WORKPLACE APPLICATIONS

Choose five clinics and call the receptionist at each. Tell the receptionist that you are studying scheduling in medical assisting school and are interested in the scheduling method that clinic uses. Tally the results each classmate obtains, then graph or chart the results for the class on one document. Discuss the frequency of the various methods of scheduling.

INTERNET ACTIVITIES

1. Research scheduling software on the Internet and select a software package that would be functional for a physician's office. Gather information about the features and benefits and present the information to the class.

2. Research information about the different types of scheduling and how effective they are in physicians' offices. Determine the type of scheduling best suited to a family practice clinic. Present the ideas to the class.

3. Research self-scheduling software and determine the advantages and disadvantages of allowing patients to schedule appointments on the Internet. Present the information to the class or write an informative report about your findings.

Copyright © 2011, 2007, 2003 by Saunders, an imprint of Elsevier Inc. All rights reserved.

11 Patient Reception and Processing

VOCABULARY REVIEW

Fill in the blanks with the correct vocabulary terms from this chapter.

1. Thomas noticed that the staff had ________________ their supplies of gauze pads, so he ordered a case using the medical supplier's online system.
2. Jerri ________________ the 1-inch syringes so that Thomas would know to order more of them for the clinic.
3. Dr. Raleigh installed a(n) ________________ system so that he could speak to the medical assistants both in the front and the back offices from the examination rooms.
4. Medical assistants must be aware of the ________________ patients have of the office staff and take steps to ensure it is a positive one.
5. Susan filed the laboratory reports in ________________ order.
6. ________________ information includes the patient's address, insurance information, and e-mail address.
7. Any ________________ offered to a patient should be within the physician's orders, so make sure a beverage with sugar is not offered to a diabetic.
8. Angela uses ________________ devices to help her remember the duties to complete before leaving the office.
9. Employees prefer to work in an office with a(n) ________________ environment.
10. Dr. Lawson has a(n) ________________ desire to serve his patients and promote wellness.
11. A secondary use of health information that cannot be reasonably prevented is called a(an) ________________. ________________.
12. Medical assistants may find it helpful to write a patient's name using ________________ spelling to remember its pronunciation.

SKILLS AND CONCEPTS

Part I: The Office Mission Statement

1. Create a mission statement for a fictional family practice.

____

____

____

____

____

Copyright © 2011, 2007, 2003 by Saunders, an imprint of Elsevier Inc. All rights reserved.

Part II: The Reception Area

1. Why is the first impression of the physician's office so important to patients?

2. List five items that might be found in the patient reception area.
   a.
   b.
   c.
   d.
   e.

3. If a computer is provided in the reception area, what cautionary measure should be taken to ensure patient privacy?

4. Describe the ideal receptionist for a physician's office.

Part III: Registration Procedures

1. List six items of demographic information found on a patient information sheet.
   a.
   b.
   c.
   d.
   e.
   f.

Part IV: Consideration for the Patient's Time

1. Why might a crowded waiting room be a sign of inefficiency rather than the physician's popularity?

Copyright © 2011, 2007, 2003 by Saunders, an imprint of Elsevier Inc. All rights reserved.

2. Delays longer than ________________ minutes should be explained to patients, and they should be allowed to reschedule if they want to do so.

3. No more than ________________ or ________________ patients should be waiting in the reception area at any given time.

4. What feelings do patients often experience when waiting in the physician's office?

Part V: Patient Confidentiality

1. How can the medical assistant help prevent a breach of patient confidentiality by the placement of charts in wall holders?

2. How can the medical assistant help prevent a breach of patient confidentiality while using sign-in sheets?

3. Provide two examples of incidental disclosure.

   a. ________________

   b. ________________

4. Why would some offices limit the number of people who can accompany a patient into the exam room?

5. Should the medical assistant ever discipline a disruptive child in the medical office? Why or why not?

6. How do glass partitions help keep patient information confidential? Are they useful in today's medical offices? Why or why not?

Copyright © 2011, 2007, 2003 by Saunders, an imprint of Elsevier Inc. All rights reserved.

Part VI: Patient Checkout

Write a verbal response to the following patients in the checkout process.

1. Suzanne Anton is ready to leave the clinic, and she owes a co-pay of $25 plus a past due balance of $10 that her insurance did not pay. She questions the $10 balance.

____

____

____

2. Randy Stephens is leaving the clinic but is angry about his visit with the physician, who insists that he lose 40 pounds. He reluctantly pays his co-pay. He needs to schedule a follow-up appointment for 1 month, during which time the physician wants him to have lost 5 pounds by following a strict diet.

____

____

____

3. Alfreda Williams has come to the clinic for a checkup. She is being treated by the physician for colon cancer, and she usually is cheerful, despite her prognosis. Today she seems distressed and hesitates before paying her bill of $65.

____

____

____

Part VII: The End of the Day

1. Paige is preparing for the next work day. What are some tasks that will help her prepare for tomorrow's patients?

____

____

____

2. List several routine tasks for closing an office.

____

____

____

3. How can the medical assistant gain confidence in asking for payments and co-payments?

____

____

____

Copyright © 2011, 2007, 2003 by Saunders, an imprint of Elsevier Inc. All rights reserved.

Part VIII: Evaluating Reception Areas

Visit several reception areas in physician's offices, hospitals, and/or clinics. Take note of the appearance and amenities in these facilities. Rate each reception area on a scale of 1 to 10. Total the figures to determine the "best" reception area.

AREA	Locations				
Cleanliness					
Color scheme					
Seating					
Lighting					
Comfort					
Amenities					
Noise level					
Total					

CASE STUDY

Read the case study and answer the questions that follow.

Jill is the receptionist for Dr. Boles and Dr. Bailey, who are psychiatrists. Each week Sara Ables comes to her appointments but brings her two small children, Joey and Julie, ages 8 and 6 years, respectively. When Sara goes back for her appointment, the children are almost uncontrollable in the reception area. Although there are never more than two patients waiting, the kids are a serious disruption in the clinic. When Jill mentioned the problem to Dr. Boles, he said that Sara really needed the sessions and that Jill should try to work with Sara on this issue. What can Jill do to remedy the situation?

WORKPLACE APPLICATIONS

Design a registration form for a fictional clinic that includes all information necessary for a new patient. Be creative with logos and fonts. Make the form attractive and easy to understand.

INTERNET ACTIVITIES

1. Search for innovations in patient reception on the Internet, including computers that allow patients to check themselves in for appointments. Present information on one of the systems to the class.

Copyright © 2011, 2007, 2003 by Saunders, an imprint of Elsevier Inc. All rights reserved.

2. Find examples of office mission statements online. Compare them and write a brief report about the contents of the various statements.

3. Research the Americans with Disabilities Act. Determine what accommodations must be made in reception areas to comply with this law. Present the information to the class.

Copyright © 2011, 2007, 2003 by Saunders, an imprint of Elsevier Inc. All rights reserved.

12 Office Environment and Daily Operations

VOCABULARY REVIEW

Fill in the blanks with the correct vocabulary terms from this chapter.

1. Julia noticed some ________________ in the inventory when comparing last month's totals with the current month's totals.
2. Rhonda prefers that all ________________ ________________ be initialed by the person who checks in the package.
3. Dr. Hughes is ________________ when dealing with conflicts within the office by talking with staff members and looking for ways to compromise.
4. Kayla enjoys developing a(n) ________________ for office expenditures each fiscal year.
5. Items on ________________ frustrate the office manager because of the follow-up required to make sure the item eventually arrives at the clinic.
6. When Douglas neglected to pay the supply bill by the due date, he ________________ late charges and increased the total due by 2%.
7. Elaine, the office manager, was able to ________________ a confrontation with the patient who complained about the bill by addressing his concerns in a cordial way.
8. By ________________ Web sites she uses frequently, Ann is able to find medical suppliers and research the best prices quickly.
9. Dr. Tarago received a(an) ________________ for speaking at the regional medical society meeting.
10. Physicians are constantly concerned about their ________________ when budgeting and planning salary increases.
11. Julia knew that there were ________________ circumstances involved with the patient statements being sent late during August.
12. September begins the ________________ ________________ for the clinic.
13. Dr. Hughes finally agreed to the ________________ of his medical transcription.
14. Dr. Tarago gave Kayla a(n) ________________ before she left to attend the medical assistant convention.

SKILLS AND CONCEPTS

Part I: Opening the Office

1. List six duties that should be completed before patients start to arrive.

   a. ____

   b. ____

   c. ____

   d. ____

   e. ____

   f. ____

Copyright © 2011, 2007, 2003 by Saunders, an imprint of Elsevier Inc. All rights reserved.

2. What parts of the medical record should be checked to see whether additional forms need to be added before a patient arrives for an office visit?

____

____

____

3. Explain the precautions that should be taken with prescription pads.

____

____

____

4. Why is patient traffic flow an important consideration in the office environment?

____

____

____

Part II: The Office Environment

1. List 10 expenses the physician's office incurs on a month-to-month basis.

a. ____

b. ____

c. ____

d. ____

e. ____

f. ____

g. ____

h. ____

i. ____

j. ____

2. List six tasks the medical assistant can do between patients or during slower periods.

a. ____

b. ____

c. ____

d. ____

e. ____

f. ____

3. Explain the purpose of white noise.

____

____

____

Copyright © 2011, 2007, 2003 by Saunders, an imprint of Elsevier Inc. All rights reserved.

4. List three things related to the office environment that the medical assistant can do to help the physician save money.

   a. ______________________________

   b. ______________________________

   c. ______________________________

5. Explain why the number of individuals with keys and alarm codes should be limited in the medical office.

   ____

   ____

   ____

Part III: Medical Waste and Regular Waste

Note whether each of the following items should be classified as medical waste or regular waste.

1. Gauze used to stop bleeding after venipuncture

   ____

2. Tissues used in the reception room to clean eyeglasses

   ____

3. Blood tubes containing blood that has already been tested

   ____

4. Used syringes

   ____

5. Paper towels used to clean a mirror in a restroom used by patients

   ____

Part IV: The Office Policy and Procedures Manual

1. Why is the office policy and procedures manual important?

   ____

   ____

   ____

2. List five sections that might be found in an office policy and procedures manual.

   a. ______________________________

   b. ______________________________

   c. ______________________________

   d. ______________________________

   e. ______________________________

Copyright © 2011, 2007, 2003 by Saunders, an imprint of Elsevier Inc. All rights reserved.

Part V: Equipment Inventory

Complete an inventory of either administrative or clinical equipment at the school using the form in Work Product 12-1 on p. 93 of the Procedures Checklists. Give the form to the instructor when finished.

Part VI: Supply Inventory

Complete an inventory of either administrative or clinical supplies at the school using the form in Work Product 12-2 on p. 95 of the Procedures Checklists. Give the form to the instructor when finished.

Part VII: Purchase Orders

Complete two purchase orders using an office supply catalog, newspaper ad, or the Internet. Complete one purchase order for supplies (things that are used up on a routine basis); complete the other for equipment (things that are reusable and usually of value).

Name ______________________

Date ______________________

PURCHASE ORDER

No. 1554

Bill to:

Blackburn Primary Care Associates PC
1990 Turquoise Drive
Blackburn, WI 54937

Ship to:

Blackburn Primary Care Associates, PC
1990 Turquoise Drive
Blackburn, WI 54937

Vendor: ______________________

Terms: ______________________

ORDER #	DESCRIPTION	QTY.	COLOR	SIZE	UNIT PRICE	TOTAL PRICE

SUBTOTAL	
TAX	
SHIPPING	
TOTAL	

Copyright © 2011, 2007, 2003 by Saunders, an imprint of Elsevier Inc. All rights reserved.

Name ____________________

Date ____________________

PURCHASE ORDER

No. 1554

Bill to:

Blackburn Primary Care Associates PC
1990 Turquoise Drive
Blackburn, WI 54937

Ship to:

Blackburn Primary Care Associates, PC
1990 Turquoise Drive
Blackburn, WI 54937

Vendor: ____________________

____

____

Terms: ____________________

ORDER #	DESCRIPTION	QTY.	COLOR	SIZE	UNIT PRICE	TOTAL PRICE
					SUBTOTAL	
					TAX	
					SHIPPING	
					TOTAL	

Part VIII: Maintenance Logs

Use the form in Work Product 12-3 on p. 97 of the Procedures Checklists to compile a log of the administrative equipment in your classroom. Follow the example given on the first line. Give the form to the instructor when you are finished.

Part IX: Travel Expense Reports

Complete a travel expense report using the form in Work Product 12-4 on p. 99 of the Procedures Checklists. Use the following information on the report. Allowed meal amounts are breakfast $10.00, lunch $18, and dinner $27.00. Figure the total for each expense category, the total expenses for the trip, and the amount to be reimbursed to the employee, if any.

Advance:
$200 cash

Expenses/Receipts:
Two hotel nights at the Regency Inn (May 2 & 3, 2010). Cost: $110.00 per night. Tax Rate: 8.25%
Cab from airport to hotel (May 2, 2010): $22.00 plus 18% tip.
Cab from hotel to airport (May 4, 2010): $22.00 plus 18% tip.
Breakfast: Free each day at the hotel buffet

Copyright © 2011, 2007, 2003 by Saunders, an imprint of Elsevier Inc. All rights reserved.

Lunch: Figure all tips at 18%

May 2—$12.56

May 3—$16.24

May 4—$10.54

Dinner: Figure all tips at 18%

May 2—$18.35

May 3—$22.34

Phone: Calls to office

May 2—$2.13

May 3—$3.43

A manual with examples of forms for the medical office was purchased at the seminar for $38.00.
The seminar cost was paid several months in advance.

Part X: Emergency Preparedness

Using the Internet, find at least five agencies in your region that provide emergency preparedness. Present a brief report to the class on each agency and the services it provides. Complete Work Product 12-5 (on p. 101 of the Procedures Checklists) according to instructor specifications.

CASE STUDY

Read the case study and answer the questions that follow.

Dianna had worked at the Family Clinic for 6 years in the front office. When a new medical assistant, Kiran, was hired to work the phones and schedule appointments, Dianna noticed that she was not following the office policy and caused several problems with the schedule. Some patients were very late in seeing the physician; this was unusual for the office, so complaints were made. Dianna volunteered to work with Kiran to help her schedule according to policy. She noticed that Kiran accessed the Internet and her e-mail frequently, but that did not seem to detract from setting appointments. Kiran promised to perform according to office policy, but after 3 weeks, the problems continued.

1. What should happen in this situation?

____

____

____

2. Why is the scheduler such an important position in the facility?

____

____

____

____

____

Workplace Applications

1. Set up an interview with an office manager and discuss the cost of running a medical practice from month to month. Discuss the biggest expenses that the physician pays each month. Report what you discover to the class.

2. Discuss emergency preparedness for the medical office and determine with a team of classmates the logical contents of an emergency preparedness plan for a physician's office. Outline a plan and present it to the class.

Copyright © 2011, 2007, 2003 by Saunders, an imprint of Elsevier Inc. All rights reserved.

Internet Activities

1. Find three medical suppliers on the Internet and compare their prices for each of the following items. Use local suppliers if information is available online about their products.

Item	Suppliers	Price #1	Price #2	Price #3
1 case of 4 × 4 gauze pads				
1 gallon of isopropyl alcohol				
1 case of table paper				

2. Research medical office layout designs on the Internet and design an office. Include a color scheme and floor plan. Present the design to the class using a computer presentation, poster, or handouts.

3. Research three local medical facilities on the Internet, looking for information such as company reports, financial information, company profiles, news, and current affairs. Write a report on one of the facilities to share with the class.

4. Research information on fire extinguishers, including their operation and the types for different uses. Prepare a report on the findings.

Copyright © 2011, 2007, 2003 by Saunders, an imprint of Elsevier Inc. All rights reserved.

13 Written Communications and Mail Processing

VOCABULARY REVIEW

Fill in the blanks with the correct vocabulary terms from this chapter.

1. Roberta has a(n) ________________ tone in her voice when she speaks to the office staff, and this has caused friction between her and the employees.
2. Most of the mail the Blackburn Clinic sends is classified as ________________ mail, which means it is sent within the boundaries of the United States.
3. Savannah asked Noble to ________________ a memo among all of the employees.
4. Dr. Lupez suggested that the clinic sell or donate all of the ________________ computer equipment once the new system arrived and was installed.
5. Jaci sometimes gets confused about subject and predicate ________________ when she is writing.
6. Mrs. Abernathy reminded the students to make the margins ________________ to the left when writing memorandums.
7. Dr. Lawler asked Roberta to order new stationery and specifically requested that the ________________ be of a high quality.
8. All the staff members enjoyed having Alicia as an intern because of her ________________ personality with the patients.
9. The physicians considered rearranging the drug sample shelves ________________ according to type of drug.
10. Dr. Hughes's ________________ remark was out of character, and Suzanne was certain that he was simply stressed over a patient.
11. Ellen forgot to measure the ________________ of a package before taking it to the post office to mail.
12. Jacqueline has a talent for writing ________________ documents that are easy to understand.
13. Angela was ________________ the newsletter yesterday afternoon.

Copyright © 2011, 2007, 2003 by Saunders, an imprint of Elsevier Inc. All rights reserved.

SKILLS AND CONCEPTS

Part I: Correspondence and Envelopes

Label the parts of the letter in the figure below, and write in the number of lines required between each section.

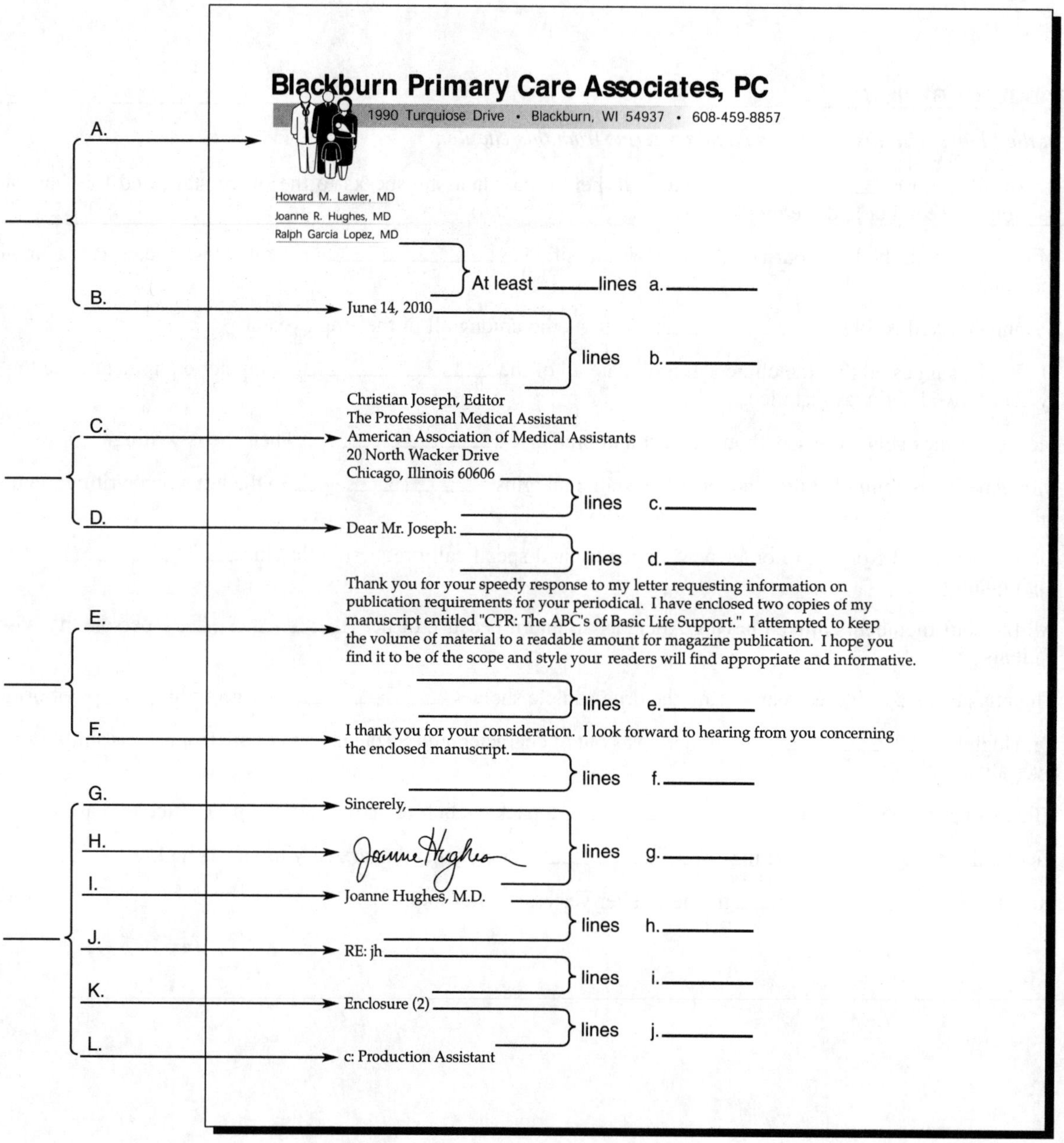

Blackburn Primary Care Associates, PC
1990 Turquiose Drive • Blackburn, WI 54937 • 608-459-8857
Howard M. Lawler, MD
Joanne R. Hughes, MD
Ralph Garcia Lopez, MD
June 14, 2010
Christian Joseph, Editor
The Professional Medical Assistant
American Association of Medical Assistants
20 North Wacker Drive
Chicago, Illinois 60606
Dear Mr. Joseph:
Thank you for your speedy response to my letter requesting information on publication requirements for your periodical. I have enclosed two copies of my manuscript entitled "CPR: The ABC's of Basic Life Support." I attempted to keep the volume of material to a readable amount for magazine publication. I hope you find it to be of the scope and style your readers will find appropriate and informative.
I thank you for your consideration. I look forward to hearing from you concerning the enclosed manuscript.
Sincerely,
Joanne Hughes
Joanne Hughes, M.D.
RE: jh
Enclosure (2)
c: Production Assistant
A.
B.
C.
D.
E.
F.
G.
H.
I.
J.
K.
L.
At least ______ lines a. ______
lines b. ______
lines c. ______
lines d. ______
lines e. ______
lines f. ______
lines g. ______
lines h. ______
lines i. ______
lines j. ______

Copyright © 2011, 2007, 2003 by Saunders, an imprint of Elsevier Inc. All rights reserved.

Complete Work Product 13-1 on p. 111 of the Procedures Checklists by writing the following addresses correctly according to OCR guidelines on the envelopes provided.

1. doctor john smith m.d. 301 west hughes street chicago illinois 54321

2. cindy johnson, physical therapist 1467 east green street suite 409b bayfield georgia 12345

3. jose kelley memorial lane number 321 west columbia florida 97654

Part II: Short Answers

1. What is a watermark?

___

___

___

2. Why is a portfolio useful in the medical office?

___

___

___

3. Explain how a ream of paper is determined.

___

___

___

4. List several pieces of equipment used for written communications.

___

___

___

5. List some of the supplies used for written correspondence.

___

___

___

6. What is standard letter-size paper?

___

___

___

Copyright © 2011, 2007, 2003 by Saunders, an imprint of Elsevier Inc. All rights reserved.

7. List the four parts of a letter.

a. ___

b. ___

c. ___

d. ___

8. Name three items that should be on a continuation page.

a. ___

b. ___

c. ___

9. What is the difference between registered and certified mail?

10. Name and briefly define the parts of speech.

a. ___

b. ___

c. ___

d. ___

e. ___

f. ___

g. ___

h. ___

11. List the four types of letter styles and the differences between each one.

a. ___

b. ___

c. ___

d. ___

12. List three things to do before answering a business letter.

a. ___

b. ___

c. ___

Copyright © 2011, 2007, 2003 by Saunders, an imprint of Elsevier Inc. All rights reserved.

Part III: Letters and Memos

Using the letterhead form in Work Products 13-2 and 13-4 (See pp. 113 and 117 in the Procedures Checklists), the memo form in Work Products 13-3 and 13-5 (see pp. 115 and 119 in the Procedures Checklists), and the fax form in Work Product 13-6, complete the following activities. Write the documents using one of the four letter styles discussed in the chapter. If allowed by the instructor, use templates for added creativity and customization.

A. Initiating Correspondence—Complete Work Product 13-2.

Write a letter from Dr. Hughes to the president of the American Medical Association suggesting a topic for the next national convention. In the letter, indicate Dr. Hughes's interest in presenting the topic.

B. Initiating a Memo—Complete Work Product 13-3.

Write a memo to all employees, making a change in office policy. The new policy should state that the new budget for continuing education per employee will change from $300 annually to $500 annually. Be sure to set an effective date.

C. Responding to Correspondence—Complete Work Product 13-4.

Respond to an invitation to speak at a local Rotary Club meeting on the subject "Health, Wellness, and Eating Well."

D. Responding to a Memo—Complete Work Product 13-5.

Respond to a memo from a supervisor who wants an update on the progress made toward arranging the drug sample area into categories as directed by the physician. Make sure to include an estimated date of completion for the project.

E. Initiating a Fax—Complete Work Product 13-6 on p. 121 of the Procedures Checklists.

Design a cover sheet for a fax message using the form in Work Product 13-6 or a template. On the cover sheet, indicate that test results for a patient are attached. Be certain to address the issue of patient confidentiality.

Copyright © 2011, 2007, 2003 by Saunders, an imprint of Elsevier Inc. All rights reserved.

WORD FIND

Find the words in the list in the following puzzle. Be sure you know the definition of each word in the list in relation to written communications and mail processing.

Z F C T Y L H U I X C I M C N D L I T T X J O Z Q A E M M A G Q Y L Y C L Y M Z
P D D P H I L H A L Z A W D D E W R Y V C C O X H Z L X U K D N F F Z Q B A J Q
P V K Y U N F R A Y V A T V F W G C R O G J J O T L M L D R I F C J J C R Y N B
R N H P S T J U E C E X R E M Y H P N M S S J G I L T V N O A M I I L G I T J G
E T D C O E Y Q O K Z B C X G Q B T H R Z F W O J E C O A F B I P D I N N P U W
V U C Q V R J Y K R P E B U B O I E T A N I M E S S I D R S E R B N A N Y N Y C
S A K F C N W W W E W R L V W N R R N K Y J P C A N X X O K Z S D F L A G A T Z
D H Q U N A T K R W P Z C A U B J I Y X E E T C J H H B M W X G A U V N F J A Q
H J N P C T B H Z B B B Z A R P L U C J F R H Q O H Z X E H F V S B Q X Y J W R
M P V A W I F X I K J I T O N X P T K A D G R Z N D A X M Z Y Y W G S W L Q Q K
O P E S D O O G W M D I Z N L Y S I K H L J H Y O B E V I J Z L U I G I H Y O K
J R K U P N L H Z R O D L Z N P L Z W U O L W R A T Q Q V R C Q Q A C Y B B O H
E M C J H A P U L N R M E N X P O I B U K V Y L B I A N N G U T Z H T Z E F V I
R G G Q I L B X X F I K S F Q W J L O L V J W O R H X O C E D G P P P Y L H W D
X Z X Z E G A Z B C H B M Y O I R Q F N B Z X I Z H I U J H K P Z J N M U E A P
V W S L R K A Z G P W F E F J F E K C Y B P J W M T G C F J C F A K R O E V Z J
T H K V L I Z C Q U V H H E C N U B I O L Y G I A Y S X U J W Q A P V O M Y R C
E N C L O S U R E O U Z C X I E C C X I F F Q T J D V K T Z I F Y Y Y A Z V R C
B W F U H K B V Q K D N W A T A H P M W J T U X B O L N U Z F F J T Q A W M A L
E K E I N M W V T C E L A M S C Y G V B D L L C W B C T Z I W J S I I W X B O J
E L E G F B C G I D C L E M E U T N R O A X X C T Y F M Z J R W O Q G I Z M Q N
Q B Q X U V R W N U P F S K M L A J P S T L A Y Z G Q L R Y M D E U E Y M G B N
X M W T O P C O R H M O I G O T O P E N I N G U T E T X H F D K Z R J X W Z O I
A R K M R N P S B U E B R K D W R O Z M E R X R X U U K P B W Q V A L Z X R D B
J M N V P S I S K S V O U T U B V K B F R G T U L P T V V T T G R P G I H P D J
K V Z L E Q A X G Q V K J Q F C B F D V H K B Y R R J W N F F E H A S L J D Q D
C U L R U I S Y R X V N L H F O B J I J O F E O F G B V E W M M L L Y C E X S S
X J R T N W N I V Y I W L S T Q L A C F E D O M N U H G W X V L E L T I Y G L H
H O U F W W I E P N G Z T Q T R O I J R J F S I U Q I J B F U R J X I L U F Y N
C D K U X R E P K U L K L K K P I I O G R K D E L E A I C C X E M Q O E T Z N C
A P M C N U D L R Y C R Y O G L I G L E Z A F G G A D M M Z O M A B P T X I Q N
K M H G I P Q O U I G P B F L B V R A S E Q M Y I A A A Q V E R G I Y T Z X V H
Q C D X M S Z O Z N C N C L T S J D C H B T O S S W S Y K K V E P O L E V N E F
C O M P L I M E N T A R Y N R O R B I S D S F O M O Z S F V D A E X H R R G W X
H E E B V U T H T R S L G X X T U E X V T U S W O W Y H E E R R P U E I J M M Q
I L I G D J V B X I I E M M O Z W L U L L S U N F N Q X E M O J R M X O H E R Z
H R R W I R T J R N L I A M E J P L W S G S O T E J X Z D R I X A R O S G D B V
I C A R P A G C M S E K Z C X V K Y H I B U J P I S G B G A A U H T U B B X E O
X N B F I G A T L I T F K B R I R S U V C G I D Q O U Q M C D C Q Z Q I G V L I
I P I H Q B T M V C L C J U A D C J L X F D W O R S R V X Y G L L T A U K V X D

Copyright © 2011, 2007, 2003 by Saunders, an imprint of Elsevier Inc. All rights reserved.

Body	Enclosure	Memorandum
Categorically	Envelope	Messages
Complimentary	Girth	Opening
Continuation	Heading	Portfolio
Correspondence	International	Postscripts
Disseminate	Intrinsic	Proofread
Domestic	Letter	Salutation
Email	Margin	ZIP code

CASE STUDY

Read the case study and answer the questions that follow.

Barbara recently graduated as a medical assistant and obtained employment at a local physician's office. She and the office manager have seemed to be at odds since Barbara redesigned several forms that had been in use at the clinic but had been copied over and over again and looked quite unprofessional. Barbara did not ask permission to redo the forms; she was attempting to help and to make a good impression. Since that incident, the office manager has given Barbara two written reprimands for minor issues.

1. What should Barbara do?

____

____

____

2. How could she have prevented this situation from the beginning?

____

____

____

3. Is the office manager at fault?

____

____

____

WORKPLACE APPLICATIONS

Collect several documents from various healthcare facilities. Compare the quality of the documents. Do they make a good first impression? Are they clearly copies that have been made over and over again? Grade the documents and revise those that are graded below a B so that they present a positive, professional image of the facility.

Copyright © 2011, 2007, 2003 by Saunders, an imprint of Elsevier Inc. All rights reserved.

INTERNET ACTIVITIES

1. Compare the services offered by companies such as FedEx, UPS, DHL, and the USPS. Determine the lowest cost for sending an overnight letter or package.

2. Research reference books that would be valuable to the medical assistant's library. Find and compare costs and make a list of several books that would be useful in the physician's office.

3. Go to the Microsoft Office home page and look for templates. Download several of the business templates and customize them for the Blackburn Primary Care Associates.

Copyright © 2011, 2007, 2003 by Saunders, an imprint of Elsevier Inc. All rights reserved.

14 The Paper Medical Record

VOCABULARY REVIEW

Fill in the blank with the correct vocabulary term from this chapter.

1. Veronica prefers a(n) ________________ filing system, in which combinations of letters and numbers are used to identify a file.
2. Julia prefers a(n) ________________ filing system, in which the letters of the alphabet are used to identify a file.
3. Paula Ann feels that only a(n) ________________ filing system provides patient confidentiality.
4. Dr. Banford uses a ________________ file to help him remember that a certain action must be taken on a certain date.
5. Teresa wants to ________________ the current software library with programs for making brochures and designing Web sites.
6. The clinic physician records ________________ information when questioning patients about their illness.
7. The clinic physician records ________________ information when examining the patient.
8. When Mira files documents into medical records, she lays one report on top of another, with the most recent on top; this filing method is called ________________.
9. The office manager is particular about the ________________ under which documents are filed, because she wants to be able to access information quickly.
10. Dr. Lawler scheduled an appointment with his accountant to discuss the ________________ of the office financial records.
11. Georgina avoids ________________ by taking care of issues and documents as they are presented to her rather than setting them aside for later.
12. Naomi has a ________________ interest in the success of the new hospital, because she owns shares in its stock.
13. The medical assistant must never remove entries in a patient's record by ________________.
14. Dr. Lupez's ________________ ________________ was irritable bowel syndrome, not colon cancer.
15. Jose read the memo about the new medical records ________________ schedule with interest, because his job includes filing.

SKILLS AND CONCEPTS

Part I: Filing Medical Records

Place the following names in the correct order for filing in the right column.

1. Cassidy Kay Hale	1. ________________
2. Candace Cassidy LeGrand	2. ________________
3. Taylor Ann Jackson	3. ________________
4. Anton Douglas Conn	4. ________________
5. Mitchel Michael Gibson	5. ________________
6. Lorienda Gaye Robison	6. ________________

Copyright © 2011, 2007, 2003 by Saunders, an imprint of Elsevier Inc. All rights reserved.

7. LaNelle Elva Crumley 7. ______
8. Allison Gaile Yarbrough 8. ______
9. Sarah Kay Haile 9. ______
10. Marie Gracelia Stuart 10. ______
11. Karry Madge Chapmann 11. ______
12. Randi Ann Perez 12. ______
13. Cecelia Gayle Raglan 13. ______
14. Sarah Sue Ragland 14. ______
15. Riley Americus Belk 15. ______
16. Starr Ellen Beall 16. ______
17. Mitchell Thomas Gibson 17. ______
18. George Scott Turner 18. ______
19. Winston Roger Murchison 19. ______
20. Sara Suzelle Montgomery 20. ______
21. Tamika Noelle Frazier 21. ______
22. Alisa Jordan Williams 22. ______
23. Alisha Dawn Chapman 23. ______
24. Bentley James Adams 24. ______
25. Montana Skye Kizer 25. ______
26. Dakota Marie LaRose 26. ______
27. Robbie Sue Metzger 27. ______
28. Thomas Charles Bruin 28. ______
29. Percevial "Butch" Adams 29. ______
30. Carlos Perez Santos 30. ______

Part II: Subjective and Objective Information

Note whether the following information is usually subjective or objective.

1. Patient's address ______
2. Yellowed eyes ______
3. Patient's e-mail address ______
4. Insurance information ______
5. Elevated blood pressure ______
6. Bloated stomach ______
7. Complaint of headache ______
8. Weight of 143 pounds ______
9. Bruises on upper arms ______
10. Patient's phone number ______

 Copyright © 2011, 2007, 2003 by Saunders, an imprint of Elsevier Inc. All rights reserved.

Part III: Short Answers

1. List four reasons medical records are kept.

   a. ______________________________

   b. ______________________________

   c. ______________________________

   d. ______________________________

2. Explain the concept of the ownership of medical records.

   ____

   ____

   ____

3. Why might color-coded files be more efficient than an alphabetic filing system?

   ____

   ____

   ____

4. What are the two major types of patient records found in a medical office?

   a. ______________________________

   b. ______________________________

5. What type of form should be completed if a patient no longer wants to allow his or her medical records to be released to a person or an organization?

   ____

   ____

   ____

Copyright © 2011, 2007, 2003 by Saunders, an imprint of Elsevier Inc. All rights reserved.

Part IV: Releasing Medical Records

Complete an Authorization to Release Medical Records form using your name as the patient.

RECORDS RELEASE AUTHORIZATION

TO ____
Doctor or Hospital

____
Address

I HEREBY AUTHORIZE AND REQUEST YOU TO RELEASE TO:

ALL RECORDS IN YOUR POSSESION CONCERNING ____________________

____ILLNESS AND/OR

TREATMENT DURING THE PERIOD FROM ______________TO ______________.

NAME ______________________________TEL. ______________________

ADDRESS____

SIGNATURE ____________________________DATE ______________________
(If relative, state relationship)

WITNESS______________________________DATE ______________________

25-8104 © 1973 BIBBERO SYSTEMS, INC., PETALUMA,, CA.

Part V: Changing or Correcting Medical Records

Correct the following medical record entries as noted, as it would be done in a medical chart. Then rewrite the entry correctly on the line provided.

1. The correct date of the appointment below was October 12, 20XX.

   10-21-20XX Patient did not arrive for scheduled appointment. *P. Smith, RMA*

   ____

2. The patient stated that the chest pain began 2 weeks ago.

   1-31-20XX Patient complained of chest pain for the last 2 months. No pain noted in arms. No nausea. Desires ECG and blood work to check for heart problems. *R. Smithee, CMA(AAMA)*

   ____

   ____

   ____

Copyright © 2011, 2007, 2003 by Saunders, an imprint of Elsevier Inc. All rights reserved.

3. The correct date for the last refill was 3-20-20XX.

   4-22-20XX Patient requested that Rx for Vicodin be refilled. Last refill was 4-20-20XX. Dr. Lawton refused refill and requested patient schedule follow-up appointment. *S. Ragland, RMA*

   ____

   ____

   ____

   What additional follow-up might be needed in this situation?

   ____

   ____

   ____

4. Mr. Eric Robertson cancelled his surgical follow-up appointment today for the third time.

   ____

   ____

   ____

5. Angela Adams called to report that she was not feeling any better since her office visit on Monday. She wants the doctor to call in a refill for her antibiotics. The chart says that she was to return to the clinic on Thursday if she was not feeling better. Today is Monday, and she says she cannot come in to the clinic this week.

   ____

   ____

   ____

6. Mary Elizabeth Smith called the physician's office to report redness around an injection site. She was in the office 3 hours ago and received an injection of penicillin. She says she also is itching quite a bit around the site and is having trouble breathing. The doctor has left the office for the day.

   ____

   ____

   ____

Part VI: Filing Procedures

1. List and explain the five basic filing steps.

   a. ____

   ____

   ____

   b. ____

   ____

   ____

   c. ____

   ____

   ____

Copyright © 2011, 2007, 2003 by Saunders, an imprint of Elsevier Inc. All rights reserved.

d. ____

____

____

e. ____

____

____

CASE STUDY

Read the information below and answer the questions.

The Blackburn Clinic is considering the purchase of new filing equipment. They currently use an open-shelf method, with the patient's names in alphabetic order. They would like to change to an alphanumeric system.

1. What must they consider before making this change?

____

____

____

2. How would the office implement this change so that it causes the least disruption to the patients and staff?

____

____

____

WORKPLACE APPLICATIONS

Visit three medical offices and determine the type of filing system each uses. Ask the receptionist about the pros and cons of each system. Share this information with the class.

INTERNET ACTIVITIES

1. Research paper-based filing systems on the Internet and determine which system you would choose for a medical office. Cite three reasons for your choice.

2. Look for special paper-based, color-coding systems on the Internet. How might these be used in a physician's office?

3. Look for filing tips on the Internet. Which of these tips might help you file faster and more efficiently in the medical office?

Copyright © 2011, 2007, 2003 by Saunders, an imprint of Elsevier Inc. All rights reserved.

15 The Electronic Medical Record

VOCABULARY REVIEW

Fill in the blanks with the correct vocabulary terms from this chapter.

1. Jennifer explained that a(n) ________________ of electronic health information usually included documents from two or more different health facilities.
2. The electronic record that originates from one facility is called the electronic ________________ record.
3. The electronic record that originates from more than one facility is called the electronic ________________ record.
4. Behavior that is generally or widely accepted is called ________________.
5. A system that is capable of interacting with another system is said to be ________________.
6. A(n) ________________-based medical record is used in combination with a paper-based record to optimize patient care.
7. Medical ________________ refers to the study of medical computing.
8. Any of a set of physical properties, the values of which determine characteristics or behavior, is its ________________.

SKILLS AND CONCEPTS

Part I: Electronic Medical Records

1. List three of the five requirements listed in President George W. Bush's order establishing the goal of having electronic medical records for most Americans by 2014.

   a. ____

   ____

   b. ____

   ____

   c. ____

   ____

2. List five advantages of the EMR system.

   a. ____

   ____

   b. ____

   ____

   c. ____

   ____

Copyright © 2011, 2007, 2003 by Saunders, an imprint of Elsevier Inc. All rights reserved.

d.

e.

3. List five disadvantages of the EMR system.

a.

b.

c.

d.

e.

Part II: EMR Capabilities

1. What is the approximate cost of implementing an EMR system for a typical physician's office with one physician?

2. Briefly describe three capabilities of an EMR system. Why do you think each capability will enhance patient care?

a.

b.

c.

Part III: The Patient and the EMR

1. Discuss how you would talk with a patient who has expressed legitimate fears about having health information in electronic form. Explain what you would say to the patient and how you would reassure the individual.

Copyright © 2011, 2007, 2003 by Saunders, an imprint of Elsevier Inc. All rights reserved.

Part IV: Nonverbal Communication and the EMR

1. List several things to remember when in the exam room with the patient and the electronic device that houses the EMR system. Specifically, what should you, as the medical assistant, do to put the patient at ease?

Part V: Nationwide Health Information Network (NHIN)

1. Briefly explain the purpose of the Nationwide Health Information Network.

2. List two goals of the Nationwide Health Information Network.

   a. ______

   b. ______

3. What are some of the governmental agencies you think will be a part of the effort to meet the goals of the Executive Order of 2006?

Part VI: Backup Systems for the EMR

1. List three backup systems for an EMR system in a physician's office.

   a. ______

   b. ______

Copyright © 2011, 2007, 2003 by Saunders, an imprint of Elsevier Inc. All rights reserved.

c. ____

____

CASE STUDY

Read the information below and answer the questions.

Dr. Adkins and Dr. Brooks want to expand their office to make sure they can take advantage of cutting-edge technology. Their goal is to use electronic equipment to perform as much of the work as possible so that all staff members can keep caring for the patients in the forefront of their minds. Dr. Adkins is fairly satisfied with the system the clinic has now. However, the medical assistant, Dr. Brooks, a "technology geek," wants the newest, greatest, and best electronics in his clinic. The office manager gives Sloan, the medical assistant, the opportunity to research electronic medical records systems to determine which are considered the best of the best.

Research what is available in your local and regional areas, make a brief report about the availabilities, and present it to the class.

1. What new possibilities did you discover in your research?

____

____

____

____

2. Why do you think many physicians are slow to adopt new technology?

____

____

____

____

3. As a medical assistant, what type of technology would make your duties easier?

____

____

____

____

WORKPLACE APPLICATIONS

Determine whether a local physician's office that uses an EMR system would allow the class to visit, perhaps on an afternoon when patients are not in the clinic. Take a list of at least five questions about using an EMR system. Observe how the system works and watch to see if the employees seem to have more or less of a workload. Watch the interaction of the employees with each other and ask whether they think the system is more of a help or a hindrance as they go about their duties.

INTERNET ACTIVITIES

1. Research the cost of an EMR system on the Internet. Find a low, moderate, and high cost system. Compare the features of each and share your information with the class.

2. Find a company that sells EMR systems. Ask a salesperson to present information to your class. Ask whether he or she can demonstrate the capabilities of the system.

3. Search for blogs used by medical assistants and look for those who have EMR systems in their clinics. What types of problems do they discuss? Are they promoting any specific systems that seem to work well?

Copyright © 2011, 2007, 2003 by Saunders, an imprint of Elsevier Inc. All rights reserved.

16 Health Information Management

VOCABULARY REVIEW

Fill in the blanks with the correct vocabulary terms from this chapter.

1. Dr. Charles received a memo from Smith-Park Hospital that reminded him to ______________ several of the medical records.
2. Janie records any ______________ ______________ that happens to a patient while he or she is in the hospital.
3. Chris asked if there was a way to ______________ outgoing e-mail messages so that they could not be altered before reaching their destination.
4. Anne knows that medical facilities must meet certain ______________ to maintain accreditation.
5. After reviewing several hundred files, Alex was concerned about the ______________ information in several patient records.
6. Betty reminded Joanne to be careful not to ______________ numbers or letters when entering information into the computer.
7. The ______________ ______________ office in a healthcare facility is concerned with providing the best and most efficient care possible to the patients.
8. Dr. Hughes knew that penicillin was a(n) ______________ for Kathleen Schultz, so he ordered a different antibiotic.
9. The new user manual has several ______________, which must be corrected.
10. The medical assistant should never attempt to ______________ the regulations that apply to medical records.
11. An injury caused by medical management rather than the underlying condition of the patient is called a(n) ______________ event.
12. A ______________ ______________ is a medical error that is corrected before it affects the patient.

SKILLS AND CONCEPTS

Part I: Short Answers

1. Define health information management in lay terms.

____

____

____

2. List five ways in which healthcare data are used.

 a. ____

 b. ____

 c. ____

 d. ____

 e. ____

Copyright © 2011, 2007, 2003 by Saunders, an imprint of Elsevier Inc. All rights reserved.

3. Explain what is meant by the underuse of medical services.

____

____

____

4. Explain what is meant by the overuse of medical services.

____

____

____

5. List five of the statistics collected by the NCHS.
   a. ____
   b. ____
   c. ____
   d. ____
   e. ____

Part II: Characteristics of High-Quality Health Data

Determine which of the nine characteristics of high-quality health data is involved in the following scenarios. Use each quality only once, and choose the one that best represents the facts presented in the scenario.

1. Janeen is concerned because the computer system did not upload the entries made the previous day.

____

2. Suzanne found a notation inside the medical record that a patient was allergic to sulfa drugs, but she noticed that the sticker on the outside of the record was marked NKA.

____

3. Sabrina brought a chart to the physician's attention in which he had written to prescribe 200 mg of Imitrex to a patient. Sabrina had heard the physician tell the patient that he was prescribing 100 mg. The physician corrected the error before writing the prescription.

____

4. Steven was unfamiliar with an abbreviation used in the medical record. He asked the office manager about the abbreviation, and she explained its use in the physician's office. In previous facilities, Steve had seen the same abbreviation used a different way.

____

5. After an employee was terminated, Chris changed applicable passwords so that the individual could no longer access the system.

____

6. Patricia researched the HIPAA Web site to make certain she understood a portion of the privacy law.

____

7. The new patient database allows several staff members to access data at the same time.

____

 Copyright © 2011, 2007, 2003 by Saunders, an imprint of Elsevier Inc. All rights reserved.

8. Joshua was reprimanded for not filing laboratory reports on a daily basis and for allowing the documents to stack up over several days.

____

9. Dr. Adams realized that some information entered into the patient database was not being used for treatment purposes, so he sent a memo to the staff and confirmed that the information no longer needed to be collected.

____

Part III: Acknowledging and Disclosing Medical Errors

1. Number the following events in the order they would be performed in the event of a medical error at the physician's office.

   a. ________ Offer a sincere apology when talking to the patient.

   b. ________ Call the patient and ask him or her to come to the office.

   c. ________ Give the patient the opportunity to ask questions.

   d. ________ Tell the physician about the error.

   e. ________ Complete an incident report and document the error in the chart.

   f. ________ Document the discussion of the error with the patient.

   g. ________ Meet with the patient in a private area where there will be no interruptions.

   h. ________ Allow the physician to explain the error to the patient.

Part IV: Medical Errors

1. Define an adverse event.

____

____

2. Define a sentinel event.

____

____

3. Define a near miss.

____

____

4. List five reasons a physician might be hesitant to disclose a medical error to the patient.

   a. ____

   b. ____

   c. ____

   d. ____

   e. ____

5. Who should be told about an error first?

____

Copyright © 2011, 2007, 2003 by Saunders, an imprint of Elsevier Inc. All rights reserved.

Part V: Incident Reports

A medical assistant gives an injection of penicillin to a patient who reported an allergy to amoxicillin. The patient complains of itching and experiences shortness of breath and wheezing while sitting in the treatment room. The physician gives the patient epinephrine and observes him for 30 minutes, during which time the itching, shortness of breath, and wheezing fully resolves. Complete an incident report for this sentinel event.

Incident Report

Do Not File in Medical Records

Confidential and privileged health care quality improvement information prepared in anticipation of litigation

Name: ______________________ Employee ☐ Patient ☐ Visitor ☐

Attending physician: ______________________
MR # ______________ SS # ______________
D.O.B. __/__/__ Sex: M[ ] F[ ]
Admission date: __/__/__
Primary diagnosis: ______________________

Facility name: ______________________
Site (if applicable) ______________________
City ______________________
Facility ID# ______________________
State ______________________
Phone # ______________________

SECTION I: General Information

General Identification (circle one)
001 Inpatient
002 Outpatient
003 Nonpatient
004 Equipment only

Location (circle one):
005 Bathroom/toilet
006 Beauty shop
007 Cafeteria/dining room
008 Corridor/hall
009 During transport
010 Emergency department
011 Exterior grounds
012 ICU/SCU/CCU
013 Labor/delivery/birthing
014 Nursery
015 Outpatient clinic
016 Patient room
017 Radiology
018 Recovery room
019 Recreation area
020 Rehab
021 Shower room
022 Surgical suite
023 Treatment/exam room

Treatment Rendered (circle one):
024 Emergency room
025 First aid
026 None
026 Transfer to other facility
027 X-ray

SECTION II: Nature of Incident (Circle all that apply):

001 Adverse outcome after surgery or anesthetic
002 Anaphylactic shock
003 Anoxic event
004 Apgar score of 5 or less
005 Aspiration
006 Assault or altercation/combative event
007 Blood or IV variance
008 Blood/body fluid exposure
009 Code/arrest
010 Damage/loss of organ
011 Death
012 Dental-related complication
013 Dissatisfaction/noncompliance*
014 Equipment operation*
015 Fall with injury*
016 Fall without injury*
017 Handling of and/or exposure to hazardous waste
018 Informed consent issue
019 Injury to other
020 Injury to self
021 Loss of limb
022 Loss of vision
023 Medication variance*
024 Needle puncture/sharp injury
025 Paralysis
026 Patient-to-patient altercation
027 Perinatal complication*
028 Poisoning
029 Suspected nonstaff-to-patient abuse
030 Suspected staff-to-patient abuse
031 Thermal burn
032 Treatment/procedure issue
033 Ulcer: nosocomial stage III/IV

** Complete appropriate area in Section III*

SECTION III: Type of Incident

If death, circle all that apply:
001 After medical equipment failure
002 After power equipment failure or damage
003 During surgery or postanesthesia
004 Within 24 hours of admission to facility
005 Within 1 week of fall in facility
006 Within 24 hours of medication error

Blood/IV Variance Issues (circle all that apply):
007 Additive
008 Administration consent
009 Contraindications/allergies
010 Equipment malfunction
011 Infusion rate
012 Labeling issue
013 Reaction
014 Solution/blood type
015 Transcription
016 Patient identification
017 Allergic/adverse reaction
018 Infiltration
019 Phlebitis

Dissatisfaction/Noncompliance (circle all that apply):
020 AMA
021 Elopement
022 Irate or angry (either family or patient)
023 Left without service
024 Noncompliant patient
025 Refused prescribed treatment

Falls (circle all that apply):*
001 Assisted fall
002 Found on floor
003 From bed
004 From chair
005 From commode/toilet
006 From exam table
007 From stretcher
008 From wheelchair
009 Patient states—unwitnessed
010 Unassisted fall
011 While ambulating
012 Witnessed fall

** For any marks in this field, Section V must be completed*

Medication Variance Issues (circle all that apply):
013 Contraindication/allergies
014 Delay in dispensing
015 Incorrect dose
016 Expired drug
017 Medication identification
018 Narcotic log variance
019 Not ordered
020 Ordered, not given
021 Patient identification
022 Reaction
023 Route
024 Rx incorrectly dispensed
025 Time of dose
026 Transcription

 Copyright © 2011, 2007, 2003 by Saunders, an imprint of Elsevier Inc. All rights reserved.

Part VI: Confidentiality Statement

Evaluate the confidentiality statement for Diamonte Hospital below. Revise the statement to make it appropriate for a medical practice setting. Use proofreader marks to indicate your proposed changes in the confidentiality statement. Rewrite the completed, revised statement on the letterhead form on the next page.

DIAMONTE HOSPITAL

Diamonte, Arizona 89104 ▪ TEL. 602-484-9991

CONFIDENTIALITY STATEMENT

I, ______________________________, understand that in the course of my activities/business at or for Diamonte Hospital, I am required to have access to and am involved in the viewing, reviewing, and/or processing of patient care data and/or health information.

I understand that I am obligated by State Law, Federal Law, and Diamonte Hospital to maintain the confidentiality of these data and information at all times.

I understand that a violation of these confidentiality considerations may result in punitive legal action against me.

I certify by my signature below that this Confidentiality Statement has been explained to me, and I agree to the principles contained herein as a condition of my activity/business at or for Diamonte Hospital.

____
Signature/date

____
Witness/date

Copyright © 2011, 2007, 2003 by Saunders, an imprint of Elsevier Inc. All rights reserved.

Blackburn Primary Care Associates
1990 Turquoise Drive
Blackburn, WI 54937
(555) 555-1234

 Copyright © 2011, 2007, 2003 by Saunders, an imprint of Elsevier Inc. All rights reserved.

CASE STUDY

Read the case study and answer the questions that follow.

Alberto discovered that three people accessed the medical records of a player on the local professional football team who had been brought to the physician's office for follow-up on injuries sustained in a car accident. He realizes that the information accessed involved the results of the player's blood alcohol level.

1. What should Alberto do?

____

____

____

2. What type of penalty, if any, is appropriate for those who accessed the information?

____

____

____

WORKPLACE APPLICATIONS

Determine how total quality management ideas can be worked into the mission statement for a physician's office. Write a mission statement that stresses quality management. How does quality management affect patients in a medical office?

INTERNET ACTIVITIES

1. Explore the NCHS website. Investigate one of the issues in the Vital Statistics area. Use information found there to write a report about any area of interest and present it to the class.

2. Explore the Joint Commission (formerly JCAHO) Web site. Peruse the sections of the site that refer to standards, patient safety, and sentinel events. Choose a fact and write a brief report.

3. Research total quality management on the Internet and write a two-page report on how quality management can improve efficiency in a physician's office.

Copyright © 2011, 2007, 2003 by Saunders, an imprint of Elsevier Inc. All rights reserved.

17 Privacy in the Physician's Office

VOCABULARY REVIEW

Fill in the blanks with the correct vocabulary terms from this chapter.

1. Dr. Lawton is considered a healthcare ________________, because he provides services and treatments to patients.
2. The ________________ against Dr. Rosales was one of his former patients, Risa Jackson, who believed that his staff had violated her privacy.
3. Byron knows that he is not allowed to ________________ any information about a patient without a release from the patient for that information.
4. Sarah could ________________ from what the patient said that he was nervous about his upcoming surgery.
5. STAT Medical Billing provides services to the Blackburn Clinic, so the company is considered a(n) ________________ ________________.
6. Julia has difficulty understanding the ________________ in which many federal documents and regulations are written.
7. Janease knew that she could ________________ two employees from guilt, because they were both at lunch when the incident happened.
8. The ________________ on the privacy statement was hard for a layperson to understand, so Annette decided to rewrite the document.
9. Roberta was assigned to be the temporary ________________ ________________ at the clinic while Maritza was on maternity leave.
10. The Office of ________________ ________________ investigates breaches of laws that pertain to HHS.
11. The Office of ________________ ________________ enforces privacy standards.
12. Dr. Hughes had to prove ________________ ________________ in that he made every attempt to notify the patient before mailing test results to her home.
13. The ________________ ________________ ________________ ________________ in a patient's record is private and must not be shared without a release from the patient.
14. Health information that is transmitted in electronic form is called ________________ ________________ ________________.
15. The patient's information that pertains to his or her health is called ________________ ________________ ________________.

SKILLS AND CONCEPTS

Part I: The Health Insurance Portability and Accountability Act

1. 1. List six benefits provided by the HIPAA Privacy Rule to patients and/or providers.

   a. ____

   b. ____

   c. ____

Copyright © 2011, 2007, 2003 by Saunders, an imprint of Elsevier Inc. All rights reserved.

d. ______

e. ______

f. ______

2. Briefly explain the Title I provision of HIPAA.

______

______

3. Briefly explain the Title II provision of HIPAA.

______

______

4. List six rights HIPAA gives to patients.

a. ______

b. ______

c. ______

d. ______

e. ______

f. ______

5. List six items of information a Notice of Privacy Policies must include.

a. ______

b. ______

c. ______

d. ______

e. ______

f. ______

Part II: Patients' Rights under HIPAA

Determine which right under HIPAA applies to each of the following scenarios. Use each right only once.

1. Susan Enlow discovered that her date of birth was incorrect when she requested her medical records from the Blackburn Clinic. She was moving to another city and wanted to take the records with her to her new provider. Susan surmised that the error might have been the reason her insurance company rejected several claims. She contacted the Blackburn Clinic in writing and asked them to correct the error and then to determine whether any claims were outstanding that might need to be resubmitted to her insurance carrier.

   Right to ______

2. Keiran requested that the clinic send a copy of his most recent physical examination and laboratory results to Dr. Ballard, who was seeing him about a long-standing problem with his knees.

   Right to ______

3. Louie requested that all communication from the physician's office be sent to his office address, because he was in the midst of a tense divorce.

   Right to ______

Copyright © 2011, 2007, 2003 by Saunders, an imprint of Elsevier Inc. All rights reserved.

4. The Blackburn Clinic gives a copy of its Notice of Privacy Policy to all patients and makes sure a signature is obtained or a note is attached to prove that the policy was offered to the patient.

   Right to ____

5. A few days after seeing Dr. Reynolds, Rita received an e-mail from a company that offered multivitamins. Dr. Reynolds had suggested that she begin taking multivitamins and mentioned that a friend sold a vitamin drink that she might be interested in trying. Rita did not give permission for release of her e-mail address at the visit. She called the clinic and asked whether her e-mail address had been distributed to anyone outside the clinic.

   Right to ____

6. Suyen made a written request to the Blackburn Clinic that no information about her treatment for drug dependency be released to anyone without her specific written permission.

   Right to ____

Part III: Incidental Disclosures

Determine which of the following situations could be classified as an incidental disclosure.

Situation		Incidental Disclosure	
		Yes	No
1.	Ms. Allen, a patient waiting in the x-ray department of a large clinic, overhears Dr. Smith mention that another patient has been diagnosed with testicular cancer, but she does not hear the patient's name during the discussion.		
2.	Bob Mitchell, a patient at Mercy Hospital, overhears a physician telling his roommate that he needs surgery for carpal tunnel syndrome.		
3.	As Zaria passes the nurses' station at a local hospital, she hears the nurses talking about the patient in room 2114. They mention that he has been diagnosed with terminal cancer. Zaria knows the patient's family and hears that the diagnosis has not been given to them yet.		
4.	Paula Stanley signs in at the front desk of the medical clinic and notices that her college professor signed in to see the physician 30 minutes ago.		

Part IV: Notice of Privacy Practices

Read the Notice of Privacy Practices in Figure 17-1 of the textbook. Based on the information in that policy, answer the following questions.

1. Can the patient obtain a copy of his or her medical record?

   ❑ Yes ❑ No

2. Can the patient request that certain information in his or her medical record not be released to certain persons or organizations?

   ❑ Yes ❑ No

3. Can the patient have a copy of the Notice of Privacy Practices?

   ❑ Yes ❑ No

4. Can the clinic use the information in the patient's medical record to compile statistics about certain diseases treated by the practice without additional permission from the patient?

   ❑ Yes ❑ No

5. Does the clinic have to honor all requests from the patient regarding the release of his or her protected health information?

   ❑ Yes ❑ No

Copyright © 2011, 2007, 2003 by Saunders, an imprint of Elsevier Inc. All rights reserved.

Part V: Privacy in the Physician's Office

Find the words on the list in the puzzle.

P R O V I D E R V E G H E Y T Y G O C O T V G P S P N O F J F R L N O I L D K C

L D I S Q A T Q R S P N Z T Z M B X W A E D B R R D I X Y B R U U E E N Y O K T

Z L A T N E D I C N I L N I O H L C I R U T B O D O H F K S Y T D G G T O H Y F

X L E N V C H L R I A S E T U Z S L B Q Z M T C S T M P C F N S I Y U A R H O U

K C J X P E L C F I F A P N F V L I K P Q E L Q R H E O O E A H O W J M L L Y C

V E W J B L D G T I P B L E K Z A Y N B C S B P C B W U M R Y T Z V N C T E K N

A O K J C N G N C R N W P Z I G H W D T D S M M T N G E G L U V I D D N Q B S L

J W A S Q G E T O D R I C N E D B U E G I E V F E B L Q W G Y S P D B G N Z Z E

K T R D M D T V C V R S Y C N J N D E G S W Y U P P D A K R H M L P Z M H O R T

T V B G I A I Q O V T R X Q U H H E A V C D X Q M R K V Y S R E Q Q I B N Q K V

O X W F W S P L J K C Y H R J E E C W I L N M I P A R P D K A K Z B S Q W D K X

E X N M I Y P N J F C I D K A E F N G Y O G F S P L J J R K Y L G Q V L O W A H

W O V O Y U K M D O O B M L J O A A G Q S I H A X G M O A V B D P J V W O F S N

C A N V V T H O T R F N T A T M O R P E U E U J V G P C P S I V U B S J A B Z I

F S N S W T I U M J E H W I S U K U T K R U M W I J V S L L J E Y I V L O R S B

W O A F J H D L U S I C R Z I F T S X W E O X X R F D F G F D C H T L M M Y X F

H S I B K P G T I N N A W M T G S N W C S W B A C S B T C O P N H E K Y A A Y E

Q K K H J K E C F B R L I W Z C X I S U Q R T B B A Z Q M G X E P Z Y Q H W O M

Z L F M N P V O W Y A R L P G M C R G C X S Y Z P S Z S Y H P G K W U H T M C M

K K F R C N R Q O P V T I S Q P Q B Z T Y H A K S U K A Y J A I E Q W E I S I A

Y F Z B J M U Q L O J P N I Q E P N V R B L I S O H C P H H L L Y X K V W G G S

F C M U A N S J I Q J R A U Z N B N U I Z Y E B E M Q K D Q K L S Q J U X F H E

T R A T N Y W V N P F F K A O W P L S M X G G J Y D T X U Y X I P Z R T Z C T O

W R I V U A F W H L K F W B N C Z I I X N W N H Y D M N M E M D W I X S D X F U

F O A B I R A Y F X C Z M B C Y C W N C U D N A P X T V E W N E U H B K Y R M M

N X I N E R H C I L W W C O M P L A I N A N T Y I K Z O S L S U V S L J R E J W

Q C K F S K P A C P X R D N Q C C D F D Z X G K E K R U L P A D J D O D G D Q W

P S N I S A K H R T J P V N P N H P F L H K Q R I K M A F H K V V D P P H P A O

C I R F E T C F J Q A Z P Q K C U L V G J Z O F C Z D B H S O D E A S A R R B Z

K J N D O L D T E H U M E F K W M D E A Y L T H L B S C X D F N F R V M C E Q E

V E J M X D G V I C B B U H S T K U M X P L B T N G V D O Y W X Y A P B J C M V

O H T F H W Y Z Y O B Z C D G R S Q X F E T A I C O S S A S S E N I S U B L Q H

W C E P M X X B I V N A N Z Z P V B G Q O P H P N Q W X R B G I E O Z P B U C B

L K L A V U Z N G X U D Q I Y I X G S L X V P E T J U O A J M N K V Q R Y D M A

V F F K A V R P F S T C X J C J L A N I Z D A J R E A K N U V X M Z K J V E R D

W S K F C X O A F Y E W S P C W N C D F I J P P J T Y Y F R B J Z W I F P M E V

Q B V Z Z V K Y E H D R R D V F N F R N I Y H H G W A F M J H M W X N I X I C F

P J Q U G M O P R Z R M M J K V Y V Z P L D X V G Q T H F U E N C N F A V C V Q

C G M G M O L X I Y U T I L B T A L A F U X R U Y X J S E O Q F A D R G B F K J

R J Y C W A V G L M Y P I G P Z L Q Q I C Q B I U V S W A Y J E I G Z B W M E E

Copyright © 2011, 2007, 2003 by Saunders, an imprint of Elsevier Inc. All rights reserved.

Accountability
Business associate
Complainant
Confidential
Disclosures
Divulge
Due diligence
Entity
Implement
Incidental
Infer
Insurance
Legalese
Preclude
Prevalent
Privacy
Protected health information
Provider
Provisions
Transaction
Verbiage

CASE STUDY

Read the case study and answer the questions that follow.

Morgan was given a copy of the Privacy Law and told to write the Notice of Privacy Practices for their clinic. After she began reading the law, she became somewhat discouraged because of the legalese and the slow pace at which she had to read to make sure she comprehended the message and requirements. She decided to attend a private training seminar on HIPAA compliance and found the instructor to be very knowledgeable.

1. How can such seminars be beneficial to the practice?

____

____

____

2. How can the medical assistant determine whether a seminar is worth attending?

____

____

____

Research seminars in your area and request information about them. Compare data with the information collected by the rest of the class.

WORKPLACE APPLICATIONS

Determine what certifications are available that relate to HIPAA. What are the requirements for obtaining these special certifications? Why might these be beneficial for the medical assistant? Is there a particular certification you are interested in obtaining?

Copyright © 2011, 2007, 2003 by Saunders, an imprint of Elsevier Inc. All rights reserved.

INTERNET ACTIVITIES

1. Research the HIPAA Web site and find information about complaints. Then write an office policy for patients that details how to make a complaint if the patient thinks that his or her privacy has been violated.

2. Find the exact Public Law number that details the Health Insurance Portability and Accountability Act.

3. Research and write a report on HIPAA's Security Standard.

4. Find five additional links, other than the HIPAA Web site, that provide useful information on HIPAA compliance.

5. Determine misleading marketing ploys that sometimes are used in promoting HIPAA training.

6. Research programs that provide a specialized certificate in HIPAA proficiency.

 Copyright © 2011, 2007, 2003 by Saunders, an imprint of Elsevier Inc. All rights reserved.

18 Basics of Diagnostic Coding

VOCABULARY REVIEW

Fill in the blanks with the correct vocabulary terms from this chapter.

1. In medical coding, assessment and diagnostic statement are synonymous with ________________.
2. ________________ is any contact between a patient and a provider of service.
3. The ________________ is the physician's determination of what is or may be wrong with the patient based on the findings from the H&P.
4. The abbreviation "CC" is a statement in the patient's own words that describes why the person sought medical attention. The letters "CC" stand for ________________ ________________ ________________.
5. ________________ is the signs and symptoms of a disease.
6. The ________________ lists conditions, injuries, and diseases in alphabetical order by main terms, modifying terms, and subterms.
7. Services that support patient diagnoses (e.g., laboratory or radiology services) are known as ________________.
8. In the context of the ICD-9-CM, the word *and* should always be interpreted as ________________.
   a. and
   b. and/or
   c. or
9. ________________ are broad sections of the ICD-9-CM coding manual grouped by disease or illness.
10. ________________ is used when one or more codes are necessary to identify a given condition.
11. Converting verbal or written descriptions into numeric and alphanumeric designations is called ________________.
12. ________________ is the abbreviations, punctuation, symbols, instructional notations, and related entities that provide guidance to the medical assistant or coder in selecting an accurate and specific code.
13. The determination of the nature of a disease, injury, or congenital defect is a(an) ________________
14. The ________________ is the information about the diagnosis or diagnoses of the patient which have been extracted from the medical documentation.
15. The cause of the disorder; a claim may be classified according to ________________.
16. ________________ terms are always written in italics, and the word ________________ is often enclosed in a box to draw particular attention to these instructions.
17. H&P or HPE is an acronym for ________________ ________________ ________________.
18. ________________ is the current system for classifying disease to facilitate collection of uniform and comparable health information, for statistical purposes, and for indexing medical records for data storage and retrieval.
19. ________________ is the initial identification of the condition or complaint the patient expresses in the outpatient medical setting.
20. The term ________________ must always be followed and is found in the Alphabetic Index, volumes 2 and 3; it is a direction given to a coder to look in another place.

Copyright © 2011, 2007, 2003 by Saunders, an imprint of Elsevier Inc. All rights reserved.

21. ________________ is a direction given to the coder to look elsewhere if the main term or subterm (or subterms) for that entry are not sufficient for coding the information.

22. ________________ is a direction given to the coder to see a specific category (three-digit code). This must always be followed.

23. SOAP notes are a system of charting that includes the following four things:

____

____

____

____

24. The term ________________ appears only in volume 1 in those subdivisions in which the user should add further information by means of an additional code to give more complete picture of the diagnosis.

25. In the context of the ICD-9-CM, the terms ________________, ________________, and ________________ dictate that both parts of the title be present in the statement of the diagnosis in order to assign the particular code.

SKILLS AND CONCEPTS

Part I: Getting to Know ICD-9-CM Coding

1. The use of ICD-9-CM codes is important for several reasons. Circle the letters of the ones that do NOT apply:
   a. Standardizing a system of diagnostic coding accepted and understood by all parties in the reimbursement cycle
   b. Creating a more convenient method of data storage and retrieval
   c. Assisting in the maximization of reimbursement
   d. Lengthening the claims processing time
   e. Facilitating and measuring regulatory compliance by use of guidelines and other instructions
   f. Assisting in measuring the appropriateness and timeliness of medical care

2. Fill in the blanks in the paragraph below:

   The ICD-9-CM code is located in volume 1, the Tabular Index, of the ICD-9-CM coding manual. The code consists of a(n) ________________ category code that represents a specific disease, illness, condition, or injury within a general disease category. For example, 250 is the disease classification, or category, for diabetes mellitus. Up to ________________ additional digits can be used, which add further definition and specificity. These additional digits are the fourth digit, or ________________; and the fifth digit, or ________________, respectively.

3. The basic ICD-9-CM manual has three volumes. Fill in the blanks regarding these three volumes:

   ________________ are used for diagnostic coding by hospitals, physicians, and all other providers of service.

   ________________, also known as the Tabular Index, contains all of the diagnostic codes grouped into 17 chapters of disease and injury. ________________ are broad sections of the ICD-9-CM coding manual grouped by disease or illness (e.g., Chapter 10 contains diagnostic codes for diseases of the genitourinary system).

   ________________ is called the Alphabetic Index and is used in the same way an alphabetic index in any textbook is used, except that it refers the user back to the category codes in the Tabular Index rather than page numbers. ________________ is used by hospitals to code procedures and services performed in the hospital environment. This volume is not used by most physician providers.

Copyright © 2011, 2007, 2003 by Saunders, an imprint of Elsevier Inc. All rights reserved.

4. Match the following:

________________	Section	a. Fourth digit
________________	Category	b. Also called a *chapter*
________________	Subcategory	c. Fifth digit
________________	Subclassification	d. Also called a *classification*

5. The ________________ ________________ is used to describe whether any disease process or manifestation exists that was caused by the disease. ________________

6. The ________________ is used on occasions when the patient is not currently ill or to explain problems that influence a patient's current illness, condition, or injury. ________________

7. The ________________ is used to classify environmental or external causes of injury, poisoning, or other adverse effects on the body. ________________

8. Match the following:

_______	Morphology of Neoplasms	a. Appendix C
_______	Glossary of Mental Disorders	b. Appendix A
_______	Classification of Drugs	c. Appendix E
_______	Classification of Industrial Accidents	d. Appendix B
_______	List of Three-Digit Categories	e. Appendix D

9. The abbreviation ________________ is the equivalent of "unspecified" and means that the diagnostic statement does not provide more specificity or definition.

10. The abbreviation ________________ is to be used only when the coder lacks the information necessary to code the term to a more specific category. ________________

11. Four basic forms of punctuation are used in the Tabular Index. Circle the letter of the one that is NOT one of those forms:

    a. Brackets

    b. Parentheses

    c. Question marks

    d. Braces

    e. Colon

12. Two other conventions found in both the Alphabetic Index and the Tabular Index are the use of ________________ and ________________ fonts.

13. ________________ type is used for all codes and titles in the Tabular Index.

14. ________________ type is used for exclusion notes and to identify any diagnosis that cannot be used as the primary diagnosis.

Instructional notations are notes included in the Tabular Index to provide additional guidance for selecting a specific diagnosis code. The following are the most common instructional notations. Fill in the blank with the appropriate term.

15. A notation indicating that under a category or other subdivision, separate terms can be found that will serve to further define, give examples of, or provide modifying adjectives and sites or conditions. ________________

16. Terms that are enclosed within a box and are printed in italics. These notations indicate that some code classifications cannot be used with the code being selected. ________________

Copyright © 2011, 2007, 2003 by Saunders, an imprint of Elsevier Inc. All rights reserved.

17. Used to define terms and give coding instructions. They often are used to list the fifth-digit subclassification or subclassifications for certain categories. ______________

18. The ______________ instruction follows a main term and indicates that a different term should be referenced.

19. This notation is a variation of the SEE instruction. ______________

20. The ______________ instruction generally is found after a main term in the Alphabetic Index and directs the coder to another area with additional index entries that may be useful.

21. This note directs the use of codes that are not normally intended to be used as a principal diagnosis or are not to be sequenced before the underlying disease. ______________

22. This word should be interpreted to mean *and* or *or*. ______________

23. This word in the Alphabetic Index is sequenced immediately after a main term. It provides additional definition or specificity to the code description. ______________

24. Match the following:

_______ Main terms	a. Are always indented two additional spaces from the level of the preceding line
_______ Modifying terms	b. Appear in bold print
_______ Subterms	c. Are found in the Alphabetic Index indented below main terms
_______ Modifiers	d. Are indented two spaces to the right under the main term

25. Three tables and one supplementary index are in the Alphabetic Index. The tables include the:

______________, ______________, and ______________.

26. The supplementary index is the Index to ______________ (E codes).

27. The ______________ Table lists the types of hypertension and the manifestations and causes of hypertension.

28. ______________ is defined as a type of hypertension in which the clinical course progresses rapidly to death.

29. ______________ hypertension is a type that does not threaten a patient's health status significantly.

30. ______________ hypertension is used only when no documentation is provided in the clinical record that the hypertension is malignant or benign.

31. The ______________ Table lists neoplasms by anatomic location.

32. A benign neoplasm is a(n) ______________.

Part II: Beginning the Encounter Process

1. Information pertinent to code selection is culled from a variety of medical documents. Circle the letter of the one that is NOT a part of the diagnostic statements:

    a. Encounter form

    b. Treatment notes

    c. Discharge summary

    d. Operative report

    e. Nurses' notes

    f. Radiology report

    g. Pathology report

    h. Laboratory report

2. The ______________ generally is a preprinted form and is also the most common form used by the medical assistant to obtain the charges and diagnosis when performing charge and payment data entry and insurance billing.

Copyright © 2011, 2007, 2003 by Saunders, an imprint of Elsevier Inc. All rights reserved.

3. ________________ are the second most common medical document from which diagnostic information can be obtained.

4. The ________________ begins with a statement in the patient's own words that describes the reason the person is seeking medical attention. This statement is called the ________________ and is often abbreviated ________________ in the History documentation in the medical record.

5. The ________________ is used primarily for extracting procedure and diagnostic information for patients who were hospitalized rather than seen in the physician's office.

6. The ________________ will also be used for extracting procedure and diagnostic information for patients who underwent surgery as an outpatient or inpatient.

7. ________________, ________________, ________________ reports are not used to obtain diagnostic statements. Any findings from these reports must be documented in the treatment notes in the medical record to be used for diagnostic coding, charge entry, or insurance billing purposes.

8. A(n) ________________ describes a disease, condition, or injury named after a person, such as Hodgkin's disease.

9. ________________ are abbreviations of words that create a new word. For example, the ________________ for gastroesophageal reflux disease is GERD. *GERD* and *gastroesophageal reflux disease* are both medical terms.

10. ________________ are slightly different; abbreviations are "shorthand" for common medical terms.

11. ________________ are words similar in meaning that can be used interchangeably.

12. A series of questions called a(n) ________________ can assist the medical assistant in navigating the Alphabetic and Tabular Index while performing the steps for diagnostic coding. The ________________ for the main text is designed to guide the selection of the appropriate ICD-9-CM diagnostic code

Part III: Coding Exercises

Code the following diagnoses to the highest level of specificity

1. The Smiths' newborn has a birthmark on his neck.

____

2. Mr. Epstein suffers from Bruck's disease.

____

3. Jenny developed bronchitis over spring break after inhaling gas fumes while sitting in a traffic jam.

____

4. Carolyn has experienced dumping syndrome periodically since her gastric bypass surgery.

____

5. Robert has experienced pain when he urinates for the past 3 weeks.

____

6. Julia has been nauseated for about a week but has not complained of vomiting.

____

7. Paul has trench foot, which is a condition of moist gangrene caused by freezing of wet skin.

____

8. Benjamin was given a health examination the night he entered prison to serve a life sentence.

____

9. Angela was classified as morbidly obese, so she qualified for gastric bypass surgery.

____

Copyright © 2011, 2007, 2003 by Saunders, an imprint of Elsevier Inc. All rights reserved.

10. Joseph was diagnosed with academic underachievement disorder and sent for counseling.

____

11. Morgan Smith had an acute myocardial infarction, commonly referred to as a heart attack.

____

12. Jessica was placed in the neonatal ICU because she was diagnosed with transient tachypnea at birth.

____

13. Terri constantly struggles with her maxillary sinus, especially in the winter.

____

14. The physician told Roger that he had epididymitis, but it was not a result of a venereal disease.

____

15. Judy has experienced neck pain for 1 week, but she does not know why the pain began.

____

16. Kevin has suffered from low back pain for years.

____

17. Brad was bitten by a brown recluse spider.

____

18. The Abbotts' child died of sudden infant death syndrome.

____

19. Mitral stenosis was Mrs. Richland's final diagnosis.

____

20. Georgia went into anaphylactic shock after drinking milk.

____

21. Joey was taken to a psychologist because he was having recurrent nightmares.

____

22. Roger has benign essential hypertension.

____

23. Susan was having trouble breathing, and her physician told her that she had a nasopharyngeal polyp that needed to be removed.

____

24. Kristy's son, Christian, suffers with croup syndrome and has been hospitalized three times because of the disorder.

____

25. Ron saw Dr. Jarrett because of an anal fissure, which resulted from a nontraumatic tear of his anus.

____

26. Griffin saw Dr. Redford for treatment of a common head cold.

____

27. A tetanus toxoid vaccination was administered to a child who stepped on a rusty nail.

____

Copyright © 2011, 2007, 2003 by Saunders, an imprint of Elsevier Inc. All rights reserved.

28. Mrs. Garrett developed a decubitus ulcer on her buttocks while she was a patient in a nursing home.

____

29. Paige has a migraine headache, and the physician did not mention intractable migraine in the medical record.

____

30. Pat has Graves' disease, and the physician did not mention thyrotoxic crisis or storm on the medical record.

____

31. Mary is in rehabilitation for episodic cocaine dependence.

____

32. Jonathan has been diagnosed with attention deficit disorder, without mention of hyperactivity.

____

33. Angelica has had chronic cystic mastitis for years.

____

34. Mr. Robertson had a TIA at home and was rushed to the hospital.

____

35. Ray noticed a ringing in his ears after working for 6 months on a construction site.

____

36. Raul has been diagnosed with iron-deficiency anemia, because he is not getting enough iron in his diet.

____

37. Camille has had recurrent earaches in the 2 years since her birth, and the physician diagnosed chronic purulent otitis media.

____

38. Sally's newborn was diagnosed with pyloric stenosis and required surgery.

____

39. Stephanie has a urinary tract infection, but the physician does not yet know what organism caused the illness.

____

40. Don has insomnia, which the physician thinks is a result of drug abuse.

____

41. Mabel Johnson has rheumatoid arthritis and takes daily medication to control the pain.

____

42. Cynthia has a plantar wart but does not want to have it removed yet.

____

43. Sebastian fractured his clavicle at the sternal end during a football game. The fracture was closed.

____

44. Peggy contracted herpes simplex with herpetic vulvovaginitis.

____

45. Eric noticed blood in his semen, and the physician diagnosed hematospermia.

____

Copyright © 2011, 2007, 2003 by Saunders, an imprint of Elsevier Inc. All rights reserved.

46. Kayla had a sore throat and fever and was diagnosed with infectious mononucleosis.

____

47. Gerald has osteoarthritis in his shoulder region and is scheduled to begin physical therapy next week.

____

48. Tray has had three headaches, not diagnosed as migraines, in the past week.

____

49. Amanda was diagnosed with multiple sclerosis.

____

50. Jeffrey has a personal history of alcoholism.

____

51. Butch had four back surgeries and developed a continuous dependence on hydrocodone.

____

52. Jake went to an ophthalmologist to have a splinter removed from his cornea.

____

53. Tammy suffered from severe pain in the temporomandibular joint area.

____

54. Josephine was struck by lightning during a thunderstorm.

____

55. Barry's alcoholism has caused cirrhosis of the liver.

____

56. The Wickers' newborn had a skin condition called *cradle cap*.

____

57. Adam has been a paraplegic since a car wreck 2 years ago.

____

58. Hudson suffered a ruptured abdominal aneurysm and had emergency surgery.

____

59. Mr. Emmett had atherosclerosis of the extremities with gangrene just before his death.

____

60. The woman with Munchausen syndrome had three children who died before law enforcement grew suspicious.

____

61. Ginger experienced dermatitis as a result of using a tanning bed.

____

62. The Lewises' first child was born with Down syndrome.

____

63. Lee Anna has experienced painful menstruation during her last three cycles.

____

64. James had one testicle removed because of seminoma. The tumor was the primary site and incident of his cancer.

____

 Copyright © 2011, 2007, 2003 by Saunders, an imprint of Elsevier Inc. All rights reserved.

65. Jacqueline has uncontrolled diabetes mellitus type 2 with ketoacidosis.

____

66. Mrs. Julius died last week from congestive heart failure.

____

67. Gary saw the physician to follow up on his previous diagnosis of cardiomegaly.

____

68. Dr. Albertez thinks that Mr. Tidwell's Parkinson's disease was drug induced.

____

69. Jerry developed Kaposi's sarcoma during the final stages of AIDS. The sarcoma was present in his lymph nodes.

____

70. Sally developed a postoperative fever because of an infection (code infection only).

____

71. Terri attempted suicide by ingesting a handful of lithium.

____

72. Beaumont's divorce affected every aspect of his life.

____

73. Mr. Maxwell's physician knew that his patient would have to be hospitalized once he diagnosed diverticulitis of the colon with hemorrhaging. Mr. Maxwell, at age 95, could not risk staying at home and allowing the bleeding to continue.

____

74. Susan was stung by a jellyfish while swimming off the coast of Mexico.

____

75. Alaydra has tunnel vision, which makes it difficult to drive safely.

____

76. The escaped criminal was cornered by the police and shot because he raised his gun and pointed it at a policeman.

____

77. Riley has acute myocarditis and was admitted to the hospital.

____

78. Alisha underwent artificial insemination in an effort to have a child.

____

79. Jackie's baby was breech and was delivered using forceps.

____

80. Ordell has acute esophagitis and complained that he had been sick for 3 days.

____

81. Robert dislocated his shoulder while playing baseball. This was a closed anterior dislocation of the humerus.

____

82. Betty has allergic gastroenteritis.

____

Copyright © 2011, 2007, 2003 by Saunders, an imprint of Elsevier Inc. All rights reserved.

83. Mrs. Ralphy was diagnosed with systemic lupus erythematosus.

____

84. Winston has synovitis of the knee.

____

85. Mrs. Radson had a skin condition known as bullous pemphigoid, in which blisters formed in patches all over her skin.

____

86. Osteomalacia made it impossible for Robbie to walk.

____

87. Henry has oral leukoplakia, which may have been caused by smoking a pipe.

____

88. Ricky was diagnosed with acute lymphocytic leukemia.

____

89. The Smithsons' 4-year-old daughter has Hurler's syndrome, which was diagnosed a few months after she was born.

____

90. Patricia has had uterine endometriosis for several years and may require a hysterectomy in the future.

____

CASE STUDY

Dr. Rogers saw Mrs. Arrant in the office this morning. Mrs. Arrant has been diagnosed in the past with congestive heart failure, diabetes mellitus type 2, and chronic myelocytic leukemia. She came to the clinic today complaining of chest pain, and she had a fever of 101.8° F. Code all these conditions. In what order would they be written on an encounter form?

____

____

____

____

WORKPLACE APPLICATIONS

Determine what certifications are available that relate to coding. What are the requirements for obtaining these special certifications? Why might these be beneficial for the medical assistant? Is there a particular certification you are interested in obtaining?

INTERNET ACTIVITIES

1. Research the AHIMA Web site and explore opportunities for a career in coding.

2. Locate a job description for a medical billing and coding specialist and determine the daily duties that coders perform in medical offices and/or large clinics.

3. Write a report on the importance of coding accurately. Share the information with the class.

4. Find five additional links other than the AHIMA Web site that provide useful information on billing and coding.

5. Research programs that provide a specialized certificate in billing and/or coding proficiency.

Copyright © 2011, 2007, 2003 by Saunders, an imprint of Elsevier Inc. All rights reserved.

19 Basics of Procedural Coding

VOCABULARY REVIEW

Fill in the blanks with the correct vocabulary terms from this chapter.

1. The primary procedure or service code selected when performing insurance billing or statistical research is a category ________________ code.
2. Jerri sometimes has difficulty with ________________ codes, which designate procedures or services that are grouped together and paid for as one procedure or service.
3. Jules prepared a(n) ________________ or summary of the diagnostic statements on Mr. Ford's medical record.
4. ________________ are found at the beginning of each of the six sections of the CPT-4 manual, and Rebecca refers to them often when coding procedures.
5. Category ________________ codes are for new or experimental procedures.
6. A procedure, service, or diagnosis named after a person is called a(n) ________________.
7. Codes in which the components of a procedure are separated and reported separately are called ________________ codes.
8. Code additions that explain circumstances that alter a provided service or provide additional clarification or detail are called ________________.
9. The main divisions of the CPT-4 manual are called ________________.
10. Abbreviations are also called ________________.

CODING EXERCISES

Code the following procedures.

1. Dr. Smith visits Eula Fairbanks, a patient with dementia, in the nursing home for less than 30 minutes.

____

2. Jessica Lundy, a newborn, was admitted to the pediatric critical care unit after her birth, where Dr. Williams provided her initial care.

____

3. Because Lucille Westerman had multiple health problems, she was admitted for observation after a fainting spell. Dr. Adams took a comprehensive history and performed a thorough examination and then made medical decisions of high complexity regarding her care.

____

4. Dr. Wray saw Tammy Luttrell in the office as a new patient. He took a detailed history and performed a detailed examination and then made medical decisions of low complexity.

____

Copyright © 2011, 2007, 2003 by Saunders, an imprint of Elsevier Inc. All rights reserved.

5. Sylvia Julius saw Dr. Bridges for her allergies. The physician took a problem-focused history, performed a problem-focused examination, and made straightforward decisions regarding her care.

____

6. Bonnie Sadler comes to the office to have blood work drawn for an obstetric panel. What is the code for the obstetric panel only?

____

7. The office charges Bonnie Sadler, a college student, for drawing a blood specimen. What is the code for venipuncture?

____

8. Terri Smithson had laparoscopic gastric bypass surgery involving the Roux-en-Y procedure.

____

9. Kim Errant had outpatient kidney imaging with vascular flow to make sure her kidneys were functioning normally.

____

10. Georgie Ebersol had blood drawn for a total bilirubin. Code the blood test only.

____

11. Roy Messing's urine was tested for total protein.

____

12. Jerry Orchard was tested for his blood alcohol level.

____

13. Andrea Adams has a bleeding disorder and has to undergo regular coagulation time tests. Her physician uses the Lee and White method.

____

14. Dr. Airheart sent Roberto's specimen to the microbiology laboratory to check for *Cryptosporidium* organisms.

____

15. The body was sent to the county medical examiner's office for a forensic autopsy, which was performed by Dr. Stein.

____

16. Jonathan Boyd was required to have a polio vaccination by his school. He received an oral dose.

____

17. Julia Anderson has a lithium level drawn to make certain that her dosage was accurate and appropriate.

____

18. Cynthia Hernandez was exposed to hepatitis, so her physician ordered an acute hepatitis panel.

____

Copyright © 2011, 2007, 2003 by Saunders, an imprint of Elsevier Inc. All rights reserved.

19. Sam Livingston, a baby in the neonatal unit, had total bilirubin tests drawn each morning.

____

20. Susan's husband has blood drawn regularly to measure his quinidine levels.

____

21. Bobby had to undergo treatment of a clavicular fracture, without manipulation, after his injury during a football game.

____

22. Betty received anesthesia for the vaginal delivery of her child.

____

23. Anesthesia was provided to Ron Smith, a brain-dead patient whose organs were being harvested for donation.

____

24. Dr. Partridge participated in a complex, lengthy telephone call regarding a patient who was scheduled for multiple surgeries.

____

25. When Terri Anderson was involved in a major car accident, the emergency department physician took a comprehensive history, performed a thorough examination, and made highly complex decisions.

____

26. Tim Taylor is a new patient with a small cyst on his back. Dr. Young took a problem-focused history and performed a problem-focused examination and then made straightforward medical decisions.

____

27. Jim Angelo, an established patient, saw the physician for a minor cut on the back of his hand. The physician spent approximately 10 minutes with Jim.

____

28. Vera Carpenter was admitted to the hospital for diabetes mellitus, congestive heart failure, and an infection of unknown origin. Dr. Antonetti performed a consultation that took about an hour, including the time spent writing orders in her medical record.

____

29. Carla had a nasal polyp removed that was hindering her ability to breathe. The excision was a simple one and was performed in Dr. Wilson's office.

____

30. Darla's son, Andy, was examined for pinworms.

____

31. The police asked the laboratory technician to perform an arsenic test on a tube of blood.

____

32. An incision was made into the newborn's pyloric sphincter to allow food to travel through his digestive system.

____

Copyright © 2011, 2007, 2003 by Saunders, an imprint of Elsevier Inc. All rights reserved.

33. Ben, a 6-year-old, had his tonsils and adenoids removed because of recurrent infections.

____

34. Edward had one testicle removed because of a growing tumor attached to it. An inguinal approach was used, and during the surgery, the physician explored the abdominal area to look for other growths.

____

35. Alex's mother insisted that she have her ears pierced by a physician so that the procedure would be as clean as possible.

____

36. Fonda was diagnosed with an abdominal ectopic pregnancy, which Dr. Tomlinson removed surgically.

____

37. The medical assistant performed a simple urinalysis, using a dipstick and a microscope to examine the specimen.

____

38. Wayne had blood drawn for a CBC with an automated WBC.

____

39. Paula had an inflammation somewhere inside her body, as evidenced by her sedimentation rate. The test was automated.

____

40. Jimmie's physician ordered computed tomography of his abdomen with contrast material.

____

41. Joan had a laparoscopic biopsy of her left ovary.

____

42. Craig had to undergo a direct repair of a ruptured aneurysm of the carotid artery, which was performed via a neck incision.

____

43. Emma was given a urine pregnancy test in the clinic before receiving x-ray examinations to diagnose her back disorder; a color comparison test kit was used.

____

44. Jennifer's child was tested for serum albumin.

____

45. Angela had a qualitative lactose test using a urine specimen.

____

46. Sarah was required to have a blood chemistry test for methadone by her probation officer.

____

47. The two children who had been lost in the woods were tested for Rocky Mountain spotted fever.

____

Copyright © 2011, 2007, 2003 by Saunders, an imprint of Elsevier Inc. All rights reserved.

48. Marcus has a total T-cell count every month.

____

49. After her needle-stick injury, Felicia was tested for the hepatitis B surface antibody.

____

50. Dr. Torrid felt that Katrina might have the Epstein-Barr virus, so he tested for the early antigen.

____

51. Dr. Battson performed a chlamydia culture on the vaginal specimen.

____

52. Juan was given a test for herpes simplex type II.

____

53. Mr. Albertson was given a blood test for uric acid.

____

54. Derrick had a Western Blot test last week. The interpretation and report are due back to the physician by tomorrow.

____

55. Roy had a urine test for total protein.

____

56. The emergency physician ordered a lead test on the small child, thinking that she had perhaps ingested some paint chips.

____

57. Joy has monthly blood tests to evaluate her iron-binding capacity.

____

58. Andi was tested for chromium yesterday and has a return appointment next week.

____

59. All gastric bypass patients are required to have a basic metabolic panel before surgery is scheduled.

____

60. June had an obstetric panel run on her second appointment with the physician.

____

61. Royce had a chest x-ray film, single frontal view, to check for pneumonia.

____

62. Dr. True suspected that Joey had fractured his sternum, so he ordered an x-ray film that would show two views of the bone.

____

Copyright © 2011, 2007, 2003 by Saunders, an imprint of Elsevier Inc. All rights reserved.

63. Jessalyn had an MRI scan of her spinal canal and its contents.

____

64. Dr. Tompkins visited a new patient at her home and spent about 20 minutes diagnosing and treating her for the flu.

____

65. Dr. Revy was on standby for about 20 minutes while the decision was made as to whether the patient would have a cesarean section.

____

66. Judge Jordan has his blood checked for potassium levels monthly.

____

67. Steven Pauly needs a chest x-ray examination, and the physician has requested four views.

____

68. Linda Ellis had a complete hip x-ray examination with two views, because her physician was considering hip replacement surgery.

____

69. Judy had blood drawn for determination of a theophylline level during her last office visit.

____

70. Joy had a closed treatment of a coccygeal fracture.

____

71. Mrs. Dickson went to see Dr. Donner for a complete radiologic examination of the scapula.

____

72. Bobbie returned to the physician's office to have a short leg walking cast applied after having worn a larger cast for 4 weeks.

____

73. Dr. Angell ordered a radiologic examination of Sylvia's mastoids, requesting two views.

____

74. Sammy had a uric acid test during his last office visit.

____

75. Peter asked his physician to repeat his CPK total, because it had been slightly high on his last visit.

____

76. Bryce has a digoxin level drawn every 3 months.

____

77. The pathologist prepared tissue for drug analysis.

____

Copyright © 2011, 2007, 2003 by Saunders, an imprint of Elsevier Inc. All rights reserved.

78. Julie was quite dehydrated for a week, so her physician ran an electrolyte panel.

____

79. Frank asked the physician how a magnesium level related to his illness.

____

80. Joel's physician believed that Joel had adrenal insufficiency, so he ordered an ACTH stimulation panel.

____

81. All three children who lived in the condemned home were subjected to a quantitative carbon monoxide test.

____

82. When Ariel turned 50, her physician recommended that she have an occult blood test annually.

____

83. Most diabetics periodically have a blood glucose test performed at the physician's office in addition to the test strip checks that they perform at home.

____

84. Selenium can be detected with a blood test.

____

85. Sarah's infant returned to the physician's office to have a PKU test a few weeks after she was born.

____

86. Van Stephens had blood work done on Monday to check his triglyceride level.

____

87. Karry has been to the physician for several days in a row to have ovulation tests, which are done by visual color comparison.

____

88. Samuel's vitamin K test results were slightly below normal.

____

89. Dr. Grant runs a spun microhematocrit on each of his pregnant patients at every prenatal visit.

____

90. Trent had a serum folic acid test run this morning at his physician's office.

Copyright © 2011, 2007, 2003 by Saunders, an imprint of Elsevier Inc. All rights reserved.

CASE STUDY

In the following text, highlight all procedures that need to be coded for billing purposes.

Roberta Sleether is a new patient who saw Dr. Morganstern. She complained of feeling tired all the time. She stated that she was exhausted even after a full 8 hours of sleep at night. Roberta said that she did not have much of an appetite and that she had been eating mostly salads and chicken, with a bowl of fruit as snacks. She is not overweight, and her blood pressure and other vital signs were normal. Dr. Morganstern decided to perform a CBC, an electrolyte panel, and a lipid panel. He also ordered a urinalysis, an iron-binding capacity, and a vitamin B_{12} test. The physician asked if she had noticed any blood in her urine or stool, and she denied blood in the urine but did mention she had several episodes of diarrhea. Dr. Morganstern added an occult blood test as well as a stool culture to check for pathogens. The physician placed Roberta on multivitamin therapy and told her to return in 1 week to discuss her laboratory test results. He spent approximately 30 minutes with Roberta, taking a detailed history, performing a detailed examination, and making low-complexity medical decisions. Roberta scheduled her appointment for the following week and left the clinic.

WORKPLACE APPLICATIONS

1. Select a medical specialty and research the procedure codes that would be commonly used in that practice.

2. Contact a practice and make an appointment to meet the person or persons who perform coding tasks. Discuss the challenges and rewards of the job. Prepare a report for the class based on the interview with the coders.

3. Design an encounter form for a fictional medical practice. Choose the specialty and make sure the codes chosen for the form are applicable to the specialty practice.

INTERNET ACTIVITIES

1. Research job postings on the Internet that relate to billing and coding.

2. Working in groups, prepare a report on the sections of the CPT-4 manual. Discuss the most common codes in each section.

3. Search for coding hints and tips online. Prepare a report for the class and discuss the tips and how to use them to code more effectively.

Copyright © 2011, 2007, 2003 by Saunders, an imprint of Elsevier Inc. All rights reserved.

20 Basics of Health Insurance

VOCABULARY REVIEW

Fill in the blanks with the correct vocabulary terms from this chapter.

1. ________________ is the maximum amount of money many third-party payers allow for a specific procedure or service.
2. A term used in managed care for an approved referral is ________________.
3. An individual entitled to receive benefits from an insurance policy or program or from a government entitlement program offering healthcare benefits is considered the ________________.
4. The amount payable by an insurance company for a monetary loss to an individual insured by that company, under each coverage, is known as ________________.
5. This rule states that when an individual is covered by two insurance policies, the insurance plan of the policyholder whose birthday comes first in the calendar year (month and day, not year) becomes the primary insurance.
6. ________________ is a payment method used by many managed care organizations in which a fixed amount of money is reimbursed to the provider for patients enrolled during a specific period of time, no matter what services were received or how many visits were made.
7. In the insurance business, companies that assume the risk of an insurance policy are considered the ________________.
8. CHAMPUS is the acronym for ____.
9. The health benefits program run by the Department of Veterans Affairs (VA) that helps eligible beneficiaries pay the cost of specific healthcare services and supplies is (give full name and acronym) ________________ ________________.
10. A(n) ________________ provision frequently is found in medical insurance policies whereby the policyholder and the insurance company share the cost of covered losses in a specified ratio.
11. This type of plan reimburses the insured for expenses resulting from illness or injury according to a specific fee schedule as outlined in the insurance policy and on a fee-for-service basis. ________________
12. A(n) ________________ is the sum of money paid at the time of medical service; a form of co-insurance.
13. Typically met on a yearly or per-incident basis, this specific amount of money, a(n) ________________, is what a patient must pay out of pocket before the insurance carrier begins paying.
14. ________________ are the spouse, children, and sometimes domestic partner or other individuals designated by the insured who are covered under a healthcare plan.
15. This type of insurance provides periodic payments to replace income when an insured person is unable to work as a result of illness, injury, or disease. ________________
16. The ________________ is the date on which an insurance policy or plan takes effect so that benefits are payable.
17. ________________ is a term that indicates whether a patient's insurance coverage is in effect and the patient is eligible for payment of insurance benefits.

Copyright © 2011, 2007, 2003 by Saunders, an imprint of Elsevier Inc. All rights reserved.

18. The term for limitations on an insurance contract for which benefits are not payable is ________________.

19. A letter or statement from the insurance carrier that describes what was paid, denied, or reduced in payment and that also contains information about amounts applied to the deductible, the patient's co-insurance, and the allowed amounts is called the ________________ ________________.

20. A letter or statement from Medicare describing what was paid, denied, or reduced in payment and that also contains information about amounts applied to the deductible, the patient's co-insurance, and the allowed amounts is called the ________________ ________________.

21. An established schedule of fees set for services performed by providers and paid by the patient is called ________________.

22. A ________________ ________________ is an organization that contracts with the government to handle and mediate insurance claims from medical facilities, home health agencies, or providers of medical services or supplies.

23. Medicaid and Medicare are examples of ________________ plans.

   a. local

   b. basic

   c. organizational

   d. government

24. Insurance written under a policy that covers a number of people under a single master contract issued to their employer or to an association with which they are affiliated would be considered a(n) ________________ policy.

25. The ________________ is the person responsible for paying a medical bill.

26. ________________ ________________ is protection in return for periodic premium payments that provides reimbursement of expenses resulting from illness or injury.

27. The Kassebaum-Kennedy Act, which was designed to improve portability and continuity of health insurance coverage; to combat waste, fraud, and abuse in health insurance and healthcare delivery; to promote the use of medical savings accounts; to improve access to long-term care services and coverage; to simplify the administration of health insurance; and to serve other purposes, is also called the (please provide the whole name and the acronym) ____ ________________________________.

28. A(n) ________________________________ is an organization that provides a wide range of comprehensive healthcare services for a specified group at a fixed periodic payment. These organizations may be sponsored by the government, medical schools, hospitals, employers, labor unions, consumer groups, insurance companies, and hospital-medical plans.

29. ________________ ________________ pay for all or a share of the cost of covered services, regardless of which physician, hospital, or other licensed ________________ provider is used. Policyholders of these plans and their dependents choose when and where to get healthcare services.

30. What type of insurance policy is designed specifically for the use of one person (and his or her dependents) and is not associated with the amenities of a group policy (e.g., lower premiums)? ________________ ________________.

31. The individual or organization covered by an insurance policy according to the policy terms, and usually the individual or group that pays the premiums, is called the ________________.

32. An umbrella term for all healthcare plans that provide healthcare in return for preset monthly payments and coordinated care through a defined network of primary care physicians and hospitals is ________________________.

Copyright © 2011, 2007, 2003 by Saunders, an imprint of Elsevier Inc. All rights reserved.

33. Tax-deferred bank or savings accounts that are combined with a low-premium, high-deductible insurance policy and designed for individuals or families who choose to fund their own healthcare expenses and medical insurance are called ______________________________.

34. Matching terms:

_______ Medicaid	a. A federally sponsored health insurance program for those over age 65 and those under age 65 who are disabled
_______ Medicare	b. A term sometimes applied to private insurance products that supplement Medicare insurance benefits
_______ Medigap	c. A federal and state sponsored health insurance program for the medically indigent

35. A(n) ______________ ______________ is a physician or other healthcare provider who enters into a contract with a specific insurance company or program and by doing so agrees to abide by certain rules and regulations set forth by that particular third-party payer.

36. The person who pays a premium to an insurance company and in whose name the policy is written in exchange for the insurance protection provided by a policy of insurance is the ______________________________.

37. ______________ is a process required by some insurance carriers in which the provider obtains permission to perform certain procedures or services or to refer a patient to a specialist.

38. The periodic (monthly, quarterly, or annual) payment of a specific sum of money to an insurance company for which the insurer, in return, agrees to provide certain benefits is called a(n) ______________.

39. The ______________________________ is a general practice or nonspecialist provider or physician responsible for the care of a patient for some health maintenance organizations; also called a *gatekeeper*.

40. An insurance term used when a primary care provider wants to send a patient to a specialist: ______________.

41. An explanation of benefits that comes from Medicaid is called a(an) ______________ ______________.

42. The fee schedule designed to provide national uniform payment of Medicare benefits after adjustment to reflect the differences in practice costs across geographic areas is called the ______________________________.

43. A(n) ______________ is a special provision or group of provisions that may be added to a policy to expand or limit the benefits otherwise payable. It may increase or reduce benefits, waive a condition or coverage, or in any other way amend the original contract.

44. A type of insurance plan funded by an organization with an employee base large enough to enable it to fund its own insurance program: ______________________________.

45. When a patient or insured individual refers himself or herself to a specialist without requesting the referral from the primary provider, this is known as ______________.

46. ______________ ______________ plans provide benefits in the form of certain surgical and medical services rendered rather than cash. This type of plan is not restricted to a fee schedule.

47. An organization that processes claims and performs other business-related functions for a health plan is a(n) ______________________________.

48. Entities that make payment on an obligation or debt but are not parties of the contract that created the debt are known as ______________________________.

49. A government-sponsored program under which authorized dependents of military personnel receive medical care; the program originally was called CHAMPUS but now is called ______________________________.

50. A(n) ______________ ______________ is a review of individual cases by a committee to make sure services are medically necessary and to study how providers use medical care resources.

Copyright © 2011, 2007, 2003 by Saunders, an imprint of Elsevier Inc. All rights reserved.

51. Insurance against liability imposed on certain employers to pay benefits and furnish care to employees who are injured and to pay benefits to dependents of employees killed in the course of or arising out of their employment is known as

________________ ________________.

FOR QUESTIONS 52-61: Read the following paragraph and then fill in the blanks.

The medical assistant's tasks related to health insurance processing are initiated when the patient encounters the provider, either by appointment, as a walk-in, or in the emergency department or hospital. To complete insurance billing and coding properly, the medical assistant must perform the following tasks.

52. Obtain information from the patient and insured, including ________________, employment, and ________________ data.

53. Verify the patient's ________________ for insurance payment with the insurance carrier or carriers, as well as ________________ available, exclusions, and whether ________________ are needed to refer patients to specialists or to perform certain services or procedures, such as surgery or diagnostic tests.

54. Perform ________________ and ________________ coding and review the encounter form or charge ticket for completeness once the patient has been seen by the provider.

55. Calculate insurance ________________ and co-insurance amounts and provide the patient with a statement showing the ________________ expense, the amount owed by the patient.

56. Obtain ________________ for referral of the patient to a specialist or for special services or procedures that require advance permission.

57. Complete an insurance claim form and submit it to the insurance company for ________________ for services and procedures performed.

58. Post payments and adjustments on the patient ledger or account and examine the ________________ (EOB), ________________ (EOMB) or the ________________ (RA) from the insurance company to identify what was paid, reduced, or denied.

59. Make adjustments to the account of the allowable amount, which is either written off (adjusted) or passed on to the patient for ________________.

60. Bill the patient for any ________________ ________________, or, if there is a secondary insurance, complete the secondary insurance claim form and submit it to the insurance company.

61. ________________ on any rejected or unpaid claims and any requests from the insurance carrier for more information about specific claims.

QUESTIONS 62-73: Match each type of insurance benefit with its description

62. ________ Hospitalization	a. Pays expenses involved in care of the teeth and gums
63. ________ Surgical	b. Provides reimbursement for all or a percentage of the cost of refraction, lenses, and frames
64. ________ Basic medical	c. Helps defray medical costs not covered by Medicare
65. ________ Major medical	d. Protects a person in the event of a certain type of accident, such as an airplane crash
66. ________ Disability	e. Provides payment of a specified amount on the insured's death
67. ________ Dental care	f. Covers a continuum of broad-ranged maintenance and health services to chronically ill, disabled, or mentally retarded individuals
68. ________ Vision care	g. Pays all or part of a surgeon's and/or assistant surgeon's fees
69. ________ Medicare supplement	h. Weekly or monthly cash benefits provided to employed policyholders who become unable to work as a result of an accident or illness

Copyright © 2011, 2007, 2003 by Saunders, an imprint of Elsevier Inc. All rights reserved.

70. _______ Special risk insurance

71. _______ Liability insurance

72. _______ Life insurance

73. _______ Long-term care insurance

i. Pays all or part of a physician's fee for nonsurgical services, including hospital, home, and office visits

j. Provides protection against especially large medical bills resulting from catastrophic or prolonged illnesses

k. Pays the cost of all or part of the insured person's hospital room and board and specific hospital services

l. Often includes benefits for medical expenses payable to individuals who are injured in the insured person's home or in an automobile accident

74. List three advantages of the managed care concept.

____

____

____

75. List three disadvantages of the managed care concept.

____

____

____

76. List 10 items of information the medical assistant should obtain from the patient before calling the insurance company for preauthorization or precertification.

a. _______________

b. _______________

c. _______________

d. _______________

e. _______________

f. _______________

g. _______________

h. _______________

i. _______________

j. _______________

77. List two types of people who would qualify for Medicare.

____

____

78. List two types of people who would qualify for Medicaid.

____

____

Copyright © 2011, 2007, 2003 by Saunders, an imprint of Elsevier Inc. All rights reserved.

79. The ________________ ________________ is the official daily publication for rules, proposed rules, and notices of federal agencies and organization, as well as Executive Orders and other presidential documents.

CASE STUDY

Survey all class members and determine the various types of insurance coverage the students have. Assign each student a different insurance company and have them call to verify benefits. Choose a medical procedure and have the students call and verify the amounts of coverage for that particular procedure. If students are uncomfortable exchanging health insurance information, allow them to verify and obtain amounts of coverage for their own insurance.

WORKPLACE APPLICATIONS

1. Working in small groups, obtain a quote for health insurance coverage for a small group. Use the Internet to research companies and choose three or four from which to obtain quotes.
2. Design a document that provides information on what should be placed in each box of the health insurance claim form. Place the document in a report cover with sheet protectors and turn it in for a special project grade.
3. Obtain encounter forms from several different physicians' offices. Use them to create mock patients, listing a diagnosis and several procedures. Complete an insurance claim form for each patient and encounter form. As an option, work in groups and present the patient to the class.

INTERNET ACTIVITIES

1. Research the various individual policies available. Obtain a quote for healthcare coverage from one company. Share the information with the class and compare the cost of individual policies with those of group policies. Discuss the differences.
2. Investigate medical savings accounts and determine how these accounts work, as well as how benefits for healthcare expenses are paid.
3. Conduct a survey of 25 physicians and ask them what insurance plans they see in the office most frequently. Research these companies on the Internet and determine their benefits and costs. Prepare a report that compares the five most frequently mentioned companies.

Copyright © 2011, 2007, 2003 by Saunders, an imprint of Elsevier Inc. All rights reserved.

21 The Health Insurance Claim Form

VOCABULARY REVIEW

Fill in the blanks with the correct term from this chapter.

1. ________________ is the transfer of the patient's legal right to collect benefits for medical expenses to the provider of those services, authorizing the payment to be sent directly to the provider.
2. The process of examining claims for accuracy and completeness before submitting the claims is called a(n) ________________, which can be performed manually or electronically with computer billing software.
3. Often referred to when tracking medical services used by patients or researching claims, a(n) ________________ ________________ is the path left by a transaction when it has been completed.
4. ________________ ________________ are insurance claim forms that have been completed correctly and that can be processed and paid promptly if they meet the restrictions on covered services and blocks.
5. A centralized facility to which insurance claims are transmitted, a(n) ________________ separates, checks, and redistributes claims electronically to various insurance carriers.
6. A method of electronic claims submission in which computer software allows a provider to submit an insurance claim directly to an insurance carrier for payment is called ________________ ________________.
7. ________________ claims are claims that contain errors or omissions that must be corrected so that the claims can be resubmitted to an insurance carrier to obtain reimbursement.
8. ________________ claims are claims that are submitted to insurance processing facilities using a computerized medium, such as direct data entry, direct wire, dial-in telephone digital fax, or personal computer download or upload.
9. The transfer of data back and forth between two or more entities using an electronic medium is called ________________, or ________________.
10. A(n) ________________ ________________ is a mark that is accepted as proof of approval of and/or responsibility for the content of an electronic document.
11. The number used by the Internal Revenue Service to identify a business or an individual functioning as a business entity for income tax reporting is known as a(n) ________________ ________________ number, or ________________.
12. A claim that is missing information and is returned to the provider for correction and resubmission is called a(n) ________________ ________________ or sometimes an *invalid claim.*
13. ________________________________ or ________________ is the electronic scanning of printed blocks as images and the use of special software to recognize these images as ASCII text for uploading into a computer database.
14. The term for the acronym NPI is ________________________________.
15. The term for the acronym PIN is ________________________________.
16. The term for the acronym UPIN is ________________________________.

Copyright © 2011, 2007, 2003 by Saunders, an imprint of Elsevier Inc. All rights reserved.

17. Hard copies of insurance claims that have been completed and sent by surface mail are known as ______________ ______________.

18. Any company, individual, or group that provides medical, diagnostic, or treatment services to a patient is considered a(n) ______________.

19. A number assigned to a provider by a carrier for use in the submission of claims is called a(n) ______________ or ______________.

20. ______________ claims are claims that have been returned unpaid to the provider for clarification of questions and that must be corrected before resubmission.

21. The number assigned by fiscal intermediaries to identify providers on claims for services is the ______________ or ______________.

22. The universal claim form was developed by the Health Care Financing Administration (HCFA) (now known as the Centers for Medicare and Medicaid Services [CMS]) and approved by the American Medical Association (AMA) for use in submitting all government-sponsored claims. It now is also known as the ______________.

23. A medical assistant may submit insurance claims to a third-party payer or an insurance carrier in one of two ways: ______________ or ______________.

24. Name two advantages of using hard copy (paper) claims.

____

____

25. Name two disadvantages of using hard copy (paper) claims.

____

____

26. List two benefits of the ICR scanning system.

____

____

27. A number of rules must be followed when completing the paper CMS-1500 form so that the insurance carrier can scan the claim. Give 10 examples of when a blank space should be used when completing a paper CMS-1500.

a. ______________________________
b. ______________________________
c. ______________________________
d. ______________________________
e. ______________________________
f. ______________________________
g. ______________________________
h. ______________________________
i. ______________________________
j. ______________________________

Copyright © 2011, 2007, 2003 by Saunders, an imprint of Elsevier Inc. All rights reserved.

28. Now list the other six rules for completing the paper CMS-1500 form so that the insurance carrier can scan the claim.

a. ______________________________

b. ______________________________

c. ______________________________

d. ______________________________

e. ______________________________

f. ______________________________

29. The transaction and code set for the CMS-1500 electronic claims submission is called the ______________.

30. Implementation Guides for each of the transaction and code sets requirements for electronic data submission can be obtained through the Center for Medicare and Medicaid Services (CMS). The data that can be submitted electronically include (list three):

a. ______________________________

b. ______________________________

c. ______________________________

31. List two ways electronic claims can be submitted.

____

____

32. Clearinghouses typically also provide additional services; list three of them.

a. ______________________________

b. ______________________________

c. ______________________________

33. Give one major advantage of electronic submission of insurance claims.

____

34. The first section of the patient registration form includes the patient information; list four items that are recorded in this section.

a. ______________________________

b. ______________________________

c. ______________________________

d. ______________________________

35. The patient registration form should be completed by the patient or the patient's guardian. The medical assistant should confirm the information by doing two things:

a. ______________________________

b. ______________________________

Copyright © 2011, 2007, 2003 by Saunders, an imprint of Elsevier Inc. All rights reserved.

QUESTIONS 36-51:

Detail the 16 steps for gathering patient information and the other information required to complete an insurance claim form.

36. ____

37. ____

38. ____

39. ____

40. ____

41. ____

42. ____

43. ____

44. ____

45. ____

46. ____

47. ____

48. ____

49. ____

50. ____

51. ____

Copyright © 2011, 2007, 2003 by Saunders, an imprint of Elsevier Inc. All rights reserved.

52. Once the patient's and the insured's demographic and insurance information has been collected, the next step is to verify the patient's eligibility and benefits. By what method or methods is this usually done?

____

____

____

____

53. If any diagnostic or therapeutic services or procedures are to be rendered by the provider that require preapproval, a(n) _______________ must be done to obtain an authorization number.

54. A CMS-1500 claim form has _______________ blocks, or items. The blocks are divided into _____ sections.

55. List the information contained in each section of a CMS-1500 claim form.

Section 1 _______________

Section 2 _______________

Section 3 _______________

56. The type of insurance the patient has is indicated in block _______________.

57. Block 1a is used for what vital piece of information?

____

58. Block 2 should contain the patient's name. This is the person receiving treatment or supplies. In what order should the patient's name be entered? _______________.

a. First, middle initial, last

b. Middle initial, last, first

c. Last, first, middle initial

59. Block 3 contains what two pieces of information?

____

____

60. Block 4 contains _______________; this is the person who owns the policy.

61. The patient's (permanent) address and phone numbered are entered in which block? _______________.

a. Block 5

b. Block 5a

c. Block 5b

62. Block 6 is Patient Relationship to Insured; explain what the following titles mean in this block.

a. Self _______________

b. Spouse _______________

c. Child _______________

d. Other _______________

Copyright © 2011, 2007, 2003 by Saunders, an imprint of Elsevier Inc. All rights reserved.

63. The insured's address and telephone number are entered in block 7. How does the information in this block differ from that in block 5?

____

____

64. Block 8 is Patient's Status; to what specifically does this refer and why is this information important?

____

____

65. In Section 3, the Patient/Insured Section, which blocks are completed for the primary insurance and which blocks are completed only if a secondary insurance claim is being submitted?

Primary insurance ______________________________

Secondary insurance ______________________________

66. Block 12 contains which signature? ______________

a. Insured's or authorized person's signature

b. Patient's or authorized person's signature

67. Block 13 contains which signature? ______________

a. Insured's or authorized person's signature

b. Patient's or authorized person's signature

68. The name of the referring provider, ordering provider, or other source that referred or ordered the service or procedure on the claim is entered in block 17. Explain the difference between a referring physician and an ordering physician.

____

____

____

____

69. Block 21 contains an important piece of information; what is it?

____

____

70. When entering the appropriate diagnosis or ICD-9-CM code or codes, what is the maximum number of codes that should be used on one claim form?

____

71. What number is placed in block 26, and who assigns this number?

____

72. What information is provided in block 28? ______________.

a. Balance due

b. Total charge

c. Amount paid

Copyright © 2011, 2007, 2003 by Saunders, an imprint of Elsevier Inc. All rights reserved.

73. What information is provided in block 29? ________________.

  a. Amount paid

  b. Balance due

  c. Total charge

74. What information is provided in block 30? ________________.

  a. Total charge

  b. Balance due

  c. Amount paid

75. Many guidelines for reviewing a claim must be followed prior to submission of the claim. List 10 of those guidelines.

  a. ____

  b. ____

  c. ____

  d. ____

  e. ____

  f. ____

  g. ____

  h. ____

  i. ____

  j. ____

76. The two main reasons for denial of payment are:

____

____

77. A clean claim is defined as ____

____.

78. A dirty (or dingy) claim is defined as ____

____.

79. A rejected claim is defined as ____

____

____.

Copyright © 2011, 2007, 2003 by Saunders, an imprint of Elsevier Inc. All rights reserved.

SKILLS AND CONCEPTS

Part I: Completing Insurance Claim Forms

Complete a claim form using the patient information in each of the following scenarios. Use the claim forms in Work Products 21-1 through 21-5.

1. Complete Claim Form 1 (Work Product 21-1) using the following information.

Today's date: 9-29-20XX

Mr. Jackson, an established patient, has suffered from situational depression since his wife of 47 years died last winter. He has a history of congestive heart failure and intermittent high blood pressure. He comes to the office on July 23, 20XX, for treatment of his depression. Dr. Swakoski sees Mr. Jackson and counsels him about medication for his condition. He is with the patient for about 25 minutes. He gives Mr. Jackson a week's worth of samples of Cymbalta and writes a prescription for the drug that is refillable for 3 months. The charge for the office visit is $85. File this claim with BC/BS.

Donald W. Jackson (patient and insured)
77834 High Road Way
Los Angeles, CA 90010
818-665-0098 (home)
SS# 567-99-0067

Insurance: BC/BS and Medicare
ID# 567990067
Employer: Retired
DOB: 3-8-1940

Diagnosis: Depression, CHF, HTN
Procedures: Office visit
Account Number: JAD0067

Family Health Center
120 E. Northwest Highway
Los Angeles, CA 90010
818-624-0112
Federal Tax ID# 75-6102034

BC/BS
11001 Spring Way, Suite 200
Sacramento, CA 90012
800-443-0033

Theodore Swakoski, MD
NPI# 6170421616
BS Provider# 621604211

 Copyright © 2011, 2007, 2003 by Saunders, an imprint of Elsevier Inc. All rights reserved.

2. Complete Claim Form 2 (Work Product 21-2) using the following information.

Today's date: 9-29-20XX

Mr. Adams, an established, married patient, comes to the office because of an episode of bronchitis. He states that he has felt poorly for about 1 week and that he now is having trouble getting a full breath of air. He has had moderate pain on coughing and admits that the cough has kept him awake or has awakened him. He says he has bronchitis about once a year in the fall. Dr. Abbott sees Mr. Adams for about 15 minutes in the office. She prescribes an antibiotic, a cough syrup, and Hycodan. Dr. Abbott knows that Mr. Adams is also diabetic, so she draws blood for a glucose test to make sure the levels are normal. She suggests that Mr. Adams stay home from work for the 2 days leading into the weekend and return to work on Monday. Dr. Abbott asks whether Mr. Adams is still having trouble sleeping, as reported on his last office visit. He admits that he is still suffering from insomnia even apart from the bronchitis. Mr. Adams also admits that his marriage is failing, and he says that the stress may be contributing to the insomnia. Dr. Abbott gives him a prescription for Ambien CR along with the other prescriptions. Mr. Adams is to return to the clinic in 1 week if he is not feeling better. The charge for the office visit is $77, and the blood sugar test is $12. Mr. Adams pays his $20 co-pay.

Benjamin C. Adams
55180 Grand Avenue Parkway
Austin, Texas 78706
512-998-1354 (home)
SS# 445-74-8363

Insurance: Humana PPO
ID# 445748363
Employer: Texas Department of Public Safety
DOB: 7-2-1954

Diagnosis: Acute bronchitis; diabetes mellitus type II, controlled; insomnia
Procedures: Office visit, blood glucose test
Account Number: ADB8363

Family Medical Clinic
1216 E. Lamar Blvd.
Austin, Texas 78704
512-624-0112
Federal Tax ID# 75-8210612

Humana
PO Box 3031103
Chicago, IL 60068
800-611-1216

Barbara Abbott, MD
NPI 4712678920

Copyright © 2011, 2007, 2003 by Saunders, an imprint of Elsevier Inc. All rights reserved.

3. Complete Claim Form 3 (Work Product 21-3) using the following information.

Today's date: 9-29-20XX

Ms. Snell comes to the office complaining of severe pain in the lower left quadrant. She states that the pain came on suddenly and that she has a history of ovarian cysts. Ms. Snell is clearly in severe pain, so Dr. Jackman gives her an injection of Toradol. Once the medication has taken effect, he performs a pelvic examination and determines that the most likely cause of her pain is a ruptured ovarian cyst. Dr. Jackman sends Ms. Snell to the hospital for an ultrasound examination and will see her in the emergency department later in the afternoon. Ms. Snell has no other significant health problems. Her office visit is $85, and the injection is $25. Dr. Jackman spent about 40 minutes with her.

Suanne L. Snell
4545 Rustic
Los Angeles, CA 90002
818-445-9970 (home)
SS# 665-76-5568

Insurance: Aetna HMO
ID# 665765568
Employer: Marriott Hotels International
DOB: 9-3-1964

Diagnosis: Ruptured ovarian cyst
Procedures: Office visit, injection
Account Number: SNS5568

Medical Surgical Clinic
4800 S. Broadway Blvd.
Los Angeles, CA 90012
818-261-1122
Federal Tax ID# 75-6120662

Aetna
PO Box 310661
Sacramento, CA 90121
800-996-8445

James Jackman, DO
NPI 8216740292

Copyright © 2011, 2007, 2003 by Saunders, an imprint of Elsevier Inc. All rights reserved.

4. Complete Claim Form 4 (Work Product 21-4) using the information below.

Today's date: 9-29-20XX

Ms. Huntington, a single female, arrives at the clinic today as a new patient. She was referred to Dr. Tyler by Dr. William R. Curry, a friend of Dr. Tyler from medical school. Ms. Huntington has been diagnosed with systemic lupus erythematosus and periodically experiences a great deal of pain. She arranged to forward her medical records to Dr. Tyler several weeks ago, and she made today's appointment before her move to New Rochelle. Dr. Tyler has worked with numerous patients who have lupus and is understanding about their needs and the challenges they face in living a normal life. Ms. Huntington states that she needs to refill her medications, and Dr. Tyler reviews them with her, agreeing to refill her prescription Motrin (800 mg), Lortab (10 mg), and Phenergan suppositories (50 mg). Ms. Huntington says that she uses the Motrin almost every day but rarely uses the Lortab, although she prefers to keep a supply on hand for times when the disease strikes aggressively. She mentions that she has not had a well-woman examination in 2 years because of the sale of her home and the purchase of a new one in New Rochelle. Dr. Tyler performs the well-woman examination and writes Ms. Huntington an order for a mammogram. She also performs a breast examination, which is included in the well-woman examination. Dr. Tyler spends about 45 minutes with the patient. She asks Ms. Huntington to return in 3 months if she does not feel the need to do so before then. Ms. Huntington is charged $179 for the new patient office visit and $55 for the Pap smear and well-woman examination. She leaves with her prescriptions.

Celeste C. Huntington
554 Georgetown Way
New Rochelle, NY 10801
914-889-6675 (home)
SS# 433-99-2364

Insurance: United Health Care PPO
ID# 433992364
Employer: Loist and Earnest Law Firm
DOB: 9-3-1960

Diagnosis: Systemic lupus erythematosus
Procedures: Office visit, Pap smear
Account Number: HUC2364

New Rochelle Family Medicine
2002 Front Street, Suite 600
New Rochelle, NY 10800
914-661-0001
Federal Tax ID# 75-6234710

United Healthcare
PO Box 292928
New York, NY 10021
212-660-1100

Rene Tyler, MD
NPI 6779354390
William R. Curry, MD
NPI 4619907217

Copyright © 2011, 2007, 2003 by Saunders, an imprint of Elsevier Inc. All rights reserved.

5. Complete Claim Form 5 (Work Product 21-5) using the following information.

Today's date: 9-29-20XX

Mrs. Saxton, a married female, has several health problems and is a frequent visitor to Dr. Handley's office. She is insured through her own policy with Unicare and also through her husband's policy with Assurant Health. She has Graves' disease, malignant HTN, bursitis of the right knee, and carpel tunnel syndrome. She arrives at the office today to have her blood pressure checked. In the waiting area, she develops mild chest pains, so the medical assistant brings her to the back office immediately and performs an ECG. Upon checking the strip, Dr. Handley believes that Mrs. Saxton may recently have had a mild heart attack, so he refers her to Dr. Stern, a cardiologist. The office sets up an immediate appointment for Mrs. Saxton, and she leaves the clinic with her husband with instructions to drive directly to Dr. Stern's office. They promise to do so. Mrs. Saxton is charged for the office visit ($165) and an ECG ($45). She is with Dr. Handley for approximately 50 minutes.

Patricia N. Saxton
13104 Highway 798 South
Tyler, TX 75701
903-882-4453 (home)
SS# 334-88-9907

Insurance: Unicare PPO
ID# 334889907
Employer: Self-employed
Husband: Levern R. Saxton
Employer: Kelly Tires
SS# 621-12-6701
ID# 621126701
DOB: 7-8-1953

Diagnosis: Malignant HTN, Graves' disease, bursitis, carpel tunnel syndrome
Procedures: Office visit, ECG
Account Number: SAP9907

South Tyler Health Clinic
120 E. West Street
Tyler, Texas 75703
903-566-1112
Federal Tax ID# 75-2162704

Unicare
12000 Walker Blvd., St. 100
Dallas, Texas 75225
800-921-0091

Wendle Handley, DO
NPI 5682103541

Assurant Health
PO Box 704
Dallas, Texas 75229
800-621-1000

Copyright © 2011, 2007, 2003 by Saunders, an imprint of Elsevier Inc. All rights reserved.

Part II: Determining Diagnosis and Procedure Codes

Determine the proper diagnosis and procedure codes.

1. Diagnosis: Lou Gehrig's disease; hydrocodone dependence

   Diagnostic code(s) ______________________________

   Procedure: Office visit, new patient (10 minutes)

   Procedure code(s) ______________________________

2. Diagnosis: Generalized osteoarthritis in the upper arm

   Diagnostic code(s) ______________________________

   Procedure: Office visit, established patient (10 minutes); basic metabolic panel; lipid panel

   Procedure code(s) ______________________________

3. Diagnosis: Foreign body in the ear

   Diagnostic code(s) ______________________________

   Procedure: Office visit, established patient (10 minutes)

   Procedure code(s) ______________________________

4. Diagnosis: Burn over 40% of body surface because of car accident with another vehicle; passenger in the car

   Diagnostic code(s) ______________________________

   Procedure: Hospital admission, new patient, physician spends approximately 50 minutes treating patient

   Procedure code(s) ______________________________

5. Diagnosis: Rosacea

   Diagnostic code(s) ______________________________

   Procedure: Office visit, established patient (15 minutes)

   Procedure code(s) ______________________________

6. Diagnosis: Sunburn, third degree

   Diagnostic code(s) ______________________________

   Procedure: Office visit, established patient (10 minutes)

   Procedure code(s) ______________________________

7. Diagnosis: Tachycardia, neonatal

   Diagnostic code(s) ______________________________

   Procedure: Hospital visit, 2 days, inpatient subsequent care (25 minutes)

   Procedure code(s) ______________________________

8. Diagnosis: Pernicious anemia

   Diagnostic code(s) ______________________________

   Procedure: Office visit, established patient (25 minutes); sedimentation rate, automated; CBC, automated

   Procedure code(s) ______________________________

Copyright © 2011, 2007, 2003 by Saunders, an imprint of Elsevier Inc. All rights reserved.

9. Diagnosis: Attention deficit disorder with hyperactivity; acute cystitis

   Diagnostic code(s) ______________________________

   Procedure: Office visit, established patient (15 minutes); urinalysis

   Procedure code(s) ______________________________

10. Diagnosis: Mastitis after delivery of a baby

    Diagnostic code(s) ______________________________

    Procedure: Office visit, established patient (5 minutes)

    Procedure code(s) ______________________________

CASE STUDY

Research the history of the CMS-1500 claim form. Determine when it was first used and the changes the form has undergone since its inception. Prepare a report that details these changes, including the most recent modifications to the CMS-1500 (08/05). Present the report to the class.

WORKPLACE APPLICATIONS

Collect several blank encounter forms from various medical specialties. Distribute the forms to classmates, sharing and trading the various forms. Mark several procedures on the forms and at least two diagnoses codes. Prepare a CMS-1500 claim based on information on the encounter forms. Share the information in class and explain the coding choices made on each claim.

INTERNET ACTIVITIES

1. Review the National Uniform Claim Committee Web site. Find the User Manual for the CMS-1500 claim form (08/05).
2. Find three companies that sell the CMS-1500 claim form. Compare costs and determine the least expensive place to order the form.
3. Research software applications available for completing CMS-1500 forms. Determine which of the applications would be good investments for a physician's office.

 Copyright © 2011, 2007, 2003 by Saunders, an imprint of Elsevier Inc. All rights reserved.

22 Professional Fees, Billing, and Collecting

VOCABULARY REVIEW

Fill in the blanks with the correct vocabulary terms from this chapter.

1. Jesse has a(n) ________________ ________________ of $464, which represents the total amount she owes after her insurance paid a portion of her bill.
2. Mrs. Ramone has a(n) ________________ on her account for an overpayment, so the office manager sent her a check for that amount.
3. Robert's mother is the ________________ of his bill, because she promised to pay the full amount for her son.
4. Julia had to ________________ collections proceedings on several accounts last month, because the patients had not made payments as promised.
5. One of the tasks Pamela enjoys is ________________ payments that arrive in the mail to patient accounts.
6. ________________ ________________ are used more and more often for payments in the physician's office.
7. An organization under contract to the government to handle insurance claims from providers is called a(n) ________________ ________________.
8. Mrs. Richland called the office to get the balance on her ________________.
9. The office staff has been debating whether they should continue to offer ________________ ________________ to other healthcare providers and their staff members.
10. A business ________________, which is any exchange or transfer of goods, services, or funds, must always be recorded.
11. Anna made several ________________ for various bills that were due last week.
12. Dr. Taylor's fee ________________ is a compilation of the fees he has charged over the past fiscal year.
13. The Peete family was considered ________________ ________________, because they could not afford medical care even though they were able to pay basic living expenses.
14. Deb sometimes confuses a credit with a(n) ________________, which is a deduction from a revenue, net worth, or liability account.
15. Jessica totaled the ________________ for the day, which came from patient and insurance payments.
16. State Farm is considered a(n) ________________ ________________ ________________, because Bethany's injuries were sustained in a car accident and State Farm will pay her medical bills.
17. Dr. Martin reviewed his fee ________________, which is a compilation of pre-established fee allowances for given services or procedures.
18. The balances due to a creditor on an account are called ________________.
19. The Blackburn Clinic uses a computer to determine patient account balances, but June remembers when they used a manual ________________ ________________.
20. When Madelyn received the denial from Mr. Paul's insurance company, she wondered if he had paid his ________________.

Copyright © 2011, 2007, 2003 by Saunders, an imprint of Elsevier Inc. All rights reserved.

SKILLS AND CONCEPTS

Part I: Fee Schedules and Billing Forms

1. Examine the fee schedule on the next page and answer the following questions.
   a. What is the charge for a consultation? ______
   b. What is the charge for a 99203? ______
   c. Why is the charge different for a 99213? ______
   d. What is the most expensive procedure on the list? CPT code ______
   e. Which injection is more expensive, insulin or vitamin B_{12}? ______

Use the same fee schedule to complete the billing forms in Work Products 22-1, 22-2, and 22-3 (See pp. 203-208 of the Procedures Checklists). Circle the codes and fill in the charges for each patient. Assume that all the patients have a previous balance of zero.

2. Work Product 22-1: Marilyn Westmoreland, established patient, straightforward, penicillin injections (75 mg), diagnosis—acute tonsillitis.

3. Work Product 22-2: Jane Wells, consultation, high complexity, ECG, diagnosis—chest pain.

4. Work Product 22-3: Paula Johnson, new patient, detailed, Solu-Medrol injection IM, diagnosis—osteoarthritis.

 Copyright © 2011, 2007, 2003 by Saunders, an imprint of Elsevier Inc. All rights reserved.

FEE SCHEDULE

BLACKBURN PRIMARY CARE ASSOCIATES, PC
1990 Turquiose Drive
Blackburn, WI 54937
608-459-8857

Federal Tax ID Number: **00-0000000**

BCBS Group Number: 14982
Medicare Group Number: 14982

OFFICE VISIT, NEW PATIENT

Focused, 99201	$45.00
Expanded, 99202	$55.00
Intermediate, 99203	$60.00
Extended, 99204	$95.00
Comprehensive, 99205	$195.00
Consultation, 99245	$250.00

OFFICE VISIT, ESTABLISHED PATIENT

Minimal, 99211	$40.00
Focused, 99212	$48.00
Intermediate, 99213	$55.00
Extended, 99214	$65.00
Comprehensive, 99215	$195.00

OFFICE PROCEDURES

EKG, 12 lead, 93000	$55.00
Stress EKG, Treadmill, 93015	$295.00
Sigmoidoscopy, Flex; 45330	$145.00
Spirometry, 94010	$50.00
Cerumen Removal, 69210	$40.00
Collection & Handling	
Lab Specimen, 99000	$9.00
Venipuncture, 35415	$9.00
Urinalysis, 81000	$20.00
Urinalysis, 81002 (Dip Only)	$12.00
Influenza Injection, 90724	$20.00
Pneumococcal Injection, 90732	$20.00
Oral Polio, 90712	$15.00
DTaP, 90700	$20.00
Tetanus Toxoid, 90703	$15.00
MMR, 90707	$25.00
HIB, 90737	$20.00
Hepatitis B, newborn to age 11 years, 90744	$60.00
Hepatitis B, 11-19 years, 90745	$60.00
Hepatitis B, 20 years and above 90746	$60.00
Intramuscular Injection, 90788	
Penicillin	$30.00
Cephtriaxone	$25.00
Solu-Medrol	$23.00
Vitamin B-12	$13.00
Subcutaneous Injection, 90782	
Epinephrine	$18.00
Susphrine	$25.00
Insulin, U-100	$15.00

COMMON DIAGNOSTIC CODES

Ischemic Heart Disease	414.9
w/o myocardial infarction	411.89
w/coronary occlusion	411.81
Hypertension, Malignant	401.0
Benign	401.1
Unspecified	401.9
w/congest. heart failure	402.91
Asthma, Bronchial	493.9
w/COPD	493.2
allergic, w/S.A.	493.91
allergic, w/o S.A.	493.90
Kyphosis	737.10
w/osteoporosis	733.0
Osteoporosis	733.00
Otitis Media, Acute	382.9
Chronic	382.9

Copyright © 2011, 2007, 2003 by Saunders, an imprint of Elsevier Inc. All rights reserved.

Part II: Ledgers and Computing Patient Balances

Work through the following information and record it on the ledger cards presented in the corresponding work product pages. Use one ledger for each exercise.

Ledger 1—Work Product 22-4 (see p. 209 of the Procedures Checklists)

Meagan Joy Reynolds
5534 Joe Pool Lake Road #233
Cedar Hill, Texas 75884
972-334-0423 (home)
972-331-0934 (cell)
meaganjoy@internet4.com
MR# REYM3341

Entry #	Transaction
1	Meagan comes to the Blackburn Primary Care Clinic on April 12 as a new patient. Her initial charge is $375, because she had a series of x-ray examinations, which were used to diagnose a blockage in her small intestine. Dr. Lupez recommends that she have surgery to correct the blockage as soon as possible. Meagan pays her bill in full with check #7110, although she has insurance coverage through her own policy with Prudential and her husband's policy through Southwest United Healthcare.
2	Meagan checks into Mercy Hospital and has surgery on April 21. Dr. Lupez charges $7,500 for the surgery. This charge will be filed with Meagan's insurances.
3	Meagan returns to the clinic on April 30 for a follow-up office visit. The charge is $150, which she pays in full with check #7261. Dr. Lupez says that she is doing very well since her surgery and asks her to return in mid-May for another checkup.
4	On May 2 the clinic receives an insurance payment from Prudential in the amount of $6,200. This money is applied to Meagan's account. The check number is 617761.
5	On May 3 the clinic receives check #7313 in the mail from Meagan for $300, which is applied to her account.
6	Meagan returns to the clinic on May 14 for an office visit. The charge is $75, and she pays $50 with check #7512.
7	Southwest United sends a check to the clinic for $800 on May 27, which is applied to her account. The check number is 8710.
8	Meagan sends a check for $125 to be put toward her account. The check, #7915, is posted on June 2.
9	Meagan returns to the clinic for an office visit and laboratory work on June 17. Her charges total $352, and she pays $150 with check #8116.
10	On June 20 the clinic receives Meagan's check toward her account for $100. Her check number is 8411.
11	Meagan visits the clinic for treatment of a migraine headache on June 26. Her charge is $85, and she pays $50 with check #8626. She schedules a follow-up visit with Dr. Lupez for June 30.
12	When Meagan returns for her follow-up visit on June 30, her office visit is $85, but she is unable to make a payment.
13	On July 5 the clinic receives a payment from Prudential on behalf of Meagan for $276. The Prudential check number is 721146.
14	On July 18 the clinic receives a check #9210 from Southwest United on behalf of Meagan for $124.
15	On July 31 the clinic refunds Meagan's credit balance to her using clinic check #9425.
16	The previous transaction brings Meagan's account to zero.

How much was the refund check? ______________________________

 Copyright © 2011, 2007, 2003 by Saunders, an imprint of Elsevier Inc. All rights reserved.

Ledger 2—Work Product 22-5 (see p. 211 of the Procedures Checklists)

Zachary Paul Staley
2324 Hill Avenue Plaza
Grosse Pointe, MI 48230
313-445-9987 (home)
313-565-6623 (cell)
zachattack@aol.com
MR# STAZ9823

Entry #	Transaction
1	Zachary Staley visited the clinic on June 6 as a new patient and was diagnosed with diabetes. His charge was $215. He paid his $15 co-pay with check #126.
2	On June 12 a check arrived from Permian Health for $180 on Zachary's account. The check number was 21617.
3	Zachary returned to the clinic on June 15 for an office visit and laboratory work. The total charge was $128, and Zachary paid his $15 co-pay with check #214.
4	On June 16 Zachary returned to the clinic without an appointment, because he felt extremely dizzy and nauseated. He was seen by Dr. Hughes, who determined that his blood sugar had dropped substantially. After his condition was stabilized, his wife picked him up and took him home. She paid his $15 co-pay with check #217. The total charge for the visit was $70.
5	On July 7 check #36171 arrived from Permian Health on Zachary's account in the amount of $142.
6	Bethany, an insurance biller, realized that a $7 charge was not allowed for a laboratory test on Zachary's account. The office policy allows disallowed charges under $10 to be written off, so Bethany adjusts his account by $7 on July 7.
7	Zachary returns to the clinic for a routine visit on July 26 and has laboratory work done. The total charge is $156, and Zachary pays his $15 co-pay with check #310.
8	On August 1 Zachary has a brief office visit and is charged $70. Zachary forgot his checkbook, so he did not pay his co-pay.
9	On August 16 Permian sends check #41217 in the amount of $102 toward Zachary's account.
10	On August 21 Permian sends check #42168 in the amount of $55 toward Zachary's account.
11	On August 30 the clinic receives check #561 from Zachary in the amount of $40 to be placed toward his account.
12	September 6 is Zachary's next office visit, and he is charged $70. He pays his $15 co-pay with check #587.
13	Zachary sends $40 toward his account, which is received by the clinic on September 9. His check number is 620.
14	Permian Health sends check #53121 in the amount of $98 to the clinic to be applied to Zachary's account on September 15.
15	On October 3 the clinic receives check #681 from Zachary, who remembers that he did not pay his co-pay on August 1. He guesses that he owes about $40 total but is unsure, so he sends $20.
16	The clinic realizes that Zachary has overpaid on his account and sends him a refund for his credit balance using check #6116 on October 4.

How much was the refund check? ______________________________

Copyright © 2011, 2007, 2003 by Saunders, an imprint of Elsevier Inc. All rights reserved.

Ledger 3—Work Product 22-6 (see p. 213 of the Procedures Checklists)

Lynn Annette Wilson
755 South Wheeley #4A
Sacramento, CA 94203
209-552-5437 (home)
209-553-7789 (cell)
lynnannw@yahoo.com
MR# WILL8845

Entry #	Transaction
1	Lynn Annette is a single mother of four who has had a difficult year. She lost a job after contracting infectious mononucleosis and missing 3 weeks of work. She had barely recovered from that illness when she was diagnosed with ulcerative colitis. Her medical bills have become increasingly difficult to pay, although she did find a new job and recently became eligible for coverage through Aetna. She is a determined woman with the best of intentions but often must put rent, utilities, and food costs before the payment of her medical bills. She comes to the clinic for a regular office visit on July 7. Her charges are $125, and she is able to pay the entire bill, since she has been saving the money for several weeks. She pays with check #1205.
2	On July 12 Lynn Annette returns to the office and has laboratory work. Her charges are $89, and she pays her $20 co-pay with check #1314.
3	Bethany in the insurance office notices that Lynn Annette was charged $9 for a single laboratory chemistry test that is not covered by her insurance. Because Bethany knows that Lynn Annette has faced financial difficulties this year, she adjusts the bill so that Lynn Annette will not be responsible for the charge. She also makes a note for the physicians that Lynn Annette's insurance does not cover that particular laboratory test and explains that an alternate chemistry test that will produce the same results is covered. The adjustment is made on July 19.
4	Aetna sends an insurance payment (check #7611493) toward Lynn Annette's account that is received on July 23. The payment is for $85.
5	Bethany processes a refund for Lynn Annette and sends her check #5612 from the clinic account on July 24. This brings her balance to zero.
6	Lynn Annette comes to the office for a regular visit on August 1. Her charges are $284, and she pays her co-pay of $20 with check #1517.
7	On August 18 the clinic receives a check from Aetna for $200 toward Lynn Annette's account. The check number is 8267484.
8	Lynn Annette sends check #1622 in the amount of $64 to clear her account on August 31.
9	On September 12 Lynn Annette's recent check payment is returned by her bank for insufficient funds. The clinic adds a charge of $30 to her account as a returned check fee.
10	Lynn Annette comes to the clinic and apologizes for her recent returned check. She explains that she missed getting her paycheck into the bank in time to cover the payment. She brings a cashier's check to cover the check and the fee. The date is September 20.
11	Lynn Annette has minor surgery in the office on October 15. The charge is $750, and she pays a co-pay of $20 in cash.
12	On February 12 Lynn Annette sends a $20 payment on her account, using check #2612. She encloses a note that says she is still having financial difficulties and will send another payment as soon as she can.
13	On April 10 Lynn Annette sends a payment of $5 using check #2711.
14	On May 12 the clinic receives a payment from Lynn Annette in the amount of $5, using check #2781.
15	In accordance with the clinic policy of reporting accounts to a collection agency after 3 months of nonpayment, Bethany reluctantly reports Lynn Annette's account to Smith Collections. The full balance is written off.
16	On September 12 a payment of $100 is received from Lynn Annette. Bethany forwards the payment to the collection agency.

How much was written off of this account? ______________________________

How is the payment noted on the account that was received after the write-off? ______________________________

____

Copyright © 2011, 2007, 2003 by Saunders, an imprint of Elsevier Inc. All rights reserved.

Completing a Day Sheet

Complete the proofs in Work Product 22-7 (see p. 215 of the Procedures Checklists) using the figures given.

Part III: Short Answers

1. Define the following terms.

   a. Usual

   ____

   ____

   b. Customary

   ____

   ____

   c. Reasonable

   ____

   ____

2. List two billing methods commonly used in the physician's office.

   a. ______________________________

   b. ______________________________

3. What notation should be made under the return address on statement envelopes?

   ____

4. Briefly explain cycle billing.

   ____

5. What are the pitfalls of fee adjustments?

   ____

6. What three values are considered in determining professional fees?

   a. ______________________________

   b. ______________________________

   c. ______________________________

7. Why are estimates useful in patient treatment?

   ____

   ____

   ____

8. List five general rules for telephone collecting.

   a. ______________________________

   b. ______________________________

   c. ______________________________

   d. ______________________________

   e. ______________________________

Copyright © 2011, 2007, 2003 by Saunders, an imprint of Elsevier Inc. All rights reserved.

9. List four ways payment for medical services is accomplished.
   a. ____
   b. ____
   c. ____
   d. ____

10. Explain why patients sometimes fail to pay their accounts.

11. What is professional courtesy, and why is it less common now than in years past?

12. Briefly explain how "skips" can be traced.

CASE STUDY

Read back through the information about Lynn Annette Wilson in Ledger 3. How could the medical assistant help Ms. Wilson keep her account out of collections? What could be said to her during a friendly phone call to encourage her to be regular with her payments? Write two collection letters to Ms. Wilson. Make the first letter a gentle reminder. The second letter should express that the account will be placed for collection if regular payments are not forthcoming. Use the stationery provided in Work Products 22-8 and 22-9 (See pp. 217-220 of the Procedures Checklists) to write the collection letters.

WORKPLACE APPLICATIONS

Mr. Sanchez comes to the desk to check out after seeing the physician. When Sarah tells him that his bill is $95, he complains that he only saw the physician for 10 minutes. The fee is in accordance with the evaluation and management guidelines. Explain the fees to Mr. Sanchez. Write what you would say to him as an explanation of his fees.

 Copyright © 2011, 2007, 2003 by Saunders, an imprint of Elsevier Inc. All rights reserved.

Write a dialog that could be used to ask a patient for payment as the person is checking out.

____

____

____

____

____

____

INTERNET ACTIVITIES

1. Research medical billing companies on the Internet and compare the costs of the various services they offer. Prepare a report or presentation for the class.

2. Search for patient accounting software and explore the options available for the physician's office. Write a brief report on one software product and present it to the class.

Copyright © 2011, 2007, 2003 by Saunders, an imprint of Elsevier Inc. All rights reserved.

23 Banking Services and Procedures

VOCABULARY REVIEW

Fill in the blanks with the correct vocabulary terms from this chapter.

1. Judy was unaware that checks were processed through ________________ before they arrived at her bank.
2. Because Alicia was the person who wrote the check, she was considered the ________________.
3. When the Blackburn Clinic purchased the ultrasound machine, they paid $10,000 toward the ________________ so that they would be charged less interest.
4. Pamela wrote a check to Samantha, so Pamela is the ________________ and Samantha is the ________________.
5. The ________________ of a check is the person who presents it for payment and may not be the person named as the payee.
6. Grace studied the ________________ ________________ ________________, which is a series of laws that regulates sales of goods, commercial paper, secured transactions in personal property, and many aspects of banking.
7. First National Bank is considered the ________________ for Dr. Lupez' business checking accounts.
8. Instruments that are legally transferable to another party are considered ________________.
9. Rhonda made several ________________ from the clinic checking account to pay monthly bills and order supplies.
10. As soon as the monthly bank statement arrives, Rhonda does a(n) ________________ ________________ to make sure the statement and checkbook balance are in agreement.

SKILLS AND CONCEPTS

Part I: Short Answers

1. List the requirements of a negotiable instrument.

   a. ____

   b. ____

   c. ____

   d. ____

2. Name several advantages to online banking.

____

____

____

Copyright © 2011, 2007, 2003 by Saunders, an imprint of Elsevier Inc. All rights reserved.

3. Why is customer service such an important aspect of today's medical offices?

____

____

____

4. List four types of checks.

   a. ____________________
   b. ____________________
   c. ____________________
   d. ____________________

5. Describe each type of endorsement.

   a. Blank

   ____

   b. Restrictive

   ____

   c. Special

   ____

   d. Qualified

   ____

6. List five reasons checks should be deposited promptly.

   a. ____________________
   b. ____________________
   c. ____________________
   d. ____________________
   e. ____________________

7. Provide five guidelines for check acceptance.

   a. ____________________
   b. ____________________
   c. ____________________
   d. ____________________
   e. ____________________

Copyright © 2011, 2007, 2003 by Saunders, an imprint of Elsevier Inc. All rights reserved.

8. List three reasons an individual might stop payment on a check.

   a. ______________________________

   b. ______________________________

   c. ______________________________

9. Explain the ABA number and what each part of the number means.

   ____

   ____

   ____

10. List the three basic steps for preparing a deposit slip.

   a. ______________________________

   b. ______________________________

   c. ______________________________

11. Where is the routing number found on a check?

   ____

Part II: Writing Checks for Disbursement of Funds

Write checks to pay the following bills. The beginning balance in the checkbook is $4,562.79. Use the checks numbered 5648 to 5651. Determine the balance after the check is written.

1. Write check #5648 to the American Medical Association for $356 for new coding books. Balance ______________
2. Write check #5649 to the Blackburn Utility Company for $46.90 to pay the water bill. Balance ______________
3. Write a check for the office mortgage payment to First National Bank in the amount of $1,700. Use check #5650. Balance ______________
4. Write check #5651 to pay a bill to United Drug and Supply of $98.34. Balance ______________
5. A deposit of $1,358 was made. Balance ______________

Copyright © 2011, 2007, 2003 by Saunders, an imprint of Elsevier Inc. All rights reserved.

Part III: Writing Refund Checks

Write checks for the following refunds. Use the ending balance from Part II, question 5, to determine the final balance in the checking account. Use the checks numbered 5652 to 5655.

1. Ms. Patty Bailey should receive a refund in the amount of $34.55 for an overpayment. Use check #5652. Balance ________________
2. Write a check for Julie Smithy for $224.12. Her insurance company paid more than expected, so she is entitled to a refund. Use check #5653. Balance ________________
3. Cindy Chan paid $10 more than she owed when she was seeing Dr. Hughes. Refund her money using check #5654. The office manager deposited $7,246.12 in checks. Balance ________________
4. Carter Graves decided to postpone his knee surgery when his wife suddenly became ill. Use check #5655 to refund his $500 deposit. Balance ________________

Part IV: Preparing a Bank Deposit

Prepare a bank deposit detail using the following information. Record your answers on the figure in Work Product 23-1.

1. Cash includes six (6) $20 bills; one (1) $100 bill; one (1) $50 bill; two (2) $10 bills; one (1) $5 bill; and one (1) $1 bill. Total cash ________________
2. Check payments were #2387 for $67 from Sue Patrick and #460 for $50 from Ronald Rodriguez. Total personal checks ________________
3. Credit card payments were $100 and $250. Total credit cards ________________
4. An insurance payment for Alejandro Sanchez arrived in the amount of $1,374.32. The payment was from Aetna and the check was #309. Total deposit ________________

Part V: Reconciling a Bank Statement

Reconcile the bank statement using the following facts and figures. Use the worksheet on page 171 to show your work. The checkbook balance is $4,616.96. The statement balance is $6,792.79 (this amount includes the deposit of $2,137.32—do not add that amount in again).

1. Three checks are outstanding: check #5648 for $356; check #5649 for $46.90; and check #5650 for $1,770. What is the total for outstanding checks? ________________
2. Does the checkbook reconcile with the statement? ________________
3. What is the ending balance? ________________

Copyright © 2011, 2007, 2003 by Saunders, an imprint of Elsevier Inc. All rights reserved.

5648

DATE ____________

TO ____________

FOR ____________

BALANCE BROUGHT FORWARD		
DEPOSITS		
BALANCE		
AMT THIS CK		
BALANCE CARRIED FORWARD		

BLACKBURN PRIMARY CARE ASSOCIATES, PC
1990 Turquoise Drive
Blackburn, WI 54937
608-459-8857

5648

94-72/1224

DATE ____________

PAY TO THE ORDER OF ____________ $ [ ]

____________ DOLLARS

DERBYSHIRE SAVINGS
Member FDIC
P.O. BOX 8923
Blackburn, WI 54937

FOR ____________ ____________

⑈055003⑈ 446782011⑈ 678800470

5649

DATE ____________

TO ____________

FOR ____________

BALANCE BROUGHT FORWARD		
DEPOSITS		
BALANCE		
AMT THIS CK		
BALANCE CARRIED FORWARD		

BLACKBURN PRIMARY CARE ASSOCIATES, PC
1990 Turquoise Drive
Blackburn, WI 54937
608-459-8857

5649

94-72/1224

DATE ____________

PAY TO THE ORDER OF ____________ $ [ ]

____________ DOLLARS

DERBYSHIRE SAVINGS
Member FDIC
P.O. BOX 8923
Blackburn, WI 54937

FOR ____________ ____________

⑈055003⑈ 446782011⑈ 678800470

5650

DATE ____________

TO ____________

FOR ____________

BALANCE BROUGHT FORWARD		
DEPOSITS		
BALANCE		
AMT THIS CK		
BALANCE CARRIED FORWARD		

BLACKBURN PRIMARY CARE ASSOCIATES, PC
1990 Turquoise Drive
Blackburn, WI 54937
608-459-8857

5650

94-72/1224

DATE ____________

PAY TO THE ORDER OF ____________ $ [ ]

____________ DOLLARS

DERBYSHIRE SAVINGS
Member FDIC
P.O. BOX 8923
Blackburn, WI 54937

FOR ____________ ____________

⑈055003⑈ 446782011⑈ 678800470

5651

DATE ____________

TO ____________

FOR ____________

BALANCE BROUGHT FORWARD		
DEPOSITS		
BALANCE		
AMT THIS CK		
BALANCE CARRIED FORWARD		

BLACKBURN PRIMARY CARE ASSOCIATES, PC
1990 Turquoise Drive
Blackburn, WI 54937
608-459-8857

5651

94-72/1224

DATE ____________

PAY TO THE ORDER OF ____________ $ [ ]

____________ DOLLARS

DERBYSHIRE SAVINGS
Member FDIC
P.O. BOX 8923
Blackburn, WI 54937

FOR ____________ ____________

⑈055003⑈ 446782011⑈ 678800470

Copyright © 2011, 2007, 2003 by Saunders, an imprint of Elsevier Inc. All rights reserved.

5652

DATE ______

TO ______

FOR ______

BALANCE BROUGHT FORWARD		
DEPOSITS		
BALANCE		
AMT THIS CK		
BALANCE CARRIED FORWARD		

BLACKBURN PRIMARY CARE ASSOCIATES, PC
1990 Turquoise Drive
Blackburn, WI 54937
608-459-8857

5652
94-72/1224

DATE ______

PAY TO THE ORDER OF ______ $

______ DOLLARS

DERBYSHIRE SAVINGS
Member FDIC
P.O. BOX 8923
Blackburn, WI 54937

FOR ______ ______

⑈055003⑈ 446782011⑈ 678800470

5653

DATE ______

TO ______

FOR ______

BALANCE BROUGHT FORWARD		
DEPOSITS		
BALANCE		
AMT THIS CK		
BALANCE CARRIED FORWARD		

BLACKBURN PRIMARY CARE ASSOCIATES, PC
1990 Turquoise Drive
Blackburn, WI 54937
608-459-8857

5653
94-72/1224

DATE ______

PAY TO THE ORDER OF ______ $

______ DOLLARS

DERBYSHIRE SAVINGS
Member FDIC
P.O. BOX 8923
Blackburn, WI 54937

FOR ______ ______

⑈055003⑈ 446782011⑈ 678800470

5654

DATE ______

TO ______

FOR ______

BALANCE BROUGHT FORWARD		
DEPOSITS		
BALANCE		
AMT THIS CK		
BALANCE CARRIED FORWARD		

BLACKBURN PRIMARY CARE ASSOCIATES, PC
1990 Turquoise Drive
Blackburn, WI 54937
608-459-8857

5654
94-72/1224

DATE ______

PAY TO THE ORDER OF ______ $

______ DOLLARS

DERBYSHIRE SAVINGS
Member FDIC
P.O. BOX 8923
Blackburn, WI 54937

FOR ______ ______

⑈055003⑈ 446782011⑈ 678800470

5655

DATE ______

TO ______

FOR ______

BALANCE BROUGHT FORWARD		
DEPOSITS		
BALANCE		
AMT THIS CK		
BALANCE CARRIED FORWARD		

BLACKBURN PRIMARY CARE ASSOCIATES, PC
1990 Turquoise Drive
Blackburn, WI 54937
608-459-8857

5655
94-72/1224

DATE ______

PAY TO THE ORDER OF ______ $

______ DOLLARS

DERBYSHIRE SAVINGS
Member FDIC
P.O. BOX 8923
Blackburn, WI 54937

FOR ______ ______

⑈055003⑈ 446782011⑈ 678800470

Copyright © 2011, 2007, 2003 by Saunders, an imprint of Elsevier Inc. All rights reserved.

THIS WORKSHEET IS PROVIDED TO HELP YOU BALANCE YOUR ACCOUNT

1. Go through your register and mark each check, withdrawal, Express ATM transaction, payment, deposit, or other credit listed on this statement. Be sure that your register shows any interest paid into your account, and any service charges, automatic payments, or Express Transfers withdrawn from your account during this statement period.
2. Using the chart below, list any outstanding checks, Express ATM withdrawals, payments, or any other withdrawals (including any from previous months) that are listed in your register but are not shown on this statement.
3. Balance your account by filling in the spaces below.

ITEMS OUTSTANDING		
NUMBER	AMOUNT	
TOTAL	$	

ENTER

The NEW BALANCE shown on this statement____________________________$

ADD

Any deposits listed in your register $
or transfers into your account $
which are not shown on this $
statement. +$ ______

TOTAL

CALCULATE THE SUBTOTAL______________**$**

SUBTRACT

The total outstanding checks and withdrawals from the chart at left___________-$

CALCULATE THE ENDING BALANCE

This amount should be the same as the current balance shown in your check register______________________$

Copyright © 2011, 2007, 2003 by Saunders, an imprint of Elsevier Inc. All rights reserved.

CASE STUDY

The Internet has changed the way business is conducted, both in the United States and beyond U. S. borders. Some individuals are quite comfortable making purchases and paying bills online. How safe are these practices? How can the medical assistant know that online bill paying services are safe and secure? Research this information and prepare a report for the class.

WORKPLACE APPLICATIONS

The more versatile the medical assistant is, the more valuable he or she will be to the physician employer. Often new graduates hesitate to ask patients to pay their accounts. However, a medical assistant who is able to collect patient accounts increases the cash flow in the office. How might the medical assistant succinctly explain the various ways a patient can make a payment?

INTERNET ACTIVITIES

1. Explore several types of billing software. Determine which seems to be the best option for a medium-sized family practice clinic. Pay special attention to software that has banking features.
2. Investigate the history of banking and prepare a report for the class.
3. Research safety measures designed to keep confidential banking information private. How do privacy policies affect Internet banking? How can the medical assistant ensure that private information remains private? Prepare a paper or report for the class on this subject.

Copyright © 2011, 2007, 2003 by Saunders, an imprint of Elsevier Inc. All rights reserved.

24 Financial and Practice Management

VOCABULARY REVIEW

Fill in the blanks with the correct vocabulary terms from this chapter.

1. Jenna told Andrea that a(n) ________________ year is often different from a calendar year.
2. Julia works with the accounts ________________ ________________, which is the money that is owed to the physicians.
3. Anna works with the accounts ________________ ________________, which is the money the physicians owe to others.
4. Once a year Dr. Medina has his accountant total his ________________ ________________, which include the entire properties subject to the payment of debts.
5. Larry is the supervisor of the ________________ ________________ department, which records all business and accounting transactions.
6. The ________________ ________________ in question was sent last month, but the equipment never arrived, so Julia questions whether she should pay the entire balance due.
7. The Rosales Clinic uses the ________________ ________________ basis of accounting, in which income is recorded when received and expenses are recorded when paid.
8. When the total ending balance of patient ledgers equals the total of accounts receivable control, the two are said to be ________________ ________________.
9. The accountant prepared a(n) ________________ ________________ sheet for December 31, which showed the total assets, liabilities, and capital for the clinic.
10. The Tyler Clinic uses the ________________ ________________ basis of accounting, in which income is recorded when earned and expenses are recorded when incurred.
11. Alice keeps a(n) ________________ ________________ on her desk that summarizes accounts paid out.
12. Each patient receives a(n) ________________ ________________ every month if the balance on his or her account is more than $5.
13. Running a(n) ________________ ________________ is one method of checking the accuracy of accounts.
14. Joy takes minor expenses, such as those for sodas and small donations, from the ________________ ________________ fund.
15. Dr. Lupez asked his accountant to prepare a statement of ________________ and ________________ for the previous fiscal year.
16. A standard of comparison to make sure answers obtained are accurate is a(n) ________________.
17. A(n) ________________ ________________ ________________ is a summary for a specific period that shows a beginning balance, an ending balance, and all the expenditures during that particular period.
18. Angelique keeps a record of all accounts paid out in a(n) ________________ ________________.
19. Something that is owed, or a debt, is called a(n) ________________.
20. The monetary value of a property or of an interest in a property in excess of claims or liens against it is called ________________.

Copyright © 2011, 2007, 2003 by Saunders, an imprint of Elsevier Inc. All rights reserved.

SKILLS AND CONCEPTS

Part I: Short Answers

1. The financial records of any business should show the following at all times:
   a. ______
   b. ______
   c. ______
   d. ______

2. When writing numbers, keep the columns straight and write ______ ______ ______.

3. The manual disbursement journal must show the following:
   a. ______
   b. ______
   c. ______

4. Name two common accounting systems used in medical offices.
   a. ______
   b. ______

5. Differentiate between accounting and bookkeeping.

______

______

______

6. List three cardinal rules of bookkeeping.
   a. ______
   b. ______
   c. ______

7. List two disadvantages of a single-entry system.
   a. ______
   b. ______

8. The IRS requires that complete records be kept on all employees, including the following:
   a. ______
   b. ______
   c. ______
   d. ______

Copyright © 2011, 2007, 2003 by Saunders, an imprint of Elsevier Inc. All rights reserved.

9. What is Form 940 used for and when must it be filed?

____

____

____

10. List seven expense categories often found in a physician's office budget.

    a. _______________

    b. _______________

    c. _______________

    d. _______________

    e. _______________

    f. _______________

    g. _______________

Part II: Bookkeeping Systems

Briefly explain the three types of bookkeeping systems.

1. Single-entry system

____

____

____

2. Double-entry system

____

____

____

3. Pegboard/write-it-once system

____

____

____

4. Which of the three systems do you think would be the easiest to work with in the medical office? Why?

____

____

____

____

Part III: Forms

Briefly explain the use of each of the following forms.

1. SS-5

____

____

____

Copyright © 2011, 2007, 2003 by Saunders, an imprint of Elsevier Inc. All rights reserved.

2. W-2

3. W-3

4. W-4

CASE STUDY

Read the case study and complete the exercise following it.

Kristy Stephens works for Dr. Mitchell, who has a small office in a suburban area just outside Birmingham, Alabama. The longer that Kristy works for Dr. Mitchell, the more she learns about accounting and the business side of running a successful medical practice. Kristy is a very organized person and wants to make sure she follows the right procedures and understands why a certain task must be done a certain way. She wants to establish a calendar that shows what duties should be done at what times.

Determine when all the forms in Part III must be turned in or filed. Add tax day to the calendar. Print the calendar, showing all filing dates on it. If a template will help, use one from the Microsoft Office home page.

WORKPLACE APPLICATIONS

Complete the following math review test. Turn it in to your instructor for grading or grade it in class.

Solve the following addition problems.

1. 99 + 104 = ___________
2. 78 + 57 = ___________
3. 98 + 128 = ___________
4. 187 + 233 = ___________
5. 284 + 440 = ___________
6. 306 + 291 = ___________
7. 204 + 278 = ___________
8. 409 + 246 = ___________
9. 15 + 74 = ___________
10. 181 + 369 = ___________

 Copyright © 2011, 2007, 2003 by Saunders, an imprint of Elsevier Inc. All rights reserved.

Solve the following subtraction problems.

1. 290 – 303 = ___________
2. 231 – 263 = ___________
3. 453 – 156 = ___________
4. 459 – 325 = ___________
5. 318 – 105 = ___________
6. 398 – 294 = ___________

Solve the following multiplication problems.

1. 46 × 24 = ___________
2. 11 × 49 = ___________
3. 48 × 17 = ___________
4. 26 × 24 = ___________
5. 42 × 15 = ___________
6. 5 × 49 = ___________
7. 47 × 12 = ___________
8. 26 × 34 = ___________
9. 45 × 21 = ___________

Solve the following division problems:

1. 1,950 ÷ 13 = ___________
2. 50,350 ÷ 53 = ___________
3. 12105 ÷ 15 = ___________
4. 9,712 ÷ 16 = ___________
5. 13,500 ÷ 20 = ___________

INTERNET ACTIVITIES

1. Investigate bookkeeping software on the Internet and use any tutorials or trial software available. Determine a good program for use in the medical office and be able to defend your decision in a class presentation.

2. Look for math worksheet sites and work through some of the sheets for practice.

Copyright © 2011, 2007, 2003 by Saunders, an imprint of Elsevier Inc. All rights reserved.

25 Medical Practice Management and Human Resources

VOCABULARY REVIEW

Fill in the blank with the correct vocabulary term from this chapter.

1. Dr. Hughes enjoys offering ________________ to employees who perform over and above the call of duty.
2. Lucia told a ________________ lie to her supervisor, which almost resulted in termination of her employment.
3. The staff enjoys ________________ talks and recently traveled to North Dallas to hear Zig Ziglar speak.
4. Employee ________________ can indicate the working conditions at a facility; when the staff is happy with their jobs, they tend to remain in their positions for a number of years.
5. Mrs. Gordon has always been a great promoter of employee ________________, never failing to offer her smile and a kind word to others.
6. Ruth Ann was written up for ________________ after she and Sue Lynn, her supervisor, had a rather loud and tense discussion last week.
7. The marketers ________________ young women in their latest advertisements to promote the hospital expansion in the labor and delivery department.
8. New employees may find it helpful to be assigned a ________________, who will assist them as they learn the office routines and responsibilities.
9. The office manager assigned several new duties to Ann, including development of meeting ________________.
10. Sandy had 17 performance ________________ to give over the course of the week.
11. People in the medical field sometimes experience ________________ and feel a need to separate themselves from the profession for a time.
12. Paul was charged with ________________ after he took money from the physical therapy clinic where he formerly worked.
13. The doctors and management personnel have worked hard to develop such a ________________ team.
14. A ________________ of ________________ is necessary in any organization, even smaller ones.
15. Barbara is ________________ with her paperwork and very seldom makes an error.

Copyright © 2011, 2007, 2003 by Saunders, an imprint of Elsevier Inc. All rights reserved.

SKILLS AND CONCEPTS

Part I: Office Managers

1. Why is it a good idea to have one person in charge of office operations?

____

____

____

2. Most management problems can be prevented by carefully defining the areas of:
   a. ____
   b. ____

3. What usually happens if a manager helps employees get what they want and need from a job?

____

____

____

4. Managers who have a group of outstanding employees are usually looked upon as _______________ _______________.

5. List the three basic types of leaders.
   a. ____
   b. ____
   c. ____

6. List and explain three types of power.
   a. ____
   b. ____
   c. ____

7. The office manager must always have enough written _______________ when terminating an employee.

8. List five ways to motivate employees.
   a. ____
   b. ____
   c. ____
   d. ____
   e. ____

9. What is a "yes" person?

____

____

10. What is one of the most effective ways to improve employee morale?

____

____

 Copyright © 2011, 2007, 2003 by Saunders, an imprint of Elsevier Inc. All rights reserved.

Part II: Hiring and Terminating Employees

Fill in the blank with the best answer.

1. One of the most effective methods of finding new employees is through word of ________________________.
2. When calling a job candidate to schedule an interview, the office manager has an opportunity to judge how well the person speaks on the ________________________.
3. The job candidate should fill out the application at the office by hand so that the applicant's ________________________ can be evaluated.
4. If the job candidate feels at ________________________, he or she will be able to share strengths and will communicate better during the interview.
5. Relationships with those who work in the medical office should, above all else, be ________________________.
6. Candidates may be required to submit to a ________________________ check, especially if they will be handling office finances.
7. One of the most critical errors in bringing a new staff member to the team is not providing fair and adequate ________________________ and ________________________.
8. Well-written job ________________________ list the essential functions of the job and specify the chain of command that should be followed in the office.
9. A dismissed employee should never be left in the office ________________________.
10. Always check at least ________________________ references when hiring a new employee.

Part III: Leading During Transitions and Change

Add the appropriate word to the following sentences about change.

1. Change ________________________.
2. ________________________ with the change.
3. ________________________ change.
4. ________________________ to change quickly.
5. ________________________ change.
6. Anticipate ________________________.

Part IV: Meeting Agendas

Number these activities in the correct order for a staff meeting.

_____ Discussion of unfinished business

_____ Adjournment

_____ Discussion of problems in the administrative area

_____ Discussion of new business

_____ Reading of the minutes from the last meeting

_____ Discussion of problems in the clinical area

_____ Discussion of problems in the common areas

Copyright © 2011, 2007, 2003 by Saunders, an imprint of Elsevier Inc. All rights reserved.

Part V: Word Find

Find the words on the list in the puzzle.

R I P B U T S S M E N T O R T Y M X H U E J I S P Z G L A M
E N C O S T Q D U V M Z P C U R M W I X H Y A E Q N A D E Y
T S K J F U I M N B N B W U O A A O Q D M Z D J I S N T Q F
E U U B C K P L N A O V V Q N L V M N C A D J G I E I M C J
N B O K G P A U I I M R T W R L D S O I E Q A A G C N J V M
T O R Z F Z M X Q M W I D I U I A M M R X R R A U Z O N C W
I R N O I T A V I T O M R I B C A I M G A P R L U U U X Q C
O D X N P B G W M V B P I P N N H Q M P P L O L X F F B H E
N I V I T J L E G R I K I E E A L Q S A W U E V O G H A E L
X N F T A Z M R E A Y W N F G R T I L A S D L I I O I N Z B
U A Y V L B O A F F A F C A X V D E H H R Z T T F N A Y G A
S T U X U X W C B U R S E R C O U H T K F N P D O I L M X R
D I E L B A F F A Y K B N V R G U F D H R T Z F J T S P D T
S O L Z N F D S O U N I T K Q J Y L Y L B B C E N R G A Z E
L N Q D F L T K T A P K I E R K F S N M C O R X U A Q D E N
X C P E X T R I N S I C V H J O B P R K M I M A M A A X Q E
P O U Q T U E J A A U C E N Q W H B Z M B H O G H Q L V Z P
K R U N I V Q Q Y C Q J S V S K Q P A R V M Y H F V N X N M
R W E X J N S T I P Y H Z Z D B W N W E W Z F F V D T S B I
L G J E G R T X N J H W P P A L D N A L S O P S C H G M Q F
Y G Z K D A H R C E K B P Y R G N A B H Y O Q L B N X K Y T
X M V F J V D N I A M G M P Q D A V Q I A G M W Q B B H D L
L U B O S G X T K N P E V E S M Z J H G C O P T G W M T H N
H F F D Y O P E U P S C L A J O J V I O B Z Z Z N T E W G J
N O I T N E V M U C R I C Z C C B X H C M Q Z O E A N R P W
L L G K N F Y R B Y A Q C X Z K S E P X X H Z S R J T X U G
P L S G Q M I C R O M A N A G E S V N D B D V S C C J A J W
B T S Q L M U T J H B B G N Z I B P B B P K S D Q U K U L O
O S H D V K Y A T B B W U I V G L M A C X V F B F T E F V B
R K X C E F X E D X D T U E B S C Q E C E G Z D Z I P B G L

Affable
Agenda
Ancillary
Appraisal
Blatant
Burnout
Chain of command
Circumvention
Cohesive
Disparaging
Embezzlement
Extrinsic
Impenetrable
Incentives
Insubordination
Intrinsic
Mentor
Meticulous
Micromanage
Morale
Motivation
Reprimands
Retention
Subordinate

Copyright © 2011, 2007, 2003 by Saunders, an imprint of Elsevier Inc. All rights reserved.

CASE STUDY

Read the case study and perform the exercise following it.

Belinda is a single mom with two children. She recently was divorced from her husband and is in the process of rebuilding her life. She enrolled in medical assisting school 8 months ago and is now preparing for graduation. Throughout her time in classes, she has researched medical facilities on the Internet and found several that are close to her apartment complex.

Belinda has several goals in life, and the most important ones involve her family. She wants to find a job that will allow her to take care of her children, provide them a good education, and save for their college education. She knows that she needs to find a job that offers health benefits. Belinda is a loyal employee and has a work history, so she is hopeful that her positions from graduation forward will be such that she is able to make steady progress toward reaching her goals.

What goals do you have for your life after graduation? Assess your own personal situation and determine five long-term (life) goals, five short-term goals (1 year or more away), and 10 immediate goals for the next 6 months. Write the goals down. For the long- and short-term goals, include a few sentences that explain why the goal is important to you. Make sure all the immediate goals are attainable in a 6-month period.

Look over your list daily. Write down all the progress you have made toward the goals and celebrate when each one is attained. It may be beneficial to keep a journal that details the progress you make toward your goals, as well as the new ones you set as the original goals are met.

WORK APPLICATIONS

1. Revise or write a new patient information booklet and assign different groups of classmates to work on different sections of the booklet. Plan a staff meeting, sending a memo to each classmate who should attend. Write an agenda for the meeting, set a time limit, and determine a general subject to discuss. Each group should discuss their part of the booklet during the meeting.

2. Compose a rough draft of your résumé. Allow three different classmates to proof the document and make suggestions. Draft a final copy and turn it in to the instructor for a grade.

INTERNET ACTIVITIES

1. Perform a job search for medical assisting positions in your area. Look for the 15 most interesting opportunities and print the job descriptions. Compare the job requirements to the skills you have learned. If appropriate, apply for the positions.

2. Research a person you consider a leader on the Internet. Read about this person's life and write a report about the individual's abilities as a leader. Share the report with the class.

3. Investigate budgeting ideas by researching the Internet. Determine what items must be included in the budget and then list all the bills and payments that must be made each month. A budget template may be available on the Microsoft Web site and can be downloaded for use. Make the estimates as close as possible to your actual income and expenses. Turn the budget in to the instructor.

Copyright © 2011, 2007, 2003 by Saunders, an imprint of Elsevier Inc. All rights reserved.

26 Medical Practice Marketing and Customer Service

VOCABULARY REVIEW

Fill in the blanks with the correct vocabulary terms from this chapter.

1. Dr. Julie Todd and Dr. Robert Todd truly enjoy ________________, because it provides an opportunity to reach and involve diverse audiences using key messages and effective programs.
2. Monica has identified several ________________ ________________ and has a strong plan for marketing efforts that she plans to implement over the next year.
3. When you are developing a marketing plan, clearly establish ________________ and think about the long- and short-term goals for the practice.
4. Monica wants to develop a(n) ________________ business plan that is workable and will be flexible if changes become necessary.
5. One area Monica hopes to improve is the ________________ laboratory, because much of the equipment is outdated and needs to be replaced.

SKILLS AND CONCEPTS

Part I: Short Answers

1. List the three steps generally followed in preparing to implement or change medical marketing strategies.

   a. ________________________________

   b. ________________________________

   c. ________________________________

2. What is meant by "reaching the target market"?

   ____

   ____

   ____

3. List five specific planning steps that are effective in developing marketing strategies.

   a. ________________________________

   b. ________________________________

   c. ________________________________

   d. ________________________________

   e. ________________________________

Copyright © 2011, 2007, 2003 by Saunders, an imprint of Elsevier Inc. All rights reserved.

4. List several phrases that should never be used with patients, especially when attempting to provide exceptional customer service.

   a. ______________________________

   b. ______________________________

   c. ______________________________

   d. ______________________________

5. Explain the concept that good customer service is a commitment.

   ____

   ____

   ____

6. What are the four Ps of marketing?

   a. ______________________________

   b. ______________________________

   c. ______________________________

   d. ______________________________

7. How does the provider determine what services to offer at the practice?

   ____

   ____

   ____

8. Provide five examples of community involvement that may help a medical practice grow.

   a. ______________________________

   b. ______________________________

   c. ______________________________

   d. ______________________________

   e. ______________________________

9. What is the difference between advertising and public relations?

   ____

   ____

   ____

10. List the four basic steps of creating a Web site.

   a. ______________________________

   b. ______________________________

   c. ______________________________

   d. ______________________________

Copyright © 2011, 2007, 2003 by Saunders, an imprint of Elsevier Inc. All rights reserved.

11. What is the goal of any business?

___

___

___

12. Why is it necessary for medical assistants to provide a high level of customer service to those who visit the physician's office?

___

___

___

Part II: Web Site Evaluation

Research various Web sites for healthcare organizations, preferably in your geographic area. Rate the Web sites from 1 to 10 (10 being the best), by putting your ranking on the line to the left of the Web site name. Then fill in the chart that follows, putting the Web sites in the order in which you ranked them.

Rank	Web Site Name	Rank	Web Site Name

Web Site	Overall Appeal	Content	Ease of Navigation	Fonts	Consistency	Comments
1						
2						
3						
4						
5						
6						
7						
8						
9						
10						

Copyright © 2011, 2007, 2003 by Saunders, an imprint of Elsevier Inc. All rights reserved.

Part III: Customers in the Physician's Office

1. Who are some of the customers who visit the medical office?

____

____

____

2. Explain how to provide patients and other guests in the office with exceptional customer service.

____

____

____

Part IV: Ethics, Marketing, and Public Relations

1. Do you think that any advertising for medical services is ethical? Why or why not?

____

____

____

2. Why has advertising become necessary in today's health industry?

____

____

____

CASE STUDY

Read the case study and answer the question at the end.

Lorendia has worked for Dr. Johnson for more than 15 years. Recently she was forced to cut her hours from 40 a week to 35, because she has been diagnosed with chronic fatigue syndrome, and she struggles toward the end of the week because of the symptoms of the disease. Lorendia has become more and more impatient with the people who come to the physician's office, and she often makes a snippy remark when she is behind in her duties. Her attitude has alienated her from most of the clinic's staff. Although her job performance is not acceptable now, for most of her career her work has been above reproach.

1. How can this situation be resolved so that Lorendia can keep her job yet improve her performance?

____

____

____

Copyright © 2011, 2007, 2003 by Saunders, an imprint of Elsevier Inc. All rights reserved.

WORKPLACE APPLICATIONS

Providing exceptional customer service can actually interfere with job duties. Some workers use customer service as an excuse to chat with patients and avoid other duties. How can the medical assistant strike a balance between providing the customer service that patients deserve and completing all the tasks required each day?

INTERNET ACTIVITIES

1. Research customer service and develop your own, original definition of the concept of customer service. Present your thoughts to the class by creating a professional presentation.

2. Research public relations and make a list of the various "free" ways publicity can be generated for the office. Choose five ideas you feel are the best. E-mail these ideas to each of your classmates. If the entire class participates, everyone will have numerous fresh ideas to use once they begin their career. Write the ideas on index cards and keep them in a box or develop a portfolio of ideas.

3. Design a fictional Web site using free software on the Internet. If appropriate, share the site with classmates and compare ideas.

Copyright © 2011, 2007, 2003 by Saunders, an imprint of Elsevier Inc. All rights reserved.

27 Infection Control

VOCABULARY REVIEW

Define the following terms.

1. anaphylaxis
2. antibody
3. antigen
4. antiseptic
5. autoimmune
6. contaminated
7. germicides
8. pathogenic
9. permeable
10. relapse
11. remission
12. vector

Copyright © 2011, 2007, 2003 by Saunders, an imprint of Elsevier Inc. All rights reserved.

Match the following terms with the correct definition.

13. _______ Disinfection
14. _______ Medical asepsis
15. _______ Surgical asepsis
16. _______ Sanitization
17. _______ Sterilization

a. Removal of disease-causing organisms or destruction of the organisms after they leave the body
b. Destruction of all microorganisms
c. Destruction of organisms before they enter the body
d. A cleansing process that reduces the number of microorganisms to a safe level as dictated by public health guidelines
e. The process of killing pathogenic organisms or rendering them inactive

Define the following terms as they relate to disease processes.

18. chronic

____

19. latent

____

20. acute

____

SKILLS AND CONCEPTS

Part I: Short Answers

1. List five groups of infectious organisms.
   a. ____
   b. ____
   c. ____
   d. ____
   e. ____

2. Label the diagram with the following terms.
   a. Reservoir host _______________
   b. Entry (any body opening) _______________
   c. Transmission mode (air, food, hand, insects, body fluid) _______________
   d. Exit mode (mouth, skin, rectum, body fluid) _______________
   e. Susceptible host _______________

3. Describe the impact of the inflammatory response on the body's ability to defend itself against infection.

____

____

____

Copyright © 2011, 2007, 2003 by Saunders, an imprint of Elsevier Inc. All rights reserved.

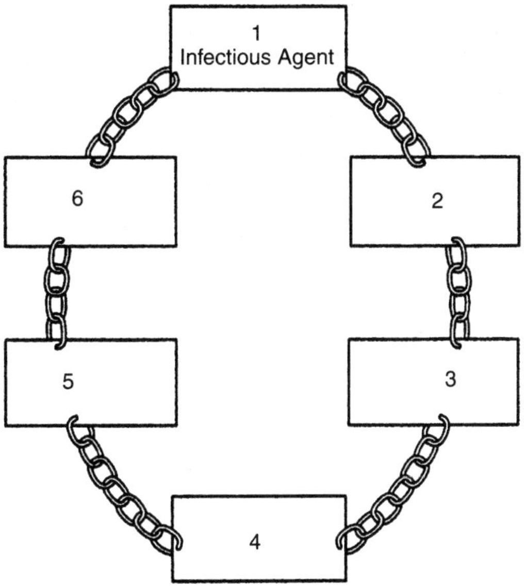

4. Explain the difference between cell-mediated immunity and humoral immunity.

____

5. List six common errors of disinfection.

a. ____

b. ____

c. ____

d. ____

e. ____

f. ____

6. Explain the five major areas included in the OSHA Compliance Guidelines.

a. ____

b. ____

c. ____

d. ____

e. ____

7. List five different bodily fluids that have been identified as potentially infectious by the CDC.

a. ____

b. ____

c. ____

d. ____

e. ____

Copyright © 2011, 2007, 2003 by Saunders, an imprint of Elsevier Inc. All rights reserved.

8. Identify four safety rules that should be followed in the ambulatory care setting to comply with OSHA's environmental protection guidelines.

   a. ______________________________

   b. ______________________________

   c. ______________________________

   d. ______________________________

9. Place a check mark beside the procedures that require the use of disposable gloves.

   ________ Assisting with a vaginal examination

   ________ Performing a routine urinalysis

   ________ Measuring a patient's temperature, pulse, and respirations

   ________ Performing a patient interview

   ________ Drawing blood from a 6-year-old child

CASE STUDIES

1. Rosa is explaining the signs and symptoms of inflammation to a patient. List the four classic symptoms.

   a. ______________________________

   b. ______________________________

   c. ______________________________

   d. ______________________________

2. A patient asks Rosa why the physician did not prescribe an antibiotic for her viral illness. What should Rosa say to the patient?

____

____

____

____

3. While performing venipuncture, Rosa receives an accidental needle stick. Describe the postexposure instructions and follow-up procedures.

____

____

____

____

4. Rosa realizes that her patient needs to be educated about proper asepsis. However, in a busy office, the staff does not have a lot of extra time. What can Rosa do during her time with the patient to educate the person properly about aseptic technique?

____

____

____

____

Copyright © 2011, 2007, 2003 by Saunders, an imprint of Elsevier Inc. All rights reserved.

5. Rosa is responsible for teaching a new member of the staff to sanitize and disinfect properly the instruments used throughout a typical day in the facility. What PPE should the employee use to protect herself from possible contamination? What are the important steps in cleaning instruments so that all biologic material is removed? What are some reasons disinfection might not occur? How can the medical assistant prevent these errors?

____

____

____

____

____

WORKPLACE APPLICATIONS

1. Employers with workers who are at risk for occupational exposure to blood or other infectious materials must implement an Occupational Safety and Health Administration (OSHA) Exposure Control Plan that details employee protection procedures. List seven items that should be included in the plan.

   a. _______________

   b. _______________

   c. _______________

   d. _______________

   e. _______________

   f. _______________

   g. _______________

2. Rosa is concerned that she may be allergic to latex. For what signs and symptoms should she look when she puts on latex gloves? Is Rosa's employer required to supply her with latex-free gloves if she does have a latex allergy? Why or why not?

____

____

____

____

3. Rosa is helping to update the OSHA Exposure Control Plan in her office. She wants to include a policy for wearing gloves. List six different times gloves should be worn.

   a. _______________

   b. _______________

   c. _______________

   d. _______________

   e. _______________

   f. _______________

Copyright © 2011, 2007, 2003 by Saunders, an imprint of Elsevier Inc. All rights reserved.

4. Review Procedure 27-4: Performing Medical Aseptic Hand Washing in your textbook. What did you learn? Practice proper hand washing for the next 24 hours. Note any new habits you have formed. Do you see any improvement? Have you noticed the hand-washing behaviors of others?

5. Rosa is assisting the physician with a dressing change when a patient suspected of having tuberculosis coughs, and mucous splatters into Rosa's eyes. Based on what you learned in Procedure 27-2, what should Rosa do?

INTERNET ACTIVITIES

1. Visit *www.osha.gov*. View the OSHA Bloodborne Pathogens Standards. What can you do in your workplace to prevent accidental exposure to blood-borne pathogens? Did you find anything surprising in the guidelines or on the Web site? Prepare to discuss your answers in class.

2. Visit the Infection Control area of the CDC site at *www.cdc.gov/ncidod/dhqp/index.html*. Investigate Infection Control Guidelines and summarize what you have learned.

Copyright © 2011, 2007, 2003 by Saunders, an imprint of Elsevier Inc. All rights reserved.

28 Patient Assessment

VOCABULARY REVIEW

Fill in the blanks with the correct vocabulary terms from this chapter.

1. Lilly's ________________ for seeing the physician today is a sore throat.
2. A(n) ________________ is the conclusion the physician reaches after evaluating all the findings, including laboratory and other test results.
3. "IBS vs. Gastroenteritis" listed under the impression is an example of a(n) ________________.
4. ________________ means pertaining to the operation of the mind by which we become aware of perceiving, thinking, and remembering.
5. ________________is the relationship of harmony and accord that exists between the patient and the healthcare provider.

SKILLS AND CONCEPTS

Part I: Short Answers

1. Describe some factors that influence a person's value system. Do you think these factors have influenced your values?

____

____

____

____

2. List and describe the three processes of active listening.

a. ____

b. ____

c. ____

3. List four important rules to remember when preparing the appropriate environment for patient interaction.

a. ____

b. ____

c. ____

d. ____

Copyright © 2011, 2007, 2003 by Saunders, an imprint of Elsevier Inc. All rights reserved.

4. List and describe the six components of the medical history.

a. ______________________________

b. ______________________________

c. ______________________________

d. ______________________________

e. ______________________________

f. ______________________________

5. List and define the three stages of the patient interview.

a. ______________________________

b. ______________________________

c. ______________________________

6. Therapeutic nonverbal behaviors are key to a successful interview process. Summarize 4 examples of nonverbal behavior that enhance therapeutic communication with patients.

a. ______________________________

b. ______________________________

c. ______________________________

d. ______________________________

7. Label the following questions as either open ended or closed ended.

______________ a. How have you been feeling?

______________ b. Do you have a headache?

______________ c. Have you ever broken a bone?

______________ d. What brings you to the physician?

______________ e. Are you feeling better?

______________ f. Do you have high blood pressure?

______________ g. Tell me about your back pain.

______________ h. When did the nausea start?

______________ i. Did your mother have a history of cancer?

______________ j. Do you smoke?

8. Label the following as "subjective" (symptom) or "objective" (sign).

a. Pain ______________

b. Nausea ______________

c. Dizziness ______________

d. Elevated blood pressure ______________

Copyright © 2011, 2007, 2003 by Saunders, an imprint of Elsevier Inc. All rights reserved.

e. Labored respirations ______________

f. Headache ______________

g. Temperature of the skin ______________

h. Back pain ______________

i. Color of the skin ______________

j. Abdominal pain ______________

9. Describe the four components of the POMR.

a. ______________

b. ______________

c. ______________

d. ______________

10. Identify and explain four questions that could be used to clarify a patient's perception of pain.

a. ______________

b. ______________

c. ______________

d. ______________

11. Identify the defense mechanism displayed by these patients.

a. A patient who refuses to believe she has breast cancer.

____

b. A 5-year-old child who starts to suck his thumb again when he is ill.

____

c. A patient who accuses you of being disrespectful when he has acted that way himself.

____

d. A patient who explains that she missed her appointment because she was so busy and she really didn't need to follow up on the biopsy results anyway.

____

12. The first letter of each part of the progress note makes up the word SOAPE. Explain the meaning of each of these letters.

S ______________

O ______________

A ______________

P ______________

E ______________

Copyright © 2011, 2007, 2003 by Saunders, an imprint of Elsevier Inc. All rights reserved.

13. What is a SOMR? How is it organized? What is the major disadvantage of this system?

____

____

____

14. What is an EMR? What are some advantages and disadvantages of this type of medical record?

____

____

____

15. Define the following abbreviations:

ac ____	bid ____
BP ____	CAD ____
CHF ____	CVA ____
CXR ____	dc ____
DVT ____	Dx ____
f/u ____	fx ____
hs ____	HTN ____
Hx ____	MI ____
NKA ____	NPO ____
prn ____	pt ____
RBC ____	R/O ____
Rx ____	stat ____
URI ____	VS ____

CASE STUDIES

In the following case studies, what types of interview barriers are indicated? Explain how these statements are dangerous and may interfere with the patient interview.

1. Mrs. Miller is expressing her concern about a changing mole in her left axillary region. Chris, the medical assistant obtaining her health history, makes the statement, "Mrs. Miller, the dysplastic nevus found in the left axillary region looks as if it could be malignant. You have not been using sunscreen, have you?"

____

____

____

2. Mr. Sunsari is being seen today for a suspicious mass in his left lung. The physician has recommended a biopsy of the mass; however, Mr. Sunsari prefers to postpone the procedure. He asks Chris what he should do about scheduling the procedure. Chris states, "I would do it right away."

____

____

____

Copyright © 2011, 2007, 2003 by Saunders, an imprint of Elsevier Inc. All rights reserved.

3. Carmen Largosi is a diabetic patient who is very concerned about her blood glucose levels. Her mother was a diabetic and had to have her left leg amputated. When Carmen expresses her fears, Chris responds with, "I wouldn't worry about that. The doctor is very good with diabetic patients."

How can you display sensitivity to the diverse influences on the patients in the following case studies? Explain the rationale behind your behavior.

1. Mrs. Nyguen Xu will not establish eye contact with you during the patient interview. Do you think this means Mrs. Xu is not telling the truth?

2. Carl Worth, a 78-year-old patient, is hard of hearing and does not appear to be paying attention when you ask questions for the patient history. His daughter is in the examination room with him. so would it be better to gather patient information from her? Why or why not?

3. Theo Lang is being seen today for a surgical follow-up visit. He asks that his partner, David, accompany him into the examination room. What should you do?

WORKPLACE APPLICATIONS

1. The receiver of a message attaches meaning to the message based on verbal and nonverbal communication. Provide examples of each and describe how the receiver may put his or her own interpretation on them.

2. Chris Isaccson, CMA (AAMA), is updating the office's policies and procedures handbook. One of the items he would like to include is communication using an age-specific approach. Create a list of the important guidelines to follow when interacting with a child.

3. Chris Isaccson, CMA (AAMA), is to present an in-service lecture, "Proper Charting Methods." What type of information should Chris include when preparing his presentation? Include both technical format and documenting patient signs and symptoms.

4. Chris has been asked by one of the physician's in the practice to summarize changes that need to be made to comply with HIPAA guidelines regarding patient confidentiality. What details should Chris include in the summary?

5. As a member of the healthcare team, Chris is responsible for practicing sound risk management principles. Summarize four principles he should consistently practice.

Copyright © 2011, 2007, 2003 by Saunders, an imprint of Elsevier Inc. All rights reserved.

INTERNET ACTIVITIES

1. EMRs are increasingly becoming part of the medical office. Visit the Web site *www.eclinicalworks.com* and choose "online demo" to view the different ways electronic medical records can be used in the medical office. What are some of the most important features? How will EMRs improve patient care?

2. Go to the Health and Human Services Web site, *www.hhs.gov/ocr/office/index.html*, to learn more about HIPAA. Click on Health Information Privacy and read more about "Understanding HIPAA Privacy." What did you learn?

MEDICAL RECORD ACTIVITIES

1. Gather a patient history from your partner in lab using the Patient History form found in the Medical Record while completing Procedure 28-1.

2. Document the following scenarios in the progress notes section of the medical record using POMR practices.
   a. Patient c/o chest pain of 4 on a 1-10 scale and sweating for the past 2 hours. The patient states taking nitroglycerin for relief of symptoms. VS are T–99°, P–68/minute, R–24/minute, with an irregular pulse and left arm pain.

      S: ____________________

      O: ____________________

   b. Patient c/o a sore throat with pain of 7 on a 1-10 scale and fever for 2 days. The patient has been taking OTCs and gargling with warm salt water for relief of symptoms. VS are T–102.4°, P–108/minute, R–20/minute. Patient also has an erythemic papular rash across the chest. Patient states exposure to strep last week.

      S: ____________________

      O: ____________________

   c. Patient c/o a headache with pain of 8 on a 1-10 scale and nausea for 3 days. The patient has been taking Lortab 5 mg for relief of symptoms. VS are T–97.6°, P–110/minute, R–20/minute. Also c/o dizziness and pain in the eyes. Patient appears pale with damp skin.

      S: ____________________

      O: ____________________

   d. Patient fell off a ladder 2 days ago and c/o low back pain of 5 on a 1-10 scale. He has been taking Advil for relief of symptoms. VS are T–98.7°, P–98/minute, R–20/minute. Patient also has ecchymosis across the flank and c/o blood in urine.

      S: ____________________

      O: ____________________

Copyright © 2011, 2007, 2003 by Saunders, an imprint of Elsevier Inc. All rights reserved.

29 Patient Education

VOCABULARY REVIEW

Fill in the blanks with the correct vocabulary terms from this chapter.

1. The holistic model suggests that healthcare workers should take into consideration all aspects of a patient's life, including patients' ________, ________, ________, ________, and ________ needs.

SKILLS AND CONCEPTS

Part I: Short Answers

1. List six guidelines for patient education.

   a ________________

   b. ________________

   c. ________________

   d. ________________

   e. ________________

   f. ________________

2. Explain seven patient factors that influence learning.

   a ________________

   b. ________________

   c. ________________

   d. ________________

   e. ________________

   f. ________________

   g. ________________

3. Summarize eight approaches to language barriers.

   a ________________

   b. ________________

   c. ________________

   d. ________________

   e. ________________

   f. ________________

   g. ________________

   h. ________________

Copyright © 2011, 2007, 2003 by Saunders, an imprint of Elsevier Inc. All rights reserved.

4. One of the most important aspects of patient teaching is to be ________________ and provide information about ________________ patients want to know ________________ patients want to know it.

5. List 10 barriers to patient learning.

   a ____________________

   b. ____________________

   c. ____________________

   d. ____________________

   e. ____________________

   f. ____________________

   g. ____________________

   h. ____________________

   i. ____________________

   j. ____________________

6. Identify five guidelines for ordering educational materials.

   a ____________________

   b. ____________________

   c. ____________________

   d. ____________________

   e. ____________________

7. The role of the medical assistant educator includes:

   a ____________________

   b. ____________________

   c. ____________________

   d. ____________________

   e. ____________________

   f. ____________________

   g. ____________________

   h. ____________________

8. Effective teaching methods include use of ________________ materials, videos, and approved ________________ sites to gather information; referral to community ________________ and experts; ________________ demonstration of medical skills; examination of patients' records of events; and involving ________________ in the education process.

Copyright © 2011, 2007, 2003 by Saunders, an imprint of Elsevier Inc. All rights reserved.

9. Use the following checklist to design and present a program for a patient during your externship or role-play with a fellow classmate.
   A. Conduct patient assessment.
      - Consider pertinent patient factors.
      - Identify barriers to learning.
      - Prioritize patient information.
      - Determine immediate and long-term needs.
      - Decide on appropriate teaching materials and methods.

      Complete ________________

   B. Prepare the teaching area and assemble necessary equipment and materials.
      - Use supplies and equipment the patient will use at home.
      - Provide positive feedback for correct display of skills.

      Complete ________________

   C. Maintain adequate, not too fast, pace.

      Complete ________________

   D. Repeatedly ask for patient feedback to confirm understanding.
      - Eliminate barriers to learning.
      - Address immediate learning needs.
      - Use repetition and rephrasing to promote understanding.

      Complete ________________

   E. Summarize the material learned or the skill mastered at the end of each teaching interaction.

      Complete ________________

   F. Outline a plan for the next meeting.

      Complete ________________

   G. Evaluate the teaching plan.
      - Was there enough time to complete the lesson?
      - Was the patient physically and psychologically ready for the information?
      - Were the goals for the session reached?

      Complete ________________

   H. Document the teaching intervention.
      - Material covered.
      - Patient response or level of skill performance.
      - Plans for next session.
      - Community referrals.

      Complete ________________

WORKPLACE APPLICATIONS

1. Gather a list of community resources for the patient in your area. To what groups are the resources geared? What is the contact information? What services do the organizations offer?

2. Taylor, a medical assistant for a family practice office, has been asked by Dr. Norberger to create patient education files for each examination room. The file should contain handouts on chronic disease, nutrition, exercise and a healthy lifestyle. Create a list of 15 topics that should be included in this file. Why did you choose them? How may they be helpful to the doctor and the patients?

Copyright © 2011, 2007, 2003 by Saunders, an imprint of Elsevier Inc. All rights reserved.

3. As Taylor begins to obtain and develop educational supplies for the patient education files, what are some guidelines she should follow as she reviews the information available? What other teaching materials should she consider using in addition to the handouts?

4. Based on what you have learned about the Health Belief Model, complete the blank spaces in the table below.

The Health Belief Model

Principles	Definition	Application to Patient Education
Perceived susceptibility		Supply information on risk level; individual risk based on ________ ________
Perceived ________	________ on the seriousness of the condition and its health risks	Outline the potential ________ of the disease
Perceived benefits	Patient's belief in ________	Emphasize the ________ that can occur if patient is compliant with health care recommendations
Perceived ________	Patient's opinion of the ________ and psychological costs of compliance	Identify ________ and work to reduce them through patient education, family outreach, ________
________	Methods developed to activate patient compliance	
Self-efficacy	Patient has the confidence to take action toward a healthier state	

5. Identify Dr. Elisabeth Kübler-Ross's stages of grief and include in your explanation a suggestion for therapeutic interaction with a patient in each stage.

a. ____

____

____

b. ____

____

____

c. ____

____

____

d. ____

____

____

e. ____

____

____

Copyright © 2011, 2007, 2003 by Saunders, an imprint of Elsevier Inc. All rights reserved.

6. Explain how the medical assistant can perform patient education for the following patients with special needs.

   a. Antonio DeMendez, a 68-year-old patient, has profound hearing loss in his left ear. He needs to be taught how to take his blood pressure medication accurately.

   ____

   ____

   ____

   b. Christina Wu, a 48-year-old patient, is legally blind. She is a new patient who is visiting the office for the first time and needs to complete a health history form. The physician recommends that she follow a low-sodium diet.

   ____

   ____

   ____

   c. Julio Gonzales is 17 and has limited English skills. He is scheduled for diagnostic testing at the hospital and must be taught how to prepare for the studies.

   ____

   ____

   ____

7. One of the roles of the medical assistant is to help patients in need of community health education and/or support services. To prepare for this role, collect a minimum of 25 community resources that are available in your area. Include in your directory the name of the group and the services provided; the contact person; telephone number, address, meeting times, and locations; and a related Web site if available. Choose one of these resources and investigate the services it provides in greater detail, either by interviewing an individual who works or volunteers in the organization and/or by attending one the group's sponsored meetings. Summarize your experience and share it with your classmates.

8. For the following scenarios, write "Yes" on the line if the medical assistant's actions are acceptable practice according to HIPAA guidelines or "No" if they are not acceptable.

   _______ The mother of a 19-year-old patient, Sue Collins, calls the office. Even though the mother is not listed as Sue's PHI, Taylor answers her questions about Sue's illness.

   _______ The patient requests that only her husband receive information about her health status. Taylor receives a call from the patient's adult daughter, who insists on learning her mother's diagnosis. Taylor feels bad for the daughter and answers her questions.

MEDICAL RECORD ACTIVITIES

1. Mary Ann has recently been diagnosed with hypercholesterolemia. As Taylor is discussing diet and exercise recommendations, Mary Ann replies that she doesn't think the cholesterol is something she should be concerned about, and what with working two jobs, she is "forced" to dine out and eat "on the run" most days. What type of barriers will Taylor need to overcome? Taylor should provide her with what type of patient education material? Document the patient education intervention.

   ____

   ____

   ____

Copyright © 2011, 2007, 2003 by Saunders, an imprint of Elsevier Inc. All rights reserved.

2. Describe how the patient's chronologic age and developmental age result in the need to adapt the teaching plan for the following patients. What changes will you make to the methods of delivery? Are any learning barriers present that must be overcome? What types of patient information will you provide to each person? Document the patient education intervention.

   a. A 74-year-old woman recently diagnosed with diabetes type 2. Before her diagnosis, she had not seen a doctor in 20 years. She loves to cook for her large family but complains of difficulty reading recipes, because the diabetes has resulted in diabetic retinopathy.

      ____

      ____

      ____

   b. An 11-year-old boy recently diagnosed with diabetes type 1. He loves to play sports and is very active. His father complains that he plays so much that getting him to eat properly is difficult. The boy is afraid of needles, and the doctor has ordered him to begin using insulin and a glucometer immediately.

      ____

      ____

      ____

 Copyright © 2011, 2007, 2003 by Saunders, an imprint of Elsevier Inc. All rights reserved.

30 Nutrition and Health Promotion

VOCABULARY REVIEW

Match the following terms with the correct definition.

_______ Turgor

_______ Cholesterol

_______ Free radicals

_______ Hydrogenated oils

_______ Vertigo

_______ Diabetes type 1

_______ Diverticulosis

_______ Digestion

_______ Triglyceride

_______ Diabetes type 2

_______ Psyllium

_______ Nutrient deficiency

_______ Amino acids

_______ Neural tube defects

a. Beta cells in the pancreas no longer produce insulin, meaning the patient must follow complicated dietary and medication treatment plans

b. Water-soluble fiber found in some cereals, dietary supplements, and bulk fiber laxatives

c. Fatty acid and glycerol compound that combines with a protein molecule to form high- or low-density lipoprotein

d. Process of converting food into chemical substances that can be used by the body

e. Conditions caused by a below-normal intake of a particular substance

f. Skin tension test that can reveal dehydration

g. Organic compounds that form the chief constituents of protein and are used by the body to build and repair tissues

h. Any of a group of congenital anomalies of the brain and spinal column caused by failure of the neural tube to close during embryonic development

i. Oils that are combined with hydrogen, making them more saturated

j. Nonessential nutrient produced by the liver that can result in atherosclerotic plaques with excessive dietary intake

k. Dizziness

l. Presence of pouchlike herniations through the muscular layer of the colon

m. Unstable compounds believed to damage cells, resulting in cancer, heart disease, and other disorders

n. In ability of the body to use glucose for energy as a result either of a lack of insulin production in the pancreas or of resistance to insulin on the cellular level

Describe the dietary imbalances that contribute to each of the following health problems.

1. Anemia

____

____

2. Cancer

____

____

Copyright © 2011, 2007, 2003 by Saunders, an imprint of Elsevier Inc. All rights reserved.

3. Constipation

____

____

4. Diabetes

____

____

5. Hypercholesterolemia

____

____

6. Hypertension

____

____

7. Osteoporosis

____

____

Fill in the blanks with the appropriate terms.

8. A(n) ____________________ nutrient, such as cholesterol, can be created in the body and does not need to be included in the diet.
9. ____________________ are chemical organic compounds composed of carbon, hydrogen, and oxygen and are primarily plant products in origin. They are divided into three groups based on the complexity of their molecules: simple sugars, complex carbohydrates (starch), and dietary fiber.
10. ____________________ is a storage form of fuel that is used to supplement carbohydrates as an available energy source.
11. ____________________ is produced by the liver and is found in animal foods; it can produce atherosclerotic plaque deposits in arteries.
12. ____________________ are composed of units known as *amino acids*, which are the materials the body uses to build and repair tissues.
13. Vitamins are divided into two groups: ____________________-soluble vitamins (A, D, E, and K) and ____________________-soluble vitamins (B complex and C).
14. The ____________________ is the amount of energy needed by fasting, resting individuals to maintain vital function.
15. Dietary fiber is commonly called ____________________.

Define the following terms.

16. metabolism

____

17. anabolism

____

18. catabolism

____

Copyright © 2011, 2007, 2003 by Saunders, an imprint of Elsevier Inc. All rights reserved.

19. high-density lipoprotein (HDL)

____

20. low-density lipoprotein (LDL)

____

21. trans fats

____

SKILLS AND CONCEPTS

Part I: Short Answers

1. How does culture influence our dietary choices? Why is this important to note when providing nutrition education to patients?

____

____

____

____

Examine the nomogram below and answer the following questions.

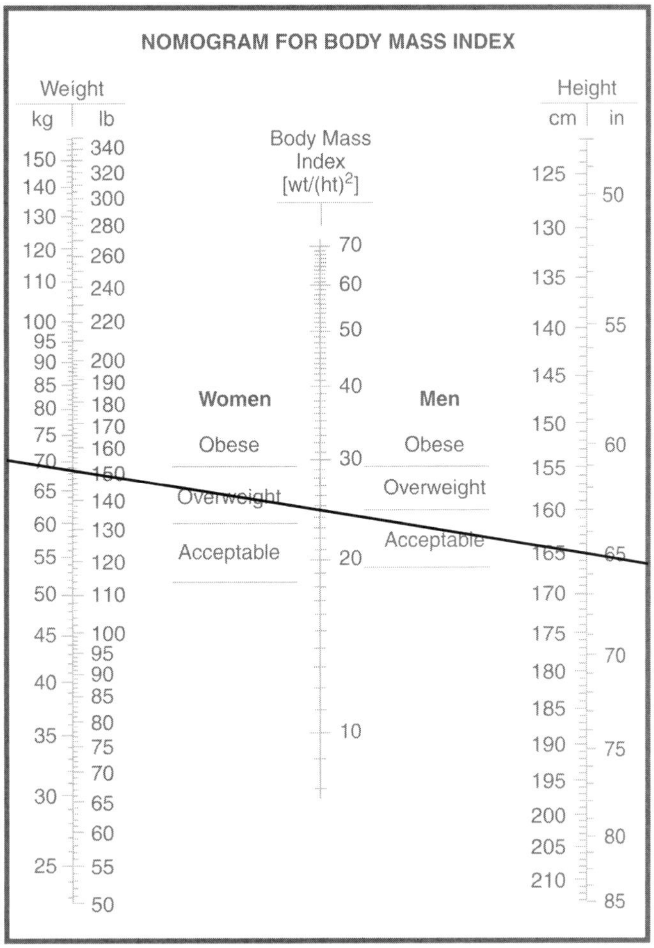

Copyright © 2011, 2007, 2003 by Saunders, an imprint of Elsevier Inc. All rights reserved.

2. What is the purpose of the nomogram?

____

____

3. How much does this patient weigh in pounds? In kilograms?

lb ____________________ kg ____________________

4. What is the height in inches? In centimeters?

in ____________________ cm ____________________

5. What is the body mass index (BMI)?

____

6. Use the nomogram to calculate your own BMI.

____

7. List four functions of water.

a. ____

b. ____

c. ____

d. ____

8. List four functions of proteins.

a. ____

b. ____

c. ____

d. ____

9. What is the Glycemic Index? How is it used to manage blood sugar levels?

____

____

____

____

10. Examine the figure that shows the anatomy of MyPyramid. Label the different sections. How does this pyramid differ from the traditional food guide pyramid? Do you think these changes will persuade individuals to lead healthier lifestyles?

____

____

____

____

Copyright © 2011, 2007, 2003 by Saunders, an imprint of Elsevier Inc. All rights reserved.

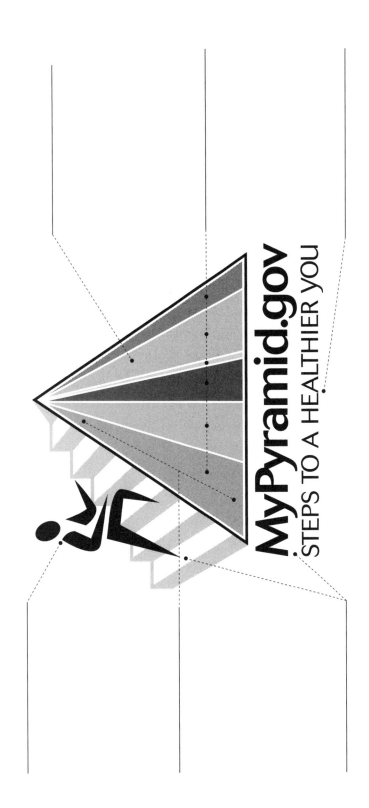

Copyright © 2011, 2007, 2003 by Saunders, an imprint of Elsevier Inc. All rights reserved.

Examine the nutrition facts label and answer the following questions.

NUTRITION FACTS
Serving size: 1¼ cups (30 g)
Servings per container: about 16

Amount per serving		**Cereal**	**Cereal with ½ cup skim milk**
Calories		110	190
Calories from fat		0	0
		% Daily value**	
Total fat 9 g*		0%	0%
Saturated fat 0 g		0%	1%
Cholesterol 0 mg		0%	1%
Sodium 270 mg		11%	14%
Total carbohydrate 26 g		9%	11%
Dietary fiber less than 1 g		0%	0%
Sugars 3 g			
Other carbohydrate 22 g			
Protein 2 g			
Vitamin A		0%	6%
Vitamin C		10%	10%
Calcium		0%	15%
Iron		50%	50%
Thiamin		25%	25%
Niacin		25%	25%
Vitamin B_6		25%	25%
Folate		25%	25%
Vitamin B_{12}		25%	30%
Amount per serving		**Cereal**	**Cereal with ½ cup skim milk**
Calories		2000	2500
Total fat	Less than	65 g	60 g
Saturated fat	Less than	20 g	25 g
Cholesterol	Less than	300 mg	300 mg
Sodium	Less than	2400 mg	2400 mg
Total carbohydrate		300 g	375 g
Dietary fiber		25 g	30 g

Calories per gram:
Fat 9 • Carbohydrate 4 • Protein 4

*Amount in cereal. One half cup skim milk adds an additional 40 calories. Less than 5 mg cholesterol, 65 mg sodium, 6 g total carbohydrate (6 g sugars), and 4 g protein.
**Percent daily values are based on 2000-calorie diet. Your daily values may be higher or lower depending on your calorie needs.

11. What is the normal serving size? ________________
12. How many calories are in one serving without milk? ________________
13. How many grams of fiber are present in one serving? ________________
14. This food is high in ________________ and ________________.
15. What is the total number of carbohydrates for 2½ cups of cereal? ________________
16. If one serving of CHO equals 15 g, then how many servings of CHO are in 1¼ cups of cereal?

Copyright © 2011, 2007, 2003 by Saunders, an imprint of Elsevier Inc. All rights reserved.

17. Examine the following table and fill in the blank spaces with the appropriate numbers.

Total Cholesterol				Low-Density Lipoprotein (LDL) Cholesterol		
Age (yr)	**Acceptable**	**Borderline**	**High**	**Acceptable**	**Borderline**	**High**
2 to 20	<170	170–199		<110	110–129	
>20			>240		130–159	

18. The main function of carbohydrate is to supply ______________________________.
19. What are the recommended ranges for percentage of daily intake for the primary nutrients?

    Carbohydrates ______________________

    Proteins ______________________

    Fats ______________________

20. The best types of oils to use in food preparation are either ____________ or ____________.
21. ____________ may interfere with the action of anticoagulant medications.
22. Patients who have had gastric bypass surgery may require certain supplements including vitamin

    ____________.

23. Adequate intakes of both ____________ and ____________ are needed to prevent osteoporosis.
24. Examine the tables below and fill in the blank spaces with the correct information about vitamins and minerals.

Vitamins

Vitamin	Best Sources	Functions	Deficiency Symptoms
A carotene		Formation and maintenance of skin, hair, and mucous membranes; aids vision in dim light; bone and tooth growth	
B_1 thiamine	Fortified cereals and oatmeal, meat, rice and pasta, whole grains, liver		Heart irregularity, fatigue, nerve disorders, mental confusion
B_2 riboflavin		Helps the body release energy from protein, fat, and carbohydrates during metabolism	
B_6 pyridoxine	Fish, poultry, lean meat, bananas, prunes, dried beans, whole grains, avocados		Convulsions, dermatitis, muscular weakness, skin cracks, anemia
B_{12} cobalamin		Aids cell development, functioning of the nervous system, and metabolism of protein and fat	
Biotin	Cereal and grain products, yeast, legumes, liver		Nausea; vomiting; depression; hair loss; dry, scaly skin
Folate folacin, folic acid			Gastrointestinal disorders, anemia, cracked lips
Niacin	Meat, poultry, fish, enriched cereals, peanuts, potatoes, dairy products, eggs	Involved in carbohydrate, protein, and fat metabolism	

Copyright © 2011, 2007, 2003 by Saunders, an imprint of Elsevier Inc. All rights reserved.

Vitamin	Best Sources	Functions	Deficiency Symptoms
Pantothenic acid	Lean meat, whole grains, legumes, vegetables, fruits		Fatigue, vomiting, stomach stress, infections, muscle cramps
C ascorbic acid		Essential for structure of bones, cartilage, muscle, and blood vessels; also helps maintain capillaries and gums and aids absorption of iron	
D		Aids bone and tooth formation; helps maintain heart action and nervous system	
E			Muscular wasting, nerve damage, anemia, reproductive failure
K			Bleeding disorders in newborns and those taking blood-thinning medications

Minerals

Functions	Sources	Deficiency Symptoms	Toxicity Symptoms
Calcium			
	Primarily found in milk and milk products; also found in dark green, leafy vegetables; tofu and other soy products; sardines; salmon with bones; and hard water		Kidney stones
Chloride			
Involved in the maintenance of fluid and acid-base balance; provides an acid medium in the form of hydrochloric acid for activation of gastric enzymes		Disturbances in acid-base balance with possible growth retardation, psychomotor defects, and memory loss	Disturbances in acid-base balance
Magnesium			
Helps build strong bones and teeth; activates many enzymes; participates in protein synthesis and lipid metabolism; helps regulate heartbeat		Rare but in disease states may lead to central nervous system problems (confusion, apathy, hallucinations, poor memory) and neuromuscular problems (muscle weakness, cramps, tremor, cardiac arrhythmia)	

Copyright © 2011, 2007, 2003 by Saunders, an imprint of Elsevier Inc. All rights reserved.

Functions	Sources	Deficiency Symptoms	Toxicity Symptoms
Phosphorus			
		Rare but with malabsorption can cause anorexia, weakness, stiff joints, and fragile bones	Hypocalcemic tetany (muscle spasms)
Potassium			
		May cause impaired growth, hypertension, bone fragility, central nervous system changes, renal hypertrophy, diminished heart rate, and death	
Sodium			
Plays a key role in the maintenance of acid-base balance; transmits nerve impulses and helps control muscle contractions; regulates cell membrane permeability		Hyponatremia (too little sodium in the blood)	
Chromium			
Activates several enzymes; enhances the removal of glucose from the blood		Weight loss, abnormalities of the central nervous system, and possible aggravation of diabetes mellitus	
Copper			
Aids in the production and survival of red blood cells; parts of many enzymes involved in respiration; plays a role in normal lipid metabolism	Shellfish (especially oysters), liver, nuts and seeds, raisins, whole grains, and chocolate		In Wilson's disease and Huntington's chorea (both hereditary diseases), copper accumulation causes neuron and liver cell damage
Fluorine			
	Fluoridated water (and foods cooked in fluoridated water), fish, tea, gelatin		Fluorosis and mottling of teeth
Iodine			
			Little toxic effect in individuals with normal thyroid gland functioning

Copyright © 2011, 2007, 2003 by Saunders, an imprint of Elsevier Inc. All rights reserved.

Functions	Sources	Deficiency Symptoms	Toxicity Symptoms
Iron			
	Heme sources: organ meats, especially liver, red meat, and other meats. Nonheme sources: iron-fortified cereals; dark green, leafy vegetables; legumes; whole grains; blackstrap molasses; dried fruit; and foods cooked in iron pans		Idiopathic hemochromatosis, which can lead to cirrhosis, diabetes mellitus, skin pigmentation, arthralgias (joint pain), and cardiomyopathy
Manganese			
		None observed in humans	Iron-deficiency anemia through inhibiting effect on iron absorption; pulmonary changes, anorexia, apathy, impotence, headaches, leg cramps, and speech impairment; in advanced stages of toxicity resembles Parkinson's disease
Selenium			
Part of an enzyme system; acts as an antioxidant with vitamin E to protect the cell from oxygen		Keshan disease (a human cardiomyopathy) and Kashin-Bek disease (an endemic human osteoarthropathy)	Physical defects of the fingernails and toenails and hair loss
Zinc			
	Whole grains, wheat germ, crabmeat, oysters, liver and other meats, brewer's yeast		Severe anemia, nausea, vomiting, abdominal cramps, diarrhea, fever, hypocupremia (low blood serum copper), malaise, fatigue

Copyright © 2011, 2007, 2003 by Saunders, an imprint of Elsevier Inc. All rights reserved.

25. In your textbook, refer to Table 30-5, which identifies the BMI for individuals as a ratio of their height and weight, and Table 30-6, which classifies disease risk based on the BMI. Determine the BMI of patients in the following scenarios and identify their disease risk.

   a. Kelly Anderson, a 12-year-old patient, is 61 inches tall and weighs 148 pounds.

   ____

   b. Anthony Noel, a 21-year-old patient, is 76 inches tall and weighs 279 pounds.

   ____

   c. Anna Garcia, 46 years old, is 64 inches tall and weighs 126 pounds.

   ____

26. Marcia is working with a teenager who shows evidence of having anorexia nervosa. What are the characteristics typically seen in patients with anorexia nervosa? How do these compare with the characteristics seen in patients with bulimia?

____

CASE STUDIES

1. Mrs. Barton has been recently diagnosed with DM type 2. At her office visit today, she tells Marcia, the medical assistant, that her glucometer readings 2 hours after eating breakfast have been running, on average, 230 to 300 mg/dL. Mrs. Barton's food diary for breakfast is as follows:

Monday Breakfast	Tuesday Breakfast	Wednesday Breakfast
1½ cup cereal 4 ounces OJ	2 pancakes 2 tablespoons syrup 4 ounces OJ	1 blueberry muffin 1 banana 1 cup of tea

What should Marcia notice from the food diary? What conclusions can Marcia draw from Mrs. Barton's breakfast choices and the resulting blood glucose readings?

____

____

____

Mrs. Barton has asked Marcia to create a sample breakfast menu for the next 3 days. Create the menu in the following chart. Why do you think this will better regulate Mrs. Barton's blood glucose level?

Thursday Breakfast	Friday Breakfast	Saturday Breakfast

2. Mr. Hawthorne is trying to make changes in his diet but is confused about how to choose a healthy type of bread at the grocery store. Based on what Marcia knows about bread labels, how should she explain the healthiest bread choice?

____

____

____

____

Copyright © 2011, 2007, 2003 by Saunders, an imprint of Elsevier Inc. All rights reserved.

3. Lucretia Lang, a 38-year-old patient who has been told to increase her fiber intake to treat chronic constipation and hypercholesterolemia, is having difficulty understanding the difference between soluble and insoluble fiber. Explain the functions of each and name good dietary sources of the two types of fiber.

____

____

____

4. Marcia has a patient on the phone who thinks he may have eaten contaminated food. What questions should Marcia ask to gather more details? What gastrointestinal symptoms occur with food poisoning? What food contaminants are most likely to cause health problems?

____

____

____

____

____

WORKPLACE APPLICATIONS

1. Marcia is gathering material for a patient education brochure describing the importance of fiber consumption. What is the function of fiber in the diet? Include the difference between soluble and insoluble fiber. What is the daily dietary recommendation for fiber intake? Create a list of foods high in fiber for Marcia to include in her brochure.

2. Marcia has been asked to assist the physician with research for a journal article, "The Importance of Antioxidants." Prepare a list of foods high in antioxidants to be included in the article.

3. The internal medicine clinic where Marcia works frequently sees patients with hypertension. The recommended treatment for lowering blood pressure is the Dietary Approaches to Stop Hypertension (DASH) diet. Describe the guidelines included in the DASH diet.

4. Obesity is at epidemic proportions in the United States. The practice where Marcia works is considering starting an obesity support program, which will include patients who are planning on or who have recently undergone bariatric surgery. Summarize the facts about obesity in the United States, the relationship to the BMI, and the facts about bariatric procedures that Marcia must understand to provide care for this patient population.

INTERNET ACTIVITIES

1. The "5 A Day for Better Health" Program is one of the nation's largest initiatives for nutrition. The goal of the program is to increase the national fruit and vegetable consumption to five per day by 2010. Visit the program's Web site at *www.5aday.org*. Why is the consumption of fruits and vegetables so important? Keep a food diary for 1 week. Have you met the goal of "5 A Day"? If not, how do you plan to add more fruits and vegetables to your diet?

2. Visit *www.mypyramid.gov*. Go to the "My Pyramid Plan" and insert your age, gender, and level of physical activity. View and print your personalized pyramid to answer the following questions.

   a. The results are based on a calorie pattern of how many calories?

   b. What is the recommended amount of grains?

   c. What tips do you find will enable you to fulfill these requirements?

   d. What is your daily recommendation for physical activity?

   e. Do your current eating habits support the results found on your personalized pyramid?

   f. What areas in your own diet need modification?

Copyright © 2011, 2007, 2003 by Saunders, an imprint of Elsevier Inc. All rights reserved.

MEDICAL RECORD ACTIVITIES

Document the following scenarios in the progress notes section of the medical record using POMR practices.

1. Suzie's recent blood work results show an LDL of 176 mg/dL and a total cholesterol of 256 mg/dL. Suzie does not seem concerned with these results and wonders why the physician wants her to follow a low-cholesterol diet. What can Marcia tell Suzie about the risks of hyperlipidemia? What are the recommended ranges for total cholesterol and LDL? Document the teaching intervention in the patient's medical record.

___

___

___

2. Ms. Lily Lu is a new patient in the practice who was recently diagnosed with hypertension and hypercholesterolemia. What culturally sensitive suggestions could Marcia make about choosing foods low in sodium and fat? Document the teaching intervention in the patient's medical record.

___

___

___

3. Tony Madaloni is a 67-year-old patient who must lose weight and restrict salt intake to lower his disease risk. What might be some of the reasons Mr. Madaloni chooses the foods he does? What suggestions could Marcia make about changes in eating habits? Document the teaching intervention in the patient's medical record.

___

___

___

4. Ajah Simone is a 22-year-old pregnant patient who is a vegan. The physician asks Marcia to reinforce his discussion on eating foods that provide a nutritionally balanced approach to incomplete proteins. What food combinations could Marcia suggest to Ms. Simone? Include this in the patient's medical record. ___

___

___

Copyright © 2011, 2007, 2003 by Saunders, an imprint of Elsevier Inc. All rights reserved.

31 Vital Signs

VOCABULARY REVIEW

Define the following medical terms.

1. apnea

____

2. arrhythmia

____

3. bradycardia

____

4. bradypnea

____

5. dyspnea

____

6. febrile

____

7. hyperlipidemia

____

8. hypertension

____

9. hyperventilation

____

10. hypotension

____

11. orthopnea

____

12. rales

____

13. rhonchi

____

14. syncope

____

Copyright © 2011, 2007, 2003 by Saunders, an imprint of Elsevier Inc. All rights reserved.

15. tachycardia

____

16. tachypnea

____

17. vertigo

____

SKILLS AND CONCEPTS

Part I: Short Answers

1. The four cardinal vital signs are:

   a. ______________________________

   b. ______________________________

   c. ______________________________

   d. ______________________________

2. Anthropometric measurements include:

   a. ______________________________

   b. ______________________________

   c. ______________________________

   d. ______________________________ and ______________________________

Part II: True or False

Indicate which statements are true (T) and which are false (F).

1. ________ A change in one or more of the patient's vital signs may indicate a change in general health.
2. ________ Sometimes vital sign measurements must be obtained a second time, after the patient is calmer or more comfortable.
3. ________ Body temperature is regulated by the hypothalamus.
4. ________ Body temperature ranges from being highest in the morning to being lowest in the late afternoon.
5. ________ Patients with a febrile condition exhibit pyrexia and can be treated with an antipyretic.
6. ________ An individual with hypertension may have a bounding pulse.
7. ________ A contraindication for taking a temporal artery temperature is bilateral impacted cerumen.
8. ________ Primary or essential hypertension is idiopathic.
9. ________ The difference between tachypnea and hyperpnea is that respirations are rapid and shallow with hyperpnea.
10. ________ A patient with orthostatic hypotension experiences a rapid drop in blood pressure when she stands too quickly.
11. ________ Otitis externa is known as "swimmer's ear."
12. ________ Frequent spirometer studies will be ordered for a patient diagnosed with COPD to determine the person's breathing capabilities.
13. ________ Individuals with advanced kidney disease always develop secondary hypertension.

Copyright © 2011, 2007, 2003 by Saunders, an imprint of Elsevier Inc. All rights reserved.

Part III: Temperatures

Use the correct terms to fill in the blanks.

1. A(n) ________________ fever rises and falls only slightly during a 24-hour period. It remains above the patient's average normal range.
2. A(n) ________________ fever comes and goes, or it spikes and then returns to the average range.
3. A(n) ________________ fever fluctuates greatly (more than 3° F) but does not return to the average range.
4. ________________ temperatures are approximately 1° F (0.6° C) lower than accurate oral readings.
5. ________________ thermometers are an accurate means of taking temperatures in adults and older children because of the closeness to the hypothalamus.
6. ________________ temperatures are an easy, noninvasive, and accurate alternative to taking rectal temperatures in infants.
7. Medication to reduce a fever is called a(an) ________________________________.
8. Tympanic thermometers should not be used if the patient has ________________ or ________________.
9. ________________ should not be used in a healthcare setting, because they are not as accurate as other methods.
10. Temperatures considered febrile include:
    a. Aural (ear) temperatures higher than ________________ ° F (38° C)
    b. Oral temperatures higher than ________________ ° F (37.5° C)
    c. Axillary temperatures higher than ________________ ° F (37° C)
11. Use the following formulas to convert the temperatures in the chart from one system to the other.

$$°C = (°F - 32) \times 5/9$$
$$°F = (°C \times 9/5) + 32$$

a. 98.6° F = ________________ ° C	f. 36° C = ________________ ° F
b. 37° C = ________________ ° F	g. 42° C = ________________ ° F
c. 97.6° F = ________________ ° C	h. 42° C = ________________ ° F
d. 99.4° F = ________________ ° C	i. 102° F = ________________ ° C
e. 43° C = ________________ ° F	j. 41° C = ________________ ° F

12. List and describe three factors that may affect body temperature.
    a. ____
    b. ____
    c. ____

Copyright © 2011, 2007, 2003 by Saunders, an imprint of Elsevier Inc. All rights reserved.

Part IV: Pulse

1. List eight pulse sites and label their correct locations on the figure below.

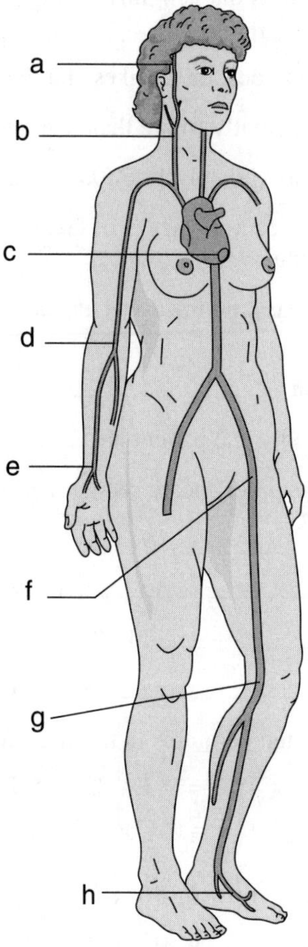

a. ______________________________

b. ______________________________

c. ______________________________

d. ______________________________

e. ______________________________

f. ______________________________

g. ______________________________

h. ______________________________

2. What three characteristics should the medical assistant note while measuring a pulse?

a. ______________________________

b. ______________________________

c. ______________________________

3. A patient with a significant difference between the apical and brachial pulse counts has a(n) ______________.

4. A well-conditioned athlete may have a pulse rate below 60 beats per minute. The medical term for this is ______________.

Copyright © 2011, 2007, 2003 by Saunders, an imprint of Elsevier Inc. All rights reserved.

5. A patient who is anxious or in pain may have an increase in the pulse rate, which is called ________________.
6. The brachial pulse, which is palpated before the blood pressure is taken, is located in the ________________ of the elbow.
7. When the heart rate varies with respirations, this is known as ________________.
8. The ________________ pulse is the most accurate method of taking the pulse of infants and of patients with an arrhythmia.
9. Pedal and popliteal pulses may be checked with a sonogram device called a(n) ________________.

Part V: Respirations

Complete the following sentences with the correct terms.

1. One full respiration includes both ________________ and ________________.
2. The exchange of oxygen and carbon dioxide in the lungs is called ________________.
3. Carlos counts eight respirations for 30 seconds. The rate is ________________ per minute.
4. A bluish discoloration of the skin caused by increased CO_2 buildup is called ________________.
5. Breathing rates are controlled by the respiratory center, which is located in the ________________ of the brain.
6. Patients typically have a ratio of ________________ pulse beat(s) to ________________ respiration(s).
7. List the three characteristics of respirations.

   a. ____

   b. ____

   c. ____

Part VI: Blood Pressure

Complete the sentences with the correct terms.

1. Blood pressure is a reflection of the pressure of the blood against the walls of the ________________.
2. The difference between the systolic and diastolic pressures is the ________________.
3. Blood pressure is recorded as a fraction; the ________________ reading is the numerator (top number) and the ________________ reading is the denominator (bottom number).
4. ________________ is the amount of blood in the arteries.
5. A(n) ________________ is the instrument used to measure the pressure of blood in the arteries.
6. ________________ is the contraction of the heart.
7. ________________ describes the relaxation of the heart.
8. Complete the following table.

Blood Pressure	Normal	Prehypertension	Hypertension
Systolic (mm Hg)	Less than	120-139	
Diastolic (mm Hg)	Less than		90 or higher

9. Describe some common signs and symptoms of hypertension.

____

____

____

Copyright © 2011, 2007, 2003 by Saunders, an imprint of Elsevier Inc. All rights reserved.

10. Summarize the American Heart Association's recommendations for the prevention and treatment of hypertension.

a. ____

____

b. ____

____

c. ____

____

d. ____

____

11. List and define the five Korotkoff phases.

a. ____

____

b. ____

____

c. ____

____

d. ____

____

e. ____

____

12. The systolic pressure may be checked by the ________________ method if the medical assistant is unable to auscultate the patient's blood pressure.

13. Explain four common causes of errors in blood pressure readings.

a. ____

b. ____

c. ____

d. ____

Part VII: Anthropometric Measurements

1. Use the following formulas to convert the weights in the chart from one system to the other.

$$1\,\text{kg} = 2.2\,\text{lb}$$
$$1\,\text{lb} = 0.45\,\text{kg}$$

a. 145 lb = ________ kg

b. 54 kg = ________ lb

c. 60 kg = ________ lb

d. 112 lb = ________ kg

e. 50 lb = ________ kg

Copyright © 2011, 2007, 2003 by Saunders, an imprint of Elsevier Inc. All rights reserved.

WORKPLACE APPLICATIONS

1. Mrs. Parker has just arrived at the office. She states that she is on her way home from work and would like to have her blood pressure checked. Should Carlos take her blood pressure right away? If he should wait, why and for how long?

____

____

____

 a. Carlos has obtained a BP reading of 150/94 mm Hg in the left arm and 160/98 mm Hg in the right arm. Concerned about the readings, Carlos decides the patient should see the physician. What type of questions might Carlos want to ask Mrs. Parker?

 ____

 ____

 ____

 b. Document the finding using the SOAPE format.

 S: _______________

 O: _______________

2. Sarah, an 18-month old patient, is being seen today for a possible ear infection. What would be the best method of taking her temperature? _______________. Her mother is concerned, because Sarah's temperature has been fluctuating between normal and high levels for 2 days; this is called a(n) _______________ fever. Carlos should take Sarah's pulse using the _______________ method. Dr. Xu recommends that Sarah's mother give her Tylenol to relieve her fever. Tylenol is classified as a(n) _______________ drug. Sarah's mother does not have a tympanic thermometer at home, so what would be the best method she could use to take the baby's temperature and why?

____

What patient education should Carlos give Sarah's mother about taking axillary temperatures accurately?

____

3. Carlos is responsible for training a new medical assistant in the OSHA guidelines for preventing disease transmission when taking vital signs. What important factors should Carlos include?

____

____

____

INTERNET ACTIVITIES

Visit *http://americanheart.org*. Under "Disease Conditions" find "High Blood Pressure." Using the "Health Risk Calculator," evaluate your risk of developing hypertension. You will need a current blood pressure reading, so work with a partner to measure your most recent blood pressure. Are you at risk? What type of lifestyle changes should you consider to avoid increasing your risk?

Copyright © 2011, 2007, 2003 by Saunders, an imprint of Elsevier Inc. All rights reserved.

MEDICAL RECORD ACTIVITIES

Vital signs are documented with temperature (T) first, pulse (P) second, and respirations (R) last; the blood pressure is recorded after the TPR. Correctly document the following information. Date and sign each entry as you would on a patient record.

1. Oral temperature of 98.7, apical pulse of 60, respirations 22, and orthostatic blood pressure of 152/98 supine and 114/76 standing.

   ____

   ____

2. Tympanic temperature of 96.8, radial pulse of 86, respirations 18, and bilateral blood pressure of 132/76 in the left arm and 128/80 in the right arm with a BMI of 29.

   ____

   ____

3. Aural temperature of 101.2, pulse of 100 and irregular, respirations 20, and blood pressure of 126/70.

   ____

   ____

4. Axillary temperature of 97.5, apical pulse of 98, respirations 24, and palpated blood pressure of 62.

   ____

   ____

5. Temporal artery temperature of 102.6, respirations 24, and apical pulse 98.

   ____

   ____

Copyright © 2011, 2007, 2003 by Saunders, an imprint of Elsevier Inc. All rights reserved.

32 Assisting with the Primary Physical Examination

VOCABULARY REVIEW

Match the following terms with their definitions.

1. ________ Bruit	a. Abnormal sound or murmur heard on auscultation
2. ________ Gait	b. White part of the eye
3. ________ Intercellular	c. Movement of the body by applied force
4. ________ Mastication	d. Physical injury caused by violence
5. ________ Trauma	e. Style of walking
6. ________ Sclera	f. Chewing
7. ________ Manipulation	g. Rhythmic contraction of involuntary GI muscles
8. ________ Peristalsis	h. Pertaining to the area between cells

Use the appropriate vocabulary word to complete each sentence.

1. The physician uses ________________ to assess the sinuses.
2. A patient with advanced heart or lung disease may develop ________________ because of a lack of oxygen to the tissues.
3. A faulty heart valve creates a(n) ________________.
4. A(n) ________________ is a small lump, lesion, or swelling felt when the skin is palpated.
5. A(n) ________________ is an abnormal sound auscultated over a blood vessel.
6. The process of ________________ creates blood cells in the bone marrow.
7. The lumen size of an artery decreases in size when ________________ occurs.
8. In a(an) ________________ procedure, the physician uses a fiberoptic instrument to view the inside of the large intestine.

SKILLS AND CONCEPTS

Part I: Short Answers

1. Histology is the study of tissues. Explain the four types of tissue in the human body.

   a. ____

   ____

   b. ____

   ____

   c. ____

   ____

Copyright © 2011, 2007, 2003 by Saunders, an imprint of Elsevier Inc. All rights reserved.

d. ______________________________

____

2. Describe the structural organization of the human body.

____

____

____

3. Identify three responsibilities of the medical assistant in room preparation.

a. ______________________________

b. ______________________________

c. ______________________________

4. Explain three responsibilities of the medical assistant in patient preparation.

a. ______________________________

b. ______________________________

c. ______________________________

5. Detail three responsibilities of the medical assistant in assisting the physician.

a. ______________________________

b. ______________________________

c. ______________________________

Part II: Assessment

Describe the following methods of assessment.

1. Inspection

____

____

2. Palpation

____

____

3. Percussion

____

____

4. Auscultation

____

____

5. Mensuration

____

____

Copyright © 2011, 2007, 2003 by Saunders, an imprint of Elsevier Inc. All rights reserved.

6. Manipulation

7. Summarize the major guidelines for proper body mechanics.

8. Outline the principles of safe lifting techniques.

9. Describe how to transfer a patient safely from a wheelchair to the examination table.

10. Describe the typical physical examination sequence.

11. Complete the following table, which outlines the organization of body systems.

Body System	Cells, Organs, and Structures	Functions
Blood	Arteries, arterioles, veins, venules, white blood cells, red blood cells, platelets, plasma	
Cardiovascular	Heart, valves, arteries, arterioles, veins, venules	
Endocrine	Pituitary, pineal, hypothalamus, thyroid, pancreas, adrenal cortex and medulla, parathyroid, thymus, ovaries, testes	
Integumentary	Skin, subcutaneous tissue, sweat and sebaceous glands, hair, nails, sense receptors	
Gastrointestinal	Mouth, tongue, teeth, pharynx, esophagus, stomach, small intestine, large intestine, liver, gallbladder, pancreas, appendix	
Lymphatic and immune	Lymph, lymph vessels, lymph nodes, thymus, tonsils, spleen, lymphocytes, antibodies	
Musculoskeletal	Bones, joints, muscles, tendons, ligaments, cartilage	

Copyright © 2011, 2007, 2003 by Saunders, an imprint of Elsevier Inc. All rights reserved.

Nervous	Brain, spinal cord, neurons, neuroglial cells, peripheral nerves, autonomic nerves	
Reproductive	*Female:* Estrogen and progesterone, ovum, ovaries, fallopian tubes, uterus, vagina, vulva, mammary glands *Male:* Testosterone, sperm, epididymis, vas deferens, prostate gland, testes, scrotum, penis, urethra	
Respiratory	Nose, sinuses, pharynx, larynx, trachea, bronchi, lungs, bronchioles, alveoli	
Sensory	Eyes, ears, taste buds, olfactory receptors, sensory receptors	
Urinary	Nephron unit, bilateral kidneys, ureters, urinary bladder, urethra	

CASE STUDIES

1. The first patient of the day is coming in for a complete physical examination; she has a suspicious breast mass. What type of equipment should the medical assistant prepare in the examination room? What method of gowning and positioning of the patient should be used?

____

____

____

____

2. Joan comes to the office today complaining of lumbar spine pain. Discuss how the patient should be gowned and positioned.

____

____

____

____

3. An adult patient complains of chest congestion, fever, and cough that have lasted for 3 days. What vital signs should be measured? Describe the gowning and positioning of the patient.

____

____

____

____

WORKPLACE APPLICATIONS

How can the medical assistant ensure patient privacy while preparing the patient for the physical examination?

____

____

____

Copyright © 2011, 2007, 2003 by Saunders, an imprint of Elsevier Inc. All rights reserved.

Identify the instruments needed for the physical examination that are shown in the following figures.

1. ______________________________

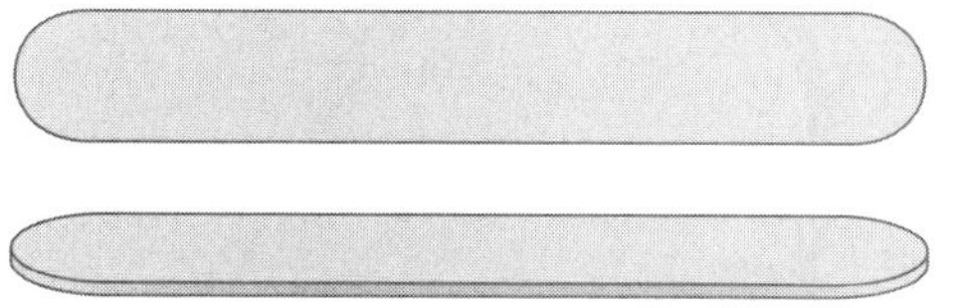

2. ______________________________

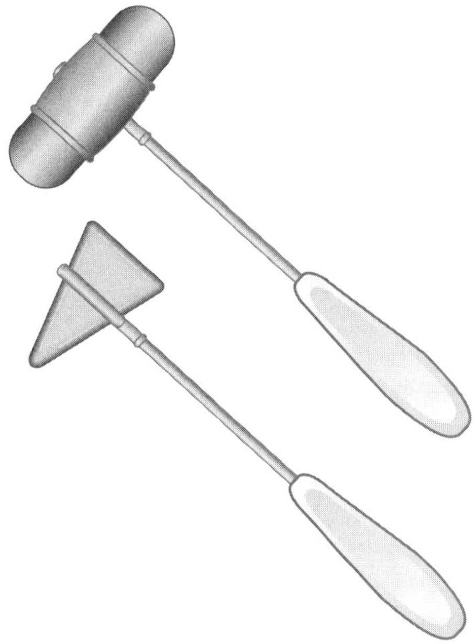

3. ______________________________

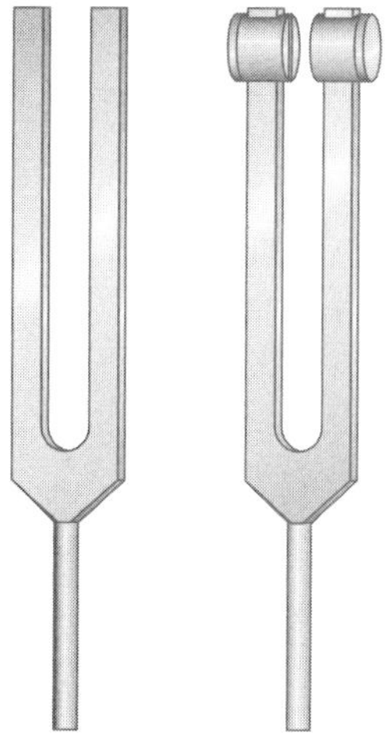

Copyright © 2011, 2007, 2003 by Saunders, an imprint of Elsevier Inc. All rights reserved.

4. ____

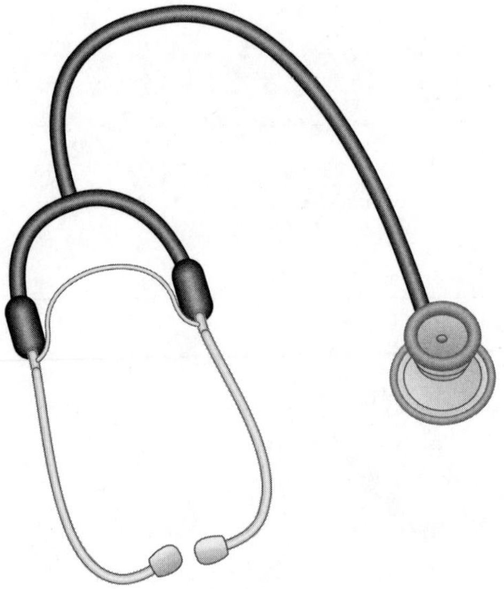

5. ____

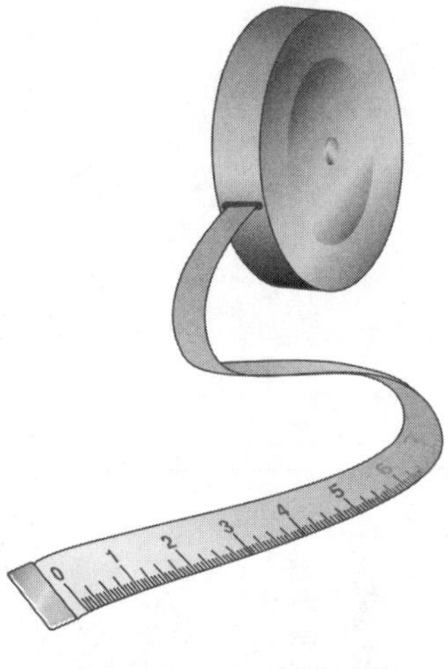

Copyright © 2011, 2007, 2003 by Saunders, an imprint of Elsevier Inc. All rights reserved.

6. ______________________________

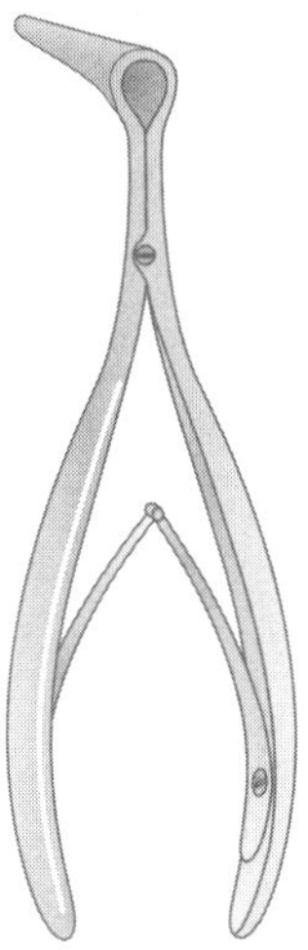

7. ______________________________

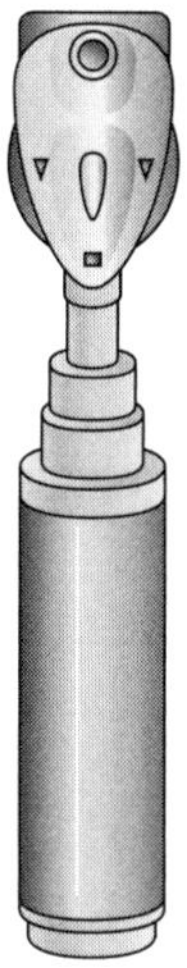

8. ______________________________

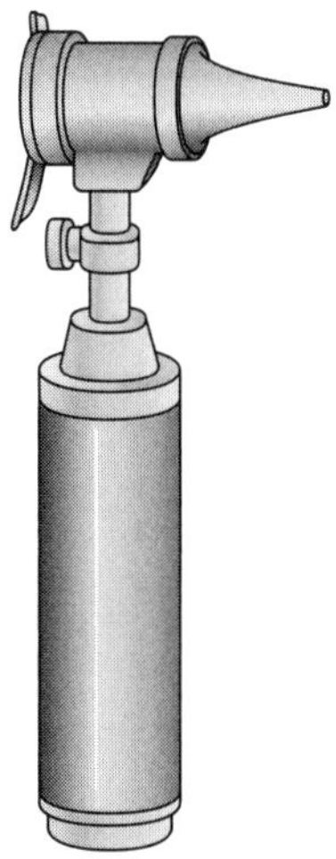

Copyright © 2011, 2007, 2003 by Saunders, an imprint of Elsevier Inc. All rights reserved.

Label each position for examination shown in the following figures.

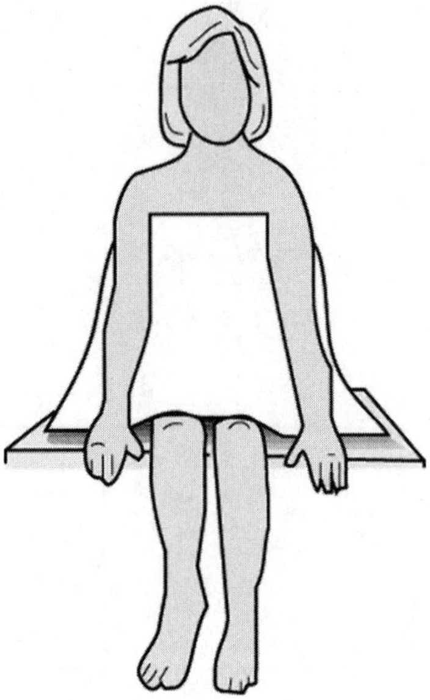

1. ____

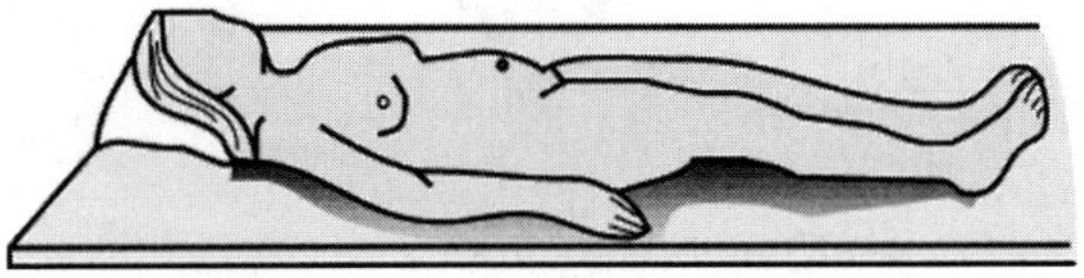

2. ____

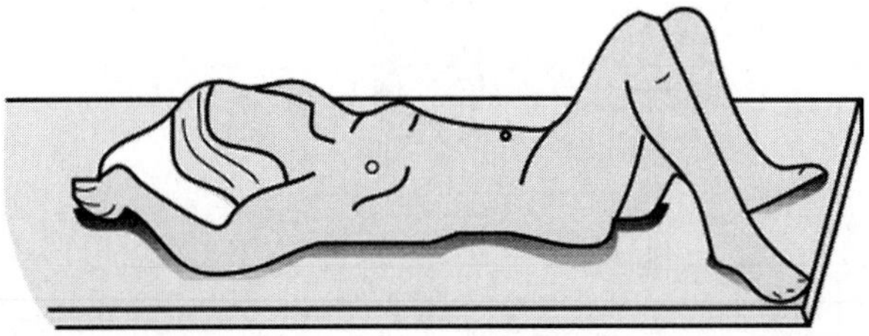

3. ____

Copyright © 2011, 2007, 2003 by Saunders, an imprint of Elsevier Inc. All rights reserved.

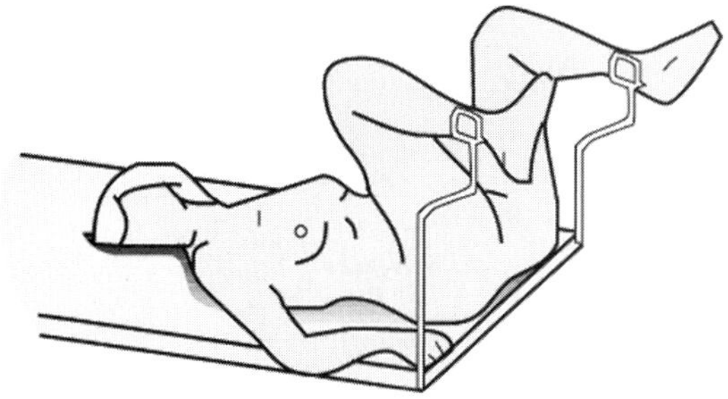

4. ______________________________

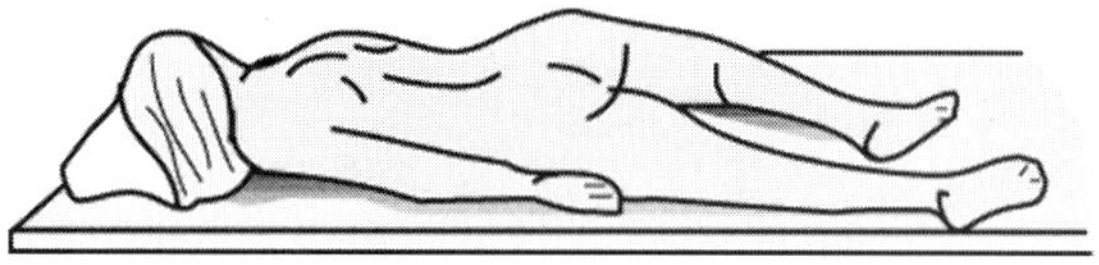

5. ______________________________

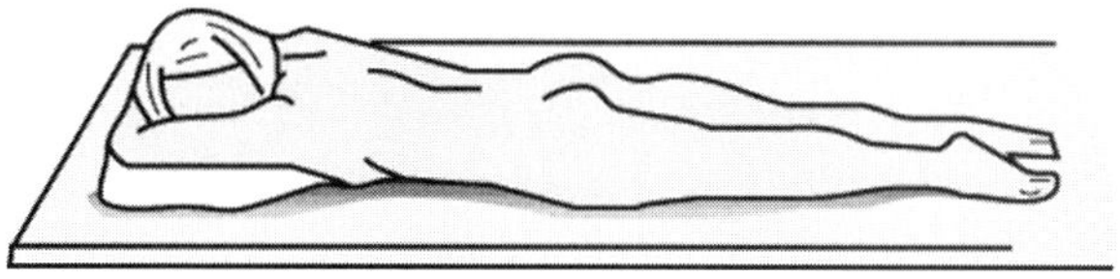

6. ______________________________

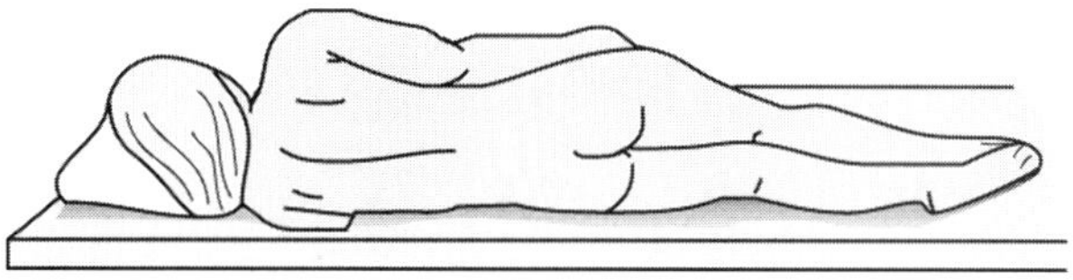

7. ______________________________

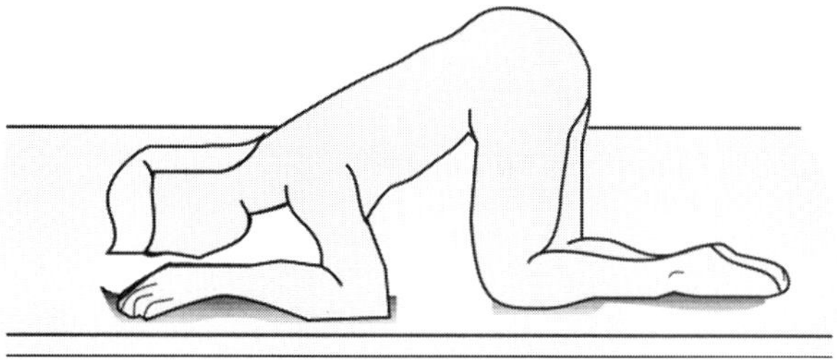

8. ______________________________

Copyright © 2011, 2007, 2003 by Saunders, an imprint of Elsevier Inc. All rights reserved.

33 Principles of Pharmacology

VOCABULARY REVIEW

Define the following medical terms.

1. angina pectoris

___

2. bronchodilator

___

3. cirrhosis

___

4. hypercholesterolemia

___

5. metabolic alkalosis

___

6. spermicide

___

7. therapeutic range

___

8. benefit-to-risk ratio

___

9. Controlled Substance Act

___

10. physical drug dependency

___

11. habituation

___

12. chemical name

___

Copyright © 2011, 2007, 2003 by Saunders, an imprint of Elsevier Inc. All rights reserved.

13. trade name

14. PDR

15. USP

16. systemic effect

17. subscription

18. inscription

19. signature

20. superscription

21. antagonism

22. synergism

23. potentiation

24. sublingual

25. intrathecal injection

26. diurnal rhythms

Copyright © 2011, 2007, 2003 by Saunders, an imprint of Elsevier Inc. All rights reserved.

Match the following definitions with the correct terms.

1. _______ Drugs used to treat and cure a disorder; for example, antibiotics cure bacterial infections
2. _______ Drugs that do not cure a disorder but relieve pain or symptoms related to the condition; for example, use of an antihistamine for allergic symptoms
3. _______ Drugs that prevent the occurrence of a condition; for example, vaccines prevent the occurrence of specific infectious diseases
4. _______ Drugs that help determine the cause of a particular health problem; for example, injection of antigen serum for allergy testing
5. _______ Drugs that provide substances the body needs to maintain health; for example, estrogen replacement therapy for menopausal women and administration of insulin to patients with diabetes
6. _______ Medications sold without prescription
7. _______ Drugs that are not protected by trademark
8. _______ Pertaining to a gluelike substance
9. _______ Denoting any medication route other than the gastrointestinal route
10. _______ Space within a vessel or tube
11. _______ Drug formulation in which tablets are coated with a special compound that does not dissolve until the tablet is exposed to the fluids of the small intestine.

a. Prophylactic
b. Therapeutic
c. Replacement
d. Palliative
e. Diagnostic
f. Parenteral
g. Colloidal
h. Generic
i. Enteric-coated
j. Over the counter
k. Lumen

SKILLS AND CONCEPTS

For each of the following terms, define the type of drug action and the typical side effects; then give an example of that type of drug.

1. Analgesic

____

____

2. Anesthetic

____

____

3. Antibiotic

____

____

4. Antidepressant

____

____

5. Antihistamine

____

____

Copyright © 2011, 2007, 2003 by Saunders, an imprint of Elsevier Inc. All rights reserved.

6. Antihypertensive

7. Antiinflammatory

8. Antimigraine

9. Antipruritics

10. Antipsychotics

11. Diuretics

12. Hypnotics

13. Lipid-lowering agents

14. Oral hypoglycemics

15. Osteoporosis treatment

16. Anticoagulants

Copyright © 2011, 2007, 2003 by Saunders, an imprint of Elsevier Inc. All rights reserved.

17. Antifungals

____

____

Fill in the blank with DEA, FDA, or FTC.

18. The ________________ regulates over-the-counter drug advertising.
19. The ________________, a division of the Department of Health and Human Services, was created in 1936 to regulate the development and sale of all prescription and over-the-counter drugs.
20. The ________________ was established in 1973 as part of the Department of Justice to enforce federal laws on the use of illegal drugs.
21. Every medical practice should have a copy of the controlled substances regulations. The medical assistant may obtain this list from a regional office of the ________________.
22. In addition to approving new drugs for the marketplace, the ________________ is also responsible for establishing standards for their purity and strength during the manufacturing process and for ensuring that generic brands are effective and safe.
23. Each physician who prescribes controlled substances or has them on site must register with the ________________ for a Controlled Substance Registration Certificate. The physician receives a specific registration number that must be included on all prescriptions for controlled substances.
24. List five specific guidelines for prescription orders for controlled substances.
    a. ____
    b. ____
    c. ____
    d. ____
    e. ____

Indicate which statements are true (T) and which are false (F).

25. ________ The chemical name represents the drug's exact formula.
26. ________ The generic drug name is assigned by the manufacturer and is protected by copyright.
27. ________ Brand names are capitalized.
28. ________ The PDR is the most commonly used drug reference book.
29. ________ A prescription is an order written by the physician for the compounding or dispensing and administration of drugs to a particular patient.
30. List six of the factors that can affect a drug's action.
    a. ____
    b. ____
    c. ____
    d. ____
    e. ____
    f. ____
31. Explain the difference between an antitussive medication and an expectorant.

____

____

____

Copyright © 2011, 2007, 2003 by Saunders, an imprint of Elsevier Inc. All rights reserved.

32. Complete the following classification of controlled substances table.

Schedule	Guidelines	Drug Examples
	No accepted medical use	
	High potential for abuse	
	Possession of these drugs is illegal.	
II		
	Accepted for medical use	
	Potential for abuse less than for schedule I or II drugs	
	May cause moderate to low physical dependence or high psychological dependence	
IV	Accepted for medical use	
	Low potential for abuse	
	May cause limited physical or psychological dependence	
		Cough medicines containing codeine, kaolin and pectin belladonna, Donnagel, Lomotil, buprenorphine

33. Complete the following pregnancy risk categories table.

Category of Risk	Category Description
A	
B	
C	
	Proven risk of fetal harm Human studies show proof of fetal damage ____________

34. Summarize the Joint Commission's (formerly JCAHO) "Do not Use" abbreviations list.

____

____

____

35. Choose five of the top 10 frequently prescribed medications shown in Table 33-5. Using a PDR, create medication cards for each, including the following information:

Indications

Precautions

Adverse Reactions

Dosage and Administration

Patient Education Factors

Copyright © 2011, 2007, 2003 by Saunders, an imprint of Elsevier Inc. All rights reserved.

36. Complete the following table of herbal products.

Name	Use	Side Effects and Cautions
Black cohosh	To relieve symptoms of menopause and to treat menstrual irregularities	
Echinacea		
	Laxative; to treat hot flashes and breast pain; arthritis; to prevent high cholesterol and cancer	
Garlic		Some evidence indicates garlic can slightly lower blood cholesterol levels and may slow development of atherosclerosis.
		Short-term use can safely relieve pregnancy-related nausea and vomiting. Side effects most often reported are gas, bloating, heartburn, and nausea.
Asian ginseng		
	To treat asthma, bronchitis, fatigue, and tinnitus; to treat Alzheimer's disease and other types of dementia; decrease intermittent claudication; to treat sexual dysfunction and multiple sclerosis	
	To treat arthritis and joint pain	
	To treat sleep disorders	
Saw palmetto		
	Traditionally used to treat mental disorders and nerve pain	

CASE STUDIES

1. The first patient of the day for Martha, the medical assistant, has some prescriptions that need to be refilled. Look up each of the following drugs in the PDR to become familiar with the drug's indications and possible side effects. Then prepare the prescriptions for the physician's signature:
   a. Crestor 10 mg; take one pill daily. Dispense 90 tablets with three refills.
   b. Atenolol 50 mg; take one and a half pills by mouth every morning. Dispense 1-month supply with one refill.
   c. Xanax 0.5 mg; take one to two tablets at bedtime as needed. Dispense 30 tablets with no refills.
   d. OxyContin 20 mg; take one tablet as needed for relief of pain. Dispense 15 tablets.

Copyright © 2011, 2007, 2003 by Saunders, an imprint of Elsevier Inc. All rights reserved.

DEA#: 8543201 John Jones, M.D. Tel: 917-544-8976
108 N. Main St.
City, State

Patient ____________________ DATE __________

ADDRESS ________________________________

Rx:

Disp:

Sig:

Refill _____ Times
Please label ☑ ____________________

DEA#: 8543201 John Jones, M.D. Tel: 917-544-8976
108 N. Main St.
City, State

Patient ____________________ DATE __________

ADDRESS ________________________________

Rx:

Disp:

Sig:

Refill _____ Times
Please label ☑ ____________________

Copyright © 2011, 2007, 2003 by Saunders, an imprint of Elsevier Inc. All rights reserved.

DEA#: 8543201 John Jones, M.D. Tel: 917-544-8976
108 N. Main St.
City, State

Patient ______________________ DATE __________

ADDRESS ____________________________________

Rx:

Disp:

Sig:

Refill _____ Times
Please label ☑ ____________________________

DEA#: 8543201 John Jones, M.D. Tel: 917-544-8976
108 N. Main St.
City, State

Patient ______________________ DATE __________

ADDRESS ____________________________________

Rx:

Disp:

Sig:

Refill _____ Times
Please label ☑ ____________________________

2. The physician has recommended OTC medication for treatment of symptoms of the common cold. What types of things should Martha encourage her patients to do when they are choosing an OTC?

3. What types of medication should the medical assistant consider when obtaining a medical history. What information about these medications should be documented in the patient's chart?

4. Simon Carmacci, age 78, has been prescribed several medications, including Tenormin, Lasix, Lipitor, and Actose. Based on what you have learned about these medications and about the physiologic changes associated with aging, summarize the potential complications of multiple prescriptions for this patient. Should you consider any patient education factors? If so, what are they?

Copyright © 2011, 2007, 2003 by Saunders, an imprint of Elsevier Inc. All rights reserved.

WORKPLACE APPLICATIONS

1. Martha has noticed that the other medical assistants in the office are unsure of the drug classifications for controlled substances. Prepare an educational handout for the office staff to use as a resource. The handout should include the definition of a controlled substance, an explanation of each schedule (I to V), the potential for abuse and/or addiction, and some examples of drugs in each schedule. Note whether the prescription can be written or oral.

2. The route of administration used for a drug depends on the intended use of the drug. What route of administration would Martha expect for each of the illnesses or medications listed below (oral, topical, inhaled, sublingual, mucous membrane, or parenteral route)? Why?

   a. Annual flu vaccination

   ____

   b. Bronchodilator for treatment of an acute asthma attack

   ____

   c. Hyperlipidemia

   ____

   d. Nitroglycerin used for angina

   ____

   e. Dermatitis

   ____

   f. Allergic rhinitis

   ____

   g. Insulin

   ____

   h. Tinea pedis

   ____

   i. Conjunctivitis

   ____

INTERNET ACTIVITIES

1. Search the Internet for articles on prescription drug abuse. What are some steps the medical assistant can take to help prevent the abuse of prescription drugs?

   ____

   ____

   ____

2. Using either the PDR or Rx List online service, look up 10 of the most prescribed medications from Table 33-5. Make medication cards for these drugs. Be prepared to discuss the indication, side effects, typical dosage levels, route of administration, and patient education factors for these drugs.

Copyright © 2011, 2007, 2003 by Saunders, an imprint of Elsevier Inc. All rights reserved.

MEDICAL RECORD ACTIVITIES

1. Mrs. Jones calls the office and states that she wants to discontinue her Diovan 80 mg because she has no prescription coverage. She states, "I feel fine and don't even know why I'm taking this medication!" What patient education can Martha provide to Mrs. Jones to make her understand the importance of continuing her current medication? Is there anything Martha can do to help Mrs. Jones obtain drug coverage? Document your conversation for the physician's review and recommendations.

2. A patient comes to the office today for a refill of Vicodin ES 7.5/500 mg, one pill every 8 hours as needed with food. After checking the medical record, you notice the patient had a prescription written 5 days ago for the same drug and was dispensed 30 pills at that time. Is it too early for this drug to be refilled? Provide your documentation to the physician. What type of information should you include?

Copyright © 2011, 2007, 2003 by Saunders, an imprint of Elsevier Inc. All rights reserved.

34 Pharmacology Math

VOCABULARY REVIEW

Define the following terms.

1. dispense

____

2. stat

____

3. unit dose

____

4. nomogram

____

5. surface area

____

6. route

____

7. numerator

____

8. denominator

____

9. proper fraction

____

10. improper fraction

____

Fill in the blanks with basic drug label terms.

11. The size or amount of the drug available in the drug package is the _______________.
12. _______________ is the potency of the drug.
13. A(n) _______________ is the pure drug that is dissolved in a liquid to form a solution.
14. Usually sterile water or saline, the _______________ is the liquid that dissolves the solute.

Copyright © 2011, 2007, 2003 by Saunders, an imprint of Elsevier Inc. All rights reserved.

SKILLS AND CONCEPTS

1. Explain the difference between proper and improper fractions.

____

____

2 Review the following examples. Identify the proper and improper fractions. If the fraction is improper perform the math to get the whole number equivalent.

$\frac{2}{3}$ ______________________ $\frac{27}{9}$ ______________________

$\frac{14}{7}$ ______________________ $\frac{5}{6}$ ______________________

$\frac{15}{5}$ ______________________ $\frac{19}{20}$ ______________________

3. Reduce the following fractions to their lowest terms.

$\frac{15}{20}$ ______________ $\frac{14}{42}$ ______________ $\frac{120}{180}$ ______________

$\frac{7}{49}$ ______________ $\frac{12}{16}$ ______________ $\frac{4}{36}$ ______________

4. Perform the following calculations and reduce the answers to the lowest terms.

$\frac{2}{3} \times \frac{9}{8} =$

$\frac{7}{9} \div \frac{3}{4} =$

$\frac{12}{14} \times \frac{1}{2} =$

$\frac{5}{12} \div \frac{6}{14} =$

5. Convert the following fractions into decimals.

$\frac{1}{3} =$ ________ $\frac{7}{23} =$ ________ $\frac{16}{84} =$ ________ $\frac{2}{9} =$ ________ $\frac{26}{34} =$ ________

6. The act of dividing a fraction results in a decimal number. Decimal numbers can then be converted to percentages by moving the decimal two spaces to the right, as follows:

0.25 = 25.0%, commonly written 25%

Convert the following decimals to percentages. Show your work in the space to the right of the questions.

0.75 = ________%

0.33 = ________%

0.25 = ________%

1.0 = ________%

0.50 = ________%

Convert the following decimals to percentages.

0.45 = ______ 1.37 = ______ 0.97 = ______ 2.59 = ______ 0.62 = ______ 1.05 = ______

7. A proportion is written as follows:

$\frac{4}{16} = \frac{1}{4}$ or 4:16::1:4

Use cross-multiplication to solve for x. Show your work in the space to the right of the questions.

$3:4 = x:12$
$1:2 = x:6$
$2:5 = x:100$
$2:6 = x:12$
$1:3 = x:75$

Copyright © 2011, 2007, 2003 by Saunders, an imprint of Elsevier Inc. All rights reserved.

Solve for x in the following problems and prove that your answer is correct.

5:4 = x:12 ____________________

3:15 = x:25 ____________________

4:28 = x:84 ____________________

9:x = 5:250 ____________________

100:x = 10:50 ____________________

8. What are the correct doses of the following medications rounded to the nearest tenth?

1.28 mL = ________ 5.76 g = ________ 14.74 mcg = ________ 3.62 mL = ________

0.18 mL = ________ 1.44 (unscored) tabs = ________ 2.11 cc = ________ 0.54 (scored) tab = ________

9. What are the three basic steps the medical assistant must complete for accurate calculation of a prescribed dose?

a. ____________________

b. ____________________

c. ____________________

Part I: Metric System

Consider the following fundamental units of the metric system:

Mass or weight: gram (g) *always lowercase*
Volume: liter (L) *always capitalized*
Length: meter (m) *always lowercase*

Consider the following equivalents:

Mass and Weight	Volume
1 kg = 1,000g	1 kL = 1,000 liters
1 g = 1,000 mg	1 L = 1,000 mL (or cc)
1 mg= 1,000 μg	1 mL (or cc) = 1,000 μL
1 dg = 0.1 g or 1/10 g	1 dL = 0.1 L or 1/10 L
1 cg = 0.01 g or 1/100 g	1 cL = 0.01 L or 1/100 L
1 mg = 0.001 g or 1/1,000 g	1 mL = 0.001 L or 1/1,000 L

Write the prefix for the following (remember to write the prefixes in lowercase).

1. ________ 1/100 of a unit
2. ________ 1/10 of a unit
3. ________ 1/1,000 of a unit
4. ________ 1/1,000,000 of a unit
5. ________ 10 units
6. ________ 100 units
7. ________ 1,000 units

Copyright © 2011, 2007, 2003 by Saunders, an imprint of Elsevier Inc. All rights reserved.

Convert the following by moving the decimals, by multiplication, or by division. Show your work in the space to the right of the questions.

8. 1.5 L = __________ mL
9. 500 mg = __________ g
10. 3 g = __________ mg
11. 2,000 mg = __________ g
12. 2.5 g = __________ mg
13. 0.5 g = __________ mg
14. 500 mL = __________ L
15. 0.75 g = __________ mg
16. 1 kg = __________ g
17. 1,000 mg = __________ g

18. Complete the following abbreviation table.

Apothecary System		Metric System	
Min (M)			gram
	dram		liter
f dr		cc	
	ounce		milliliter
fl oz			
Gr			

Part II: Apothecary System and Household Measurements

1. The basic unit of weight in the apothecary system for a solid measurement is the __________________.
2. The basic unit of volume in the apothecary system for a liquid measurement is __________________.
3. Household measurements are not precisely accurate, so they should never be used in the medical setting.
   a. True
   b. False
4. The household measurement for weight is __________________.
5. In household measurements, liquid oral medications are taken by the drop, teaspoon, or tablespoon and are supplied in bottles labeled in ounces or pints.
   a. True
   b. False
6. Supply the abbreviations or symbols for these metric, apothecary system, and common household units.
   a. ounce __________________
   b. teaspoon __________________
   c. milligram __________________
   d. grain __________________
   e. pint __________________
   f. dram __________________
   g. tablespoon __________________

Copyright © 2011, 2007, 2003 by Saunders, an imprint of Elsevier Inc. All rights reserved.

Use the conversions to complete the questions that follow.

Mass and Weight	Volume
1 cup = 8 oz	1 tsp = 5 mL (cc)
1 oz = 2 Tbsp	1 Tbsp = 15 mL (cc)
1 Tbsp = 3 tsp	1 fl oz = 30 mL (cc)
1 tsp = 60 drops	1 grain = 60 mg

7. A standard teaspoon equals 5 mL. If a liquid drug has 100 mg/teaspoon, how many milligrams are in each milliliter?

____

How did you determine your answer?

____

____

____

8. You are asked to give 2 teaspoons of cough medicine to a child. How many milliliters will you give?

____

9. How many teaspoons are in 1 oz? ____________

10. Now that you know that 5 mL is the same as 1 tsp, how many milliliters are in 1 oz? ____________

11. Complete the following household equivalents table.

60	gtt	=			
3		=	1 T		
180	gtt	=		=	½ oz
	T	=	1 oz	=	6 t (or tsp)
360	gtt	=			
1	oz	=			
	oz	=	1 tsp		
8	oz	=			
2	c	=	1 pt	=	oz
	pt	=	1 qt	=	32 oz
4	c	=	1 qt	=	oz
	qt	=	1 gal	=	128 oz

Part III: Conversion between Systems of Measurement

Conversions between units of measurements can also be done by using the following formula:

$$\text{Have} \times \frac{\text{Wanted}}{\text{Have (conversion)}} = \text{Unit Wanted in New System}$$

Copyright © 2011, 2007, 2003 by Saunders, an imprint of Elsevier Inc. All rights reserved.

Perform the following conversions. The conversion factor is 1 kg = 2.2 lb. Show your work in the space to the right of the questions.

1. 150 lb = ________________ kg
2. 78 lb = ________________ kg
3. 18 kg = ________________ lb
4. 210 lb = ________________ kg
5. 71 kg = ________________ lb
6. 198 lb = ________________ kg
7. 112 lb = ________________ kg
8. 163 lb = ________________ kg
9. 21 kg = ________________ lb
10. 4.4 lb = ________________ kg
11. 6 lb 10 oz = ________________ kg

Convert inches to centimeters. The conversion factor is 2.5 cm/inch. Show your work in the space to the right of the questions.

12. 62 inches = ________________ cm
13. 34 inches = ________________ cm
14. 97 inches = ________________ cm
15. 5′0″ = ________________ inches = ________________ cm
16. 6′2″ = ________________ inches = ________________ cm
17. The following formula provides a method of converting drug orders from the ordered unit of measurement to the label unit:

$$\text{Drug have} \times \frac{\text{Wanted}}{\text{Have}} = \text{Unit Wanted in New System}$$

    Use this formula to convert the following drug orders. Show your work next to the problem.

    30 gr = __________ g

    0.25 gr = __________ mg

    8 fl oz = __________ mL

    12 mL = __________ fl dr

    180 mg = __________ gr

    60 mg = __________ gr

18. The standard formula for calculating dosage is:

$$\frac{\text{Available strength}}{\text{Ordered strength}} = \frac{\text{Available amount}}{\text{Amount to give}}$$

    Using the standard formula, calculate the following dosages. Show your work.

    Physician's order: Bicillin 400,000 units IM; Label: 1,200,000 units per 2 mL

    Physician's order: 75 mg Demerol IM stat; Label: 100 mg per cc

    Physician's order: 200 mcg Vitamin B_{12} SC; Label: 1000 mcg per mL

    Physician order: Amoxicillin solution 250 mg; Label: 0.5 g per 2 cc

Copyright © 2011, 2007, 2003 by Saunders, an imprint of Elsevier Inc. All rights reserved.

19. An alternative formula for calculating drug dosages is: D/H × Q
    - **D**—Desired dose (the physician's order)
    - **H—**What is on hand (the dosage strength listed on the medication label)
    - **Q**—Quantity in the unit (identified on the label as one tablet, 5 mL, and so on)

    Using this formula, calculate the following dosages. Show your work.

    Physician's order: Compazine 12 mg IM. On hand is a 15 mL vial that contains 4 mg/mL.

    Physician's order: Depro-Medrol 25 mg IM. On hand is a 10 mL vial that contains 80 mg/mL.

    Physician's order: 250 mg Amoxil PO. On hand are 500 mg scored tablets.

    Physician's order: 15 mg Coumadin PO. On hand are 7.5 mg tablets.

CASE STUDIES

Calculate the following doses of medication. Remember the following standard formula:

$$\frac{\text{Available strength}}{\text{Ordered strength}} = \frac{\text{Available amount}}{\text{Amount to give}}$$

Physician's Order	Label Reads	Amount to Give	Practice Charting
Keflex 500 mg	250 mg capsule		
Lasix 40 mg	20 mg tablet		
Zoloft 75 mg	25 mg tablet		
Claritin 30 mg	10 mg tablet		
Prilosec 40 mg	10 mg capsule		
Celebrex 200 mg	100 mg capsule		
Vioxx 12.5 mg	25 mg		
Lanoxin 0.125 mg	0.25 mg tablet		
Coumadin 20 mg	5 mg tablet		
Augmentin 250 mg	500 mg per 5 mL		
Prednisone 40 mg	5 mg tablet		
Prozac 20 mg	10 mg capsule		
Synthroid 0.44 mg	88 μg per tablet		
Zocor 60 mg	20 mg tablet		
Glucophage 1 g	500 mg tablet		
Zestril 2.5 mg	5 mg tablet		
Norvasc 10 mg	2.5 mg tablet		
Cipro 750 mg	250 mg tablet		
Zyrtec syrup 4 mg	5 mg/5 mL		
Zovirax 200 mg	400 mg tablet		

Pediatric Dosages

Clark's Rule

Clark's rule is based on the weight of the child. It uses 150 lb (70 kg) as the average adult weight and assumes that the child's dose is proportionately less. The formula is as follows:

$$\text{Pediatric dose} = \frac{\text{Child's weight in pounds}}{150\ \text{lb}} \times \text{Adult dose}$$

Copyright © 2011, 2007, 2003 by Saunders, an imprint of Elsevier Inc. All rights reserved.

Order	Adult Dose	Child's Weight	Amount to Give
Penicillin	100,000 units	22 lb	
Benadryl	50 mg	13 lb	
Tylenol	500 mg	54 lb	
Sudafed	60 mg	37 lb	

West's Nomogram

West's nomogram uses a calculation of the body surface area (BSA) of infants and young children to determine the pediatric dose.

$$\text{Pediatric dose} = \frac{\text{(BSA) of child in m}^2}{1.7\ \text{m}^2\ \text{(average adult BSA)}} \times \text{Adult dose}$$

Order	Adult Dose	Child's BSA	Amount to Give
Penicillin	100,000 U	0.5 m^2	
Benadryl	50 mg	0.3 m^2	
Tylenol	500 mg	0.6 m^2	
Sudafed	60 mg	0.7 m^2	

WORKPLACE APPLICATIONS

Use Clark's rule, West's nomogram, or the body weight method to answer the following questions:

1. A child weighs 42 lb. The physician orders 1 mg of medication per kilogram. How many kilograms does the child weigh? How many milligrams of medication do you need to give?

   ____

2. An infant weighs 14 lb. The adult dose is 100 mg. When Clark's rule is used, how much is the pediatric dose?

   ____

3. The physician orders 5 mg of medication per kilogram of body weight. The patient weighs 145 lb. How many milligrams do you give?

   ____

4. The child has a BSA of 0.9 m^2, and the adult dose is 200 mg. According to West's nomogram, what is the pediatric dose?

   ____

5. The nurse practitioner orders 250 mg of Rocephin to be given by injection. The vial contains Rocephin at a concentration of 500 mg/mL. How much medication will the medical assistant draw into the syringe?

   ____

6. The patient takes 5,000 units of heparin by injection each day. The vial contains heparin, 10,000 units/mL. How much heparin does the home health nurse need to draw up into the syringe?

   ____

7. The patient weighs 163 lb. The order is for 2 mg/kg. How much medicine does the patient need?

   ____

Copyright © 2011, 2007, 2003 by Saunders, an imprint of Elsevier Inc. All rights reserved.

8. The physician orders Phenergan 12.5 mg by mouth. You have Phenergan syrup in a concentration of 25 mg/5 mL. How many milliliters will you give?

____

9. You need to give a 500-unit injection of vitamin B_{12}. You have on hand vitamin B_{12} at a concentration unit of 1,000 units/mL. How much will you measure in the syringe?

____

MEDICAL RECORD ACTIVITIES

Document the following scenarios in the progress notes section of the medical record using POMR practices.

1. An infant who weighs 11 lb is ordered Amoxil q 6 hr. The label reads 250 mg in 5 cc of suspension. The recommended range of the medication for an infant is 15 mg/kg/day. How much should the child receive per dose? Document the administration of this medication.

____

____

____

2. An infant who weighs 12 lb 5 oz is ordered Diflucan qid for the treatment of thrush. The label reads 150 mg in 3 cc of suspension. The recommended range of the medication is 3 mg/kg/day. How much should the child receive per dose? Document the administration of this medication.

____

____

____

3. An infant is ordered Zantac bid. The infant weighs 35 lb. The label reads 300 mg in 5 cc of suspension. The recommended range of the medication is 10 mg/kg/day. How much should the child receive per dose? Document the administration of this medication.

____

____

____

INTERNET ACTIVITY

Use the Internet or a drug reference book to collect information and make index cards for 20 commonly used drugs. Include the following information:

Brand name
Generic name
Type of drug
Usual dose
Uses

Copyright © 2011, 2007, 2003 by Saunders, an imprint of Elsevier Inc. All rights reserved.

35 Administering Medications

VOCABULARY REVIEW

Match the following terms with their definitions.

________ 1.	Angled tip of a needle	a. Bevel
________ 2.	Narrowing of the bronchiole tubes	b. Scored tablet
________ 3.	Abnormal accumulation of fluid in the interstitial spaces of tissues	c. Hypotension
________ 4.	A coating added to an oral medication that resists the effects of stomach juices; designed so that medicine is absorbed in the small intestine	d. Polyuria
________ 5.	Sealed so that no air is allowed to enter	e. Volatile
________ 6.	Low blood pressure	f. Wheal
________ 7.	Administering repeated injections of diluted extracts of the substance that causes an allergy; also called *desensitization*	g. Viscosity
________ 8.	An abnormally hard, inflamed area	h. Vasodilation
________ 9.	Administering a double dose for the first dose of the medication; usually done with antibiotic therapy to reach therapeutic blood levels quickly	i. Immunotherapy
________ 10.	Inflammation of a vein; may lead to thrombus formation	j. Loading dose
________ 11.	The curved formation of liquids in a container	k. Edema
________ 12.	Excretion of an unusually large amount of urine	l. Meniscus
________ 13.	Drug in pill form manufactured with an indentation for division through the center	m. Bronchoconstriction
________ 14.	Increase in the diameter of a blood vessel	n. Induration
________ 15.	The quality of being thick; property of resistance to flow in a fluid	o. Enteric coated
________ 16.	Referring to an explosive substance's capacity to vaporize at a low temperature	p. Phlebitis
________ 17.	Localized area of edema or a raised lesion	q. Hermetically sealed

Solid Oral Forms

Define the following terms.

1. scored

____

2. tablet

____

3. buffered

____

Copyright © 2011, 2007, 2003 by Saunders, an imprint of Elsevier Inc. All rights reserved.

4. capsule

5. caplet

6. time released

Liquid Oral Forms

Define the following terms.

1. syrup

2. aromatic waters

3. liquors

4. suspension

5. emulsion

6. gel or magma

7. tinctures

8. elixirs

Mucous Membrane Forms

List the site of absorption indicated by the following terms.

1. buccal

2. sublingual

3. inhalation

Copyright © 2011, 2007, 2003 by Saunders, an imprint of Elsevier Inc. All rights reserved.

Topical Forms

Describe or define the following.

1. lotion

____

2 liniment

____

3. ointment

____

4. transdermal

____

Parenteral Forms

Define or describe the following.

1. vial

____

2. ampule

____

3. multiuse

____

4. prefilled

____

5. cartridge system

____

SKILLS AND CONCEPTS

1. List and explain the seven rights of drug administration.

   a. _______________

   b. _______________

   c. _______________

   d. _______________

Copyright © 2011, 2007, 2003 by Saunders, an imprint of Elsevier Inc. All rights reserved.

e. ______________________________

____

f. ______________________________

____

g. ______________________________

____

2. When should the medical assistant check the drug label?

____

____

____

3. List four things the medical assistant can do to ensure safety of medication administration.

a. ______________________________

b. ______________________________

c. ______________________________

d. ______________________________

Label the following statements as either "ampule" or "vial."

4. Has a rubber stopper ______________________________
5. Has sharp edges after it is opened ______________________________
6. Is always single use ______________________________
7. Air must be injected into it before medicine can be removed ______________________________
8. Can be multiuse ______________________________
9. A filtered needle is required to avoid getting glass in the syringe ______________________________
10. Has a vacuum after it is opened ______________________________
11. Extra care is required to prevent contamination ______________________________
12. Always discarded in a sharps container ______________________________
13. Gauze or an unopened alcohol prep should be used to prevent injury as the neck breaks away ______________________________
14. List four routes of parenteral administration; include approved abbreviations and how to locate the sites anatomically.

a. ______________________________

b. ______________________________

c. ______________________________

d. ______________________________

Parenteral Medication Equipment

Indicate which statements about needles are true (T) and which are false (F).

1. ________ Needles may be purchased separately or as part of a needle-syringe unit.
2. ________ The diameter or lumen size of a needle is called its *gauge*.
3. ________ The larger the gauge number, the smaller the diameter of the needle.

Copyright © 2011, 2007, 2003 by Saunders, an imprint of Elsevier Inc. All rights reserved.

4. ________ Gauges 25 and 26 are commonly used for subcutaneous injections.

5. ________ Gauges 20 to 23 usually are necessary for intramuscular injections when the medication is thick (e.g., penicillin).

6. ________ Needles that are ½- or ⅝-inch long are used for intramuscular injections.

7. ________ Needles that are ½- or ⅝-inch long are used for subcutaneous injections.

8. ________ A contaminated needle should be recapped before disposal in a sharps container.

9. ________ The parts of the needle are the barrel, calibrated scale(s), plunger, and tip.

10. ________ Longer needles are necessary for depositing drugs intradermally.

11. Label the syringes in the figure below.

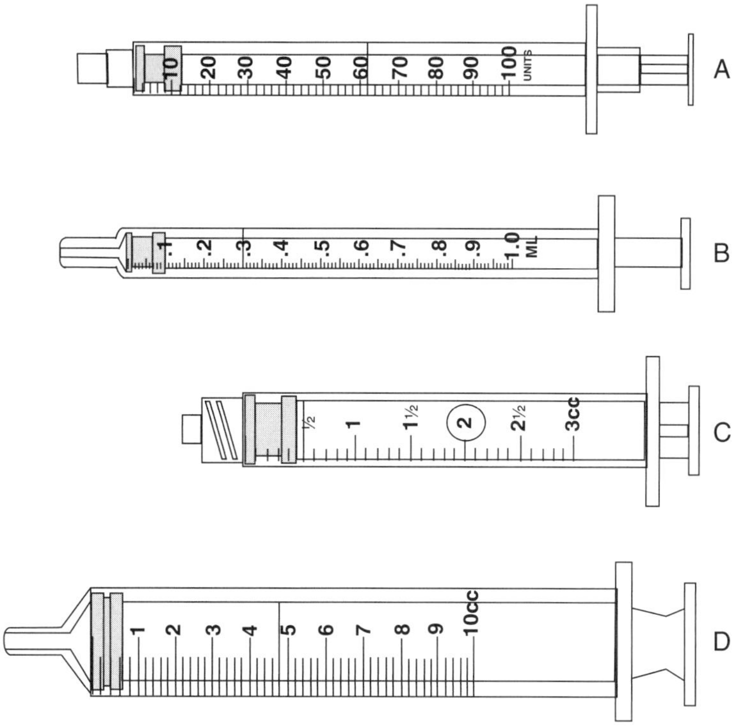

a. On the insulin syringe, draw a line at 62 units.

b. On the tuberculin syringe, draw a line at 0.3 mL.

c. On the 3 cc Luer-Lok syringe, draw a line at ½ cc.

d. On the 10 cc slip-tip syringe, draw a line at 4.8 cc.

e. Insulin syringes can be purchased in 30 U, 50 U, and 100 U sizes. Which is the one pictured?

f. The angle of an insulin injection is ________________, and the angle of injection for an ID administration is ________________.

g. What gauge and length of needle would be used for a TB skin test? ________________ For an insulin injection? ________________ For an IM injection? ________________

h. The 1 mL TB syringe is calibrated at _____ mL per line. The 3 mL syringe is calibrated at ________________ mL per line.

Copyright © 2011, 2007, 2003 by Saunders, an imprint of Elsevier Inc. All rights reserved.

Injection Sites

1. Label the intramuscular, intradermal, and subcutaneous injection sites correctly on the following figure.

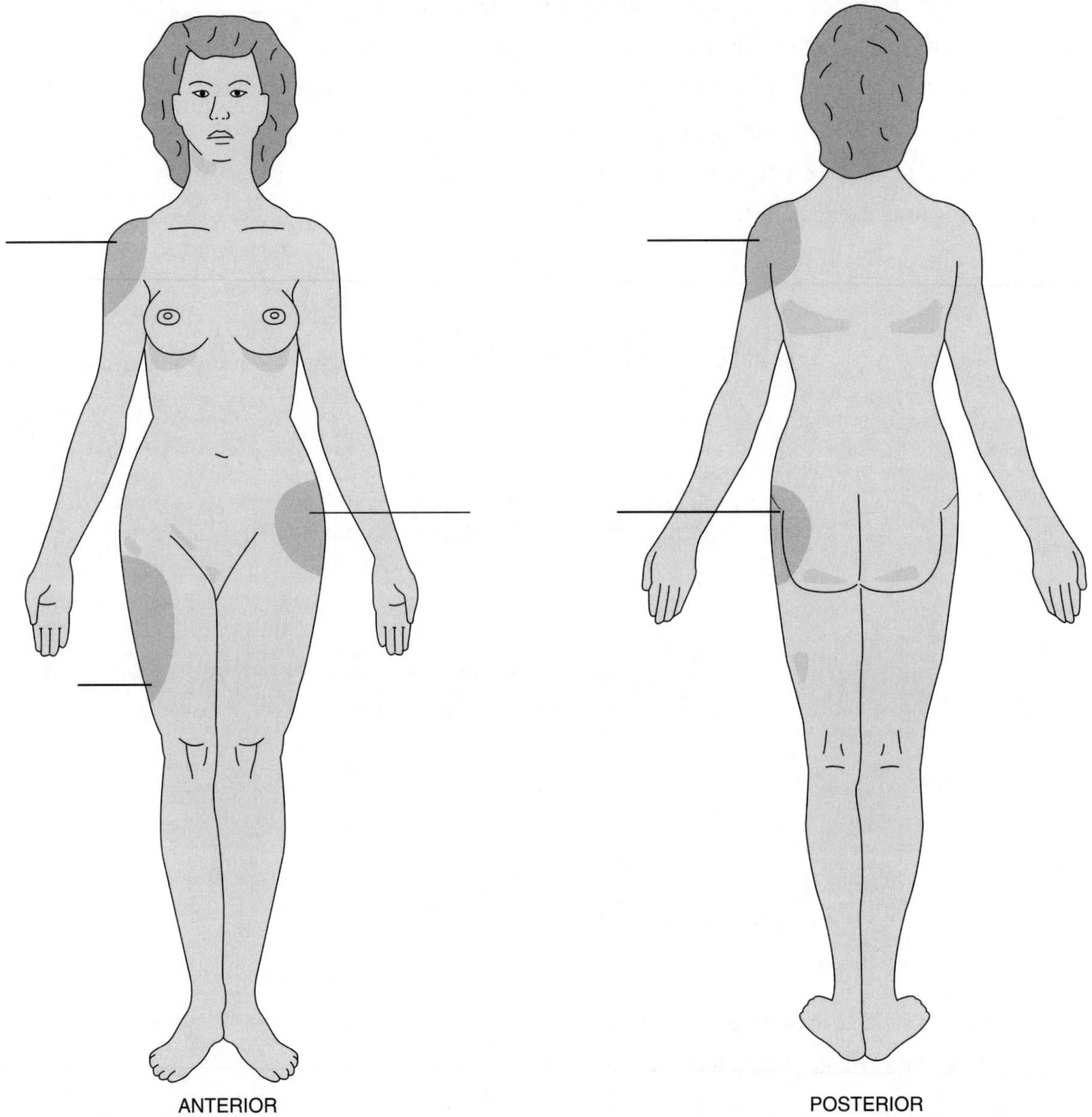

a. Deltoid

b. Ventrogluteal

c. Adult vastus lateralis

d. Gluteal (dorsogluteal)

e. TB skin test

f. Insulin injection site

Copyright © 2011, 2007, 2003 by Saunders, an imprint of Elsevier Inc. All rights reserved.

Pediatric Sites

1. On the following figure, label and name the appropriate IM injection site for a small child who is too young to walk.

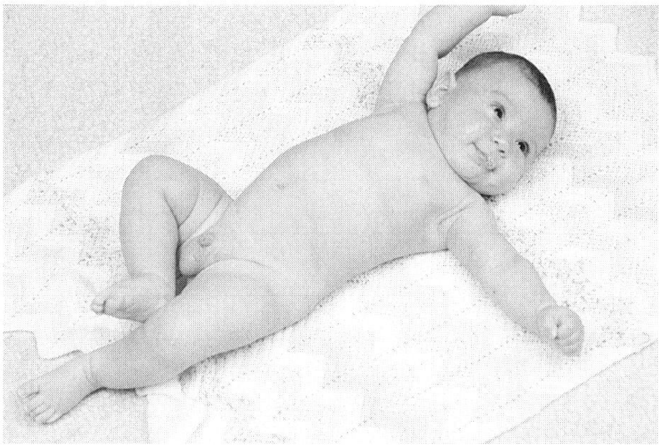

2. Explain why infant IM injections are limited to the vastus lateralis site.

____

____

____

WORKPLACE APPLICATIONS

1. Dorothy, the medical assistant, has been asked by Dr. Thau to update the medication abbreviation list to be included as part of the policy and procedures manual. Use the list below to spell out each.

   a. q 4 hr ____________________
   b. tid ____________________
   c. qid ____________________
   d. bid ____________________
   e. q 3 hr ____________________
   f. HS ____________________
   g. AC ____________________
   h. PC ____________________
   i. PRN ____________________
   j. PO ____________________
   k. NPO ____________________
   l. PR ____________________
   m. IV ____________________
   n. SC (SQ) ____________________
   o. IM ____________________
   p. SL ____________________

Copyright © 2011, 2007, 2003 by Saunders, an imprint of Elsevier Inc. All rights reserved.

q. QD ______________________________

r. QAM ______________________________

s. QPM ______________________________

2. Dorothy is in charge of organizing a newly constructed examination room. The room will be used for medication administration, and Dorothy wants to make sure it is fully equipped. What supplies must Dorothy order to fulfill OSHA guidelines? What are some other items she may want to make sure are in the room to make patients as comfortable as possible?

____

____

____

____

3. Dorothy has been asked to perform a two-step tuberculin skin test on a new employee. Why is this being done? Explain the procedure to the new co-worker.

____

____

____

____

4. Dorothy is responsible for reading and documenting the outcome of a Mantoux test that was administered 2 days ago. Explain the criteria for a positive test result, including the reasons a result may be considered positive even if the induration is less than 15 mm.

____

____

____

____

MEDICAL RECORD ACTIVITIES

1. Dorothy is administering DTaP 0.5 mL intramuscularly to a 5-year-old patient. What site should she use? Document the procedure.

2. You have just administered allergy injections to a patient. As you are informing the patient that he must wait in the office for 20 minutes for monitoring for any reactions, the patient informs you that he is unable to remain in the office. What should you do? Document your answer.

3. You are providing instruction on the use of an Epipen to a patient who is allergic to bee venom. Provide step-by-step instructions for the patient. Using your knowledge of patient education, what are some points to remember with demonstration? What types of materials should you give the patient to take home? Document your session with the patient in the medical record.

4. You are getting ready to administer IM penicillin to a patient as ordered. Just as you are about to inject the medication, the patient tells you she is allergic to penicillin. What should you do? Provide the appropriate documentation in the patient record.

5. You are gathering a new patient history for Dr. Thau. What types of questions should you ask the patient about his or her use of medications? Role-play with a partner, interviewing each other about medication use. Document your findings.

Copyright © 2011, 2007, 2003 by Saunders, an imprint of Elsevier Inc. All rights reserved.

36 Emergency Preparedness and Assisting with Medical Emergencies

VOCABULARY REVIEW

Define the following terms.

1. cyanosis

___

2. dyspnea

___

3. ecchymosis

___

4. emetic

___

5. fibrillation

___

6. hematuria

___

7. mediastinum

___

8. myocardium

___

9. necrosis

___

10. photophobia

___

11. polydipsia

___

12. polyuria

___

13. transient ischemic attack

___

Copyright © 2011, 2007, 2003 by Saunders, an imprint of Elsevier Inc. All rights reserved.

Fill in the blanks with the correct terms.

14. ________________________ is defined as the immediate care given to a person who has been injured or has suddenly become ill.

15. AED stands for ________________________.

16. CPR stands for ________________________.

17. CVA stands for ________________________.

18. TIA stands for ________________________.

19. MI stands for ________________________.

20. ______________ is the most dangerous form of heat-related injury and results in a shutdown of body systems.

21. ______________ are the initial signs of a heat-related emergency.

22. Patients with ______________ appear flushed and report headaches, nausea, vertigo, and weakness.

23. ______________ are medications that may be administered to dissolve a blood clot.

24. A patient who has experienced a sudden cardiac arrest will show a(n) ______________ pattern on the ECG.

25. The medical term for extensive bruising of the skin is ______________.

26. If the physician diagnoses a disease that has no known cause, it is called ______________.

27. ______________ is a pulse rate below 60 beats per minute.

SKILLS AND CONCEPTS

1. List five classic symptoms of a heart attack.
   a. ________________________
   b. ________________________
   c. ________________________
   d. ________________________
   e. ________________________

2. What is the difference between classic myocardial signs and symptoms and those that may be experienced by female patients?

   ____

3. List and explain seven types of shock.
   a. ________________________
   b. ________________________
   c. ________________________
   d. ________________________
   e. ________________________
   f. ________________________
   g. ________________________

Copyright © 2011, 2007, 2003 by Saunders, an imprint of Elsevier Inc. All rights reserved.

4. Sprains and strains are treated with:

a. ______

b. ______

c. ______

d. ______

5. Give five examples of situations in which patients with abdominal pain should be seen by a healthcare provider immediately.

a. ______

b. ______

c. ______

d. ______

e. ______

6. Screening emergency telephone calls is an important role of the medical assistant in the ambulatory care setting. List below a minimum of two questions the medical assistant should ask for the following health problems.

a. Syncope

______

______

b. Head injury

______

______

c. Insect bites or stings

______

______

d. Burns

______

______

e. Wounds

______

______

7. Summarize a minimum of four methods of maintaining a safe environment for both staff and patients.

______

______

______

______

8. Explain the procedure for effectively discharging a fire extinguisher.

______

______

______

Copyright © 2011, 2007, 2003 by Saunders, an imprint of Elsevier Inc. All rights reserved.

9. List the criteria that should be included in a healthcare facility's evacuation plan.

10. Ambulatory care practitioners should be prepared to contact community emergency services as needed. Identify five resources available in your community for emergency preparedness. Include the services provided and contact information for each.

a.

b.

c.

d.

e.

11. Standard Precautions are crucial for preventing the transmission of diseases associated with bioterrorism. Summarize infection control procedures that should be implemented in the event a bioterrorism incident may have occurred.

12. Summarize the CDC's recommendations to help minimize the negative psychological effects of an emergency situation on both staff members and patients.

13. OSHA recommends multiple factors that can help promote staff safety. Explain six accident prevention behaviors that should be followed in a healthcare setting.

a.

b.

c.

d.

e.

f.

Copyright © 2011, 2007, 2003 by Saunders, an imprint of Elsevier Inc. All rights reserved.

14. You are responsible for placing and labeling biohazard waste containers in the physician's office where you work. Explain the methods for proper disposal of hazardous material in the physician's office.

____

____

____

____

15. Discuss the role of medical assistants in emergency preparedness and the ways they can help if a natural disaster or other emergency occurs in their community.

____

____

____

____

____

CASE STUDIES

1. Sally calls the office complaining of lumbar pain that has been present for the past 2 weeks. What type of screening questions should you ask the patient? When should the patient be seen in the office? Provide the appropriate documentation.
2. Mr. Walker, a 64-year-old patient of Dr. Bendt, calls the office complaining of shortness of breath, pressure in the chest, and sweating for the past hour. Upon checking the patient's chart, you find that Mr. Walker is a smoker and obese. What advice should you give the patient? Show your documentation.

   The physician refers Mr. Walker to the emergency department, but he refuses to go, stating, "I don't feel well enough to drive to the hospital." What should be done to meet the needs of the patient? Document your conversation.
3. A patient calls, stating that she has found a tick on her left forearm. Explain the proper technique for removal of the tick. Also, you should advise the patient to watch for what signs and symptoms? Document your conversation.
4. A 19-year-old patient sitting in the waiting room experiences a grand mal seizure. What should Cheryl, the medical assistant, do to prevent injury to the patient? After the seizure the patient needs to be placed in the recovery position to maintain her airway. Explain how to place her in this position.

WORKPLACE APPLICATIONS

1. You learned in your text about factors that are crucial for patient safety and a few of the most common mistakes that can be made by healthcare workers that result in injury to a patient. Develop a handout that summarizes patient safety factors and share it with the class.
2. At a recent office meeting, telephone screening difficulties were addressed. Dr. Bendt asks you to review the current procedures and policies that are followed when patients call the office with emergencies and offer suggestions on how possible questions might be improved. In addition, the physician would like you to make a list of "home care advice" to go along with the symptoms. The work should also include "if" and "how soon" the patient should be seen in the office or under what circumstances the patient should be referred to the emergency department. Include the following situations in your project.

Asthma	Insect bites and stings
Wounds	Head injuries
Burns	Chest pain
Diabetic coma	Hypoglycemia
Back pain	Dysuria
Burns	Syncope
Hyperglycemia	High blood pressure

Copyright © 2011, 2007, 2003 by Saunders, an imprint of Elsevier Inc. All rights reserved.

3. As a medical assistant, you understand that medical emergencies have many different signs and symptoms. Dr. Bendt has asked you to create an informative brochure to educate patients about the importance of early detection and treatment. The brochure should include the following:
   a. Definition of illness
   b. Importance of early detection
   c. Signs and symptoms
   d. Risk factors
   e. Prevention recommendations
   f. What patients should do if they think they are experiencing this condition

4. Cheryl is in charge of establishing the office crash cart. What type of supplies should the cart have? What medications should be included? How should the cart and supplies be maintained? Where should the cart be kept?

5. The medical assistant can play an integral role in a community's response to natural or human-created disasters. Summarize how the medical assistant can contribute to the community response to an emergency.

INTERNET ACTIVITIES

1. You notice that your CPR certification is about to expire. Search for a list of certification sites in your area. Make a list of the contact information and share the locations with your classmates.
2. Perform a search for the Poison Control Center in your area. Search for and create a list of ideas for ways to prevent poisoning. Create an informative poster to display in your physician's office.
3. Investigate the CDC's site for emergency preparedness planning: *www.bt.cdc.gov/planning/#healthcare*
4. Search the CDC's site for coordinating emergency response: *www.bt.cdc.gov/cotper/*

MEDICAL RECORD ACTIVITIES

Documentation of an on-site emergency includes the following:

- Patient's name, address, age, and health insurance information
- Allergies, current medications, and pertinent health history
- Name and relationship of any person with the patient
- Vital signs and chief complaint
- Sequence of events, beginning with how the problem occurred, any changes in the patient's overall condition, and any observations made regarding the patient's condition
- Details of procedures or treatments performed on the patient

Document the details of the following cases.

1. Charise Mourning calls at 4 PM, just after the physician has left for the day, and reports that her husband, Sam, fell going down the steps and can't bear weight on his left leg. Mrs. Mourning is 78 years old and does not know how to drive. What questions should you ask? How should you handle the situation? Document pertinent information in Mr. Mourning's medical record.

____

____

____

____

____

Copyright © 2011, 2007, 2003 by Saunders, an imprint of Elsevier Inc. All rights reserved.

2. Lynne Franklin, the 17-year-old mother of a 9-month-old son, calls, hysterical and crying. She states that the baby is "jerking and shaking all over the crib." She states, "I tried to hold him down, and I heard something snap! What should I do? He looks like he is turning blue!" Lynne tells you he had a fever all night. The last time she took his temperature it was 103° F axillary. She is alone with the baby. How should the situation be handled? Document the details in the baby's medical record.

____

____

____

____

____

3. Charles Drysden, a 42-year-old patient, calls when the rest of the office is out to lunch. He is at work and is experiencing heaviness in his chest, difficulty breathing, indigestion, sweating, and minor jaw discomfort. He reports that the discomfort in his chest started about 30 minutes ago, after he ate a large lunch. Mr. Drysden took Mylanta for the indigestion but is not feeling any better. He wants to drive himself to the office even though a co-worker has offered to take him to the emergency department (ED). His pain is getting worse, but he doesn't think he needs to go to the ED. What should you do? Document the important details in Mr. Drysden's medical record.

____

____

____

____

____

4. You are working in the administrative area of the office when a patient enters the waiting room screaming for attention. She insists the physician ordered her the wrong medication, and she wants to talk to the doctor immediately. The physician is not in the office today, so you attempt to handle this very angry patient. Using the skills discussed in Procedure 36-3, try to work out a solution with the patient. Document the patient interaction in the woman's health record.

____

____

____

____

____

Copyright © 2011, 2007, 2003 by Saunders, an imprint of Elsevier Inc. All rights reserved.

37 Assisting in Ophthalmology and Otolaryngology

VOCABULARY REVIEW

Match the term with the correct definition.

1. _______ Adjustment of the eye for seeing various sizes of objects at different distances
2. _______ Reduction or dimness of vision with no apparent organic cause; often referred to as *lazy eye syndrome*
3. _______ An allied healthcare professional specializing in evaluation of hearing function, detection of hearing impairment, and determination of the anatomic site of impairment
4. _______ Structures found in the retina that make the perception of color possible
5. _______ A small pit in the center of the retina that is considered the center of clearest visiony
6. _______ Any substance or medication that causes constriction of the pupil
7. _______ A region at the back of the eye where the optic nerve meets the retina; considered the blind spot of the eye because it contains only nerve fibers and no rods or cones and therefore is insensitive to light
8. _______ The second cranial nerve, which carries impulses for the sense of sight
9. _______ The formation of spongy bone in the labyrinth of the ear, often causing the auditory ossicles to become fixed and unable to vibrate when sound enters the ear
10. _______ A substance or medication that damages the eighth cranial nerve or the organs of hearing and balance
11. _______ Abnormal sensitivity to light
12. _______ A usually chronic, recurrent skin disease marked by bright red patches covered with silvery scales
13. _______ Structures located in the retina of the eye and forming the light-sensitive elements
14. _______ An excessive discharge of sebum from the sebaceous glands, forming greasy scales or cheesy plugs on the body
15. _______ An instrument used to measure intraocular pressure
16. _______ A topical ophthalmic medication that dilates the pupil; used in diagnostic procedures of the eye and treatment for glaucoma
17. _______ A noise sensation of ringing heard in one or both ears

a. Cones
b. Accommodation
c. Seborrhea
d. Psoriasis
e. Rods
f. Audiologist
g. Amblyopia
h. Photophobia
i. Optic nerve
j. Otosclerosis
k. Ototoxic
l. Fovea centralis
m. Optic disc
n. Miotic
o. Mydriatic
p. Tinnitus
q. Tonometer

Copyright © 2011, 2007, 2003 by Saunders, an imprint of Elsevier Inc. All rights reserved.

Fill in the blanks with the correct terms.

18. A(n) ________________ is a licensed medical physician who can diagnose eye disorders, prescribe medication, conduct eye screenings, prescribe glasses or contact lenses, and perform otic surgery.
19. ________________ are trained to fill prescriptions written for corrective lenses by grinding the lenses and dispensing eyewear.
20. A(n) ________________ can perform eye examinations, diagnose vision problems and eye diseases, and treat visual defects through corrective lenses and eye exercises.

SKILLS AND CONCEPTS

1. On the following figure, label the structures of the outer eye.

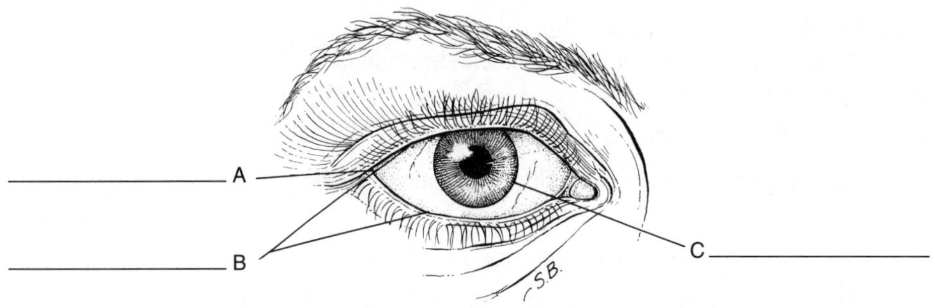

2. Name the two disorders of the outer eye pictured in the following figures.

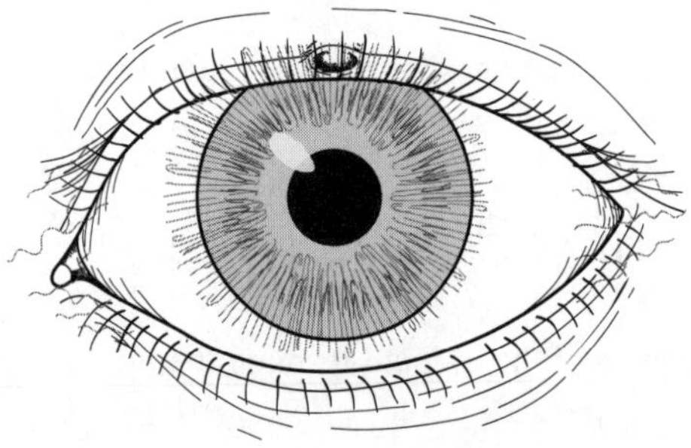

a. ____

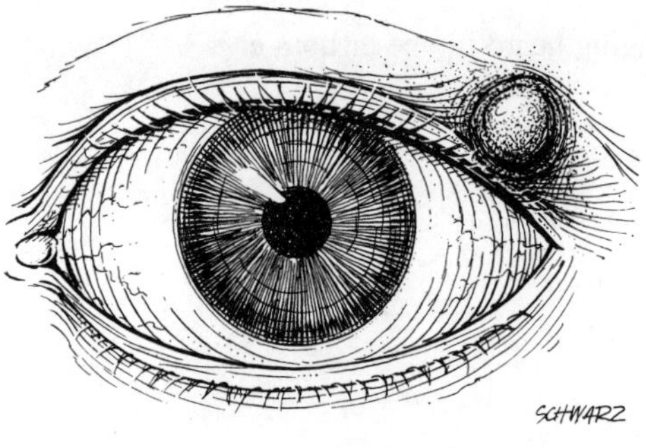

Copyright © 2011, 2007, 2003 by Saunders, an imprint of Elsevier Inc. All rights reserved.

b. ______

3. List and define three refractive errors.

a. ______

b. ______

c. ______

4. List three signs and symptoms of refractive errors.

a. ______

b. ______

c. ______

5. Compare and contrast strabismus and amblyopia.

______

______

______

6. Differentiate between otitis media and otitis externa.

______

______

______

7. Explain how a corneal abrasion is diagnosed and treated.

______

______

______

Copyright © 2011, 2007, 2003 by Saunders, an imprint of Elsevier Inc. All rights reserved.

CASE STUDIES

1. Amy, the medical assistant, has a patient who is interested in a surgical procedure to correct her myopia. What can Amy tell her patient about the different types of corrective procedures?

2. Joe, a 5-year-old patient, is brought to the office with itchy, watery eyes with a purulent discharge. His mother states that Joe's older brother recently was seen in the office with the same symptoms. What type of problem do you think Joe has? Is it contagious? With what education can Amy provide Joe and his mother to stop the spread of infection? Document the patient education intervention.

3. Kiasha Johnson, 4 years old, is being seen today for suspected otitis media. The physician decides to delay prescribing antibiotics to see how the child does in the next day or so. Mrs. Johnson doesn't understand why her child is not being given an antibiotic. Help reinforce the physician's recommendations and document the patient education intervention.

WORKPLACE APPLICATIONS

1. Kim asks Amy to create a list of common disorders of the eyeball. Prepare the list, defining the disorder, identifying the common signs and symptoms of the disorder, and describing the treatment involved.

2. Amy is learning to perform a Snellen examination. What type of guidelines should she keep in mind while performing this procedure?

3. After learning how to perform a throat swab, Amy attempts to gather a specimen from a 4-year-old patient. The young child appears scared and apprehensive. What can Amy do to calm the patient's fears? Explain the verbal and nonverbal communication Amy can use with the child to perform the procedure.

INTERNET ACTIVITIES

Use a drug reference book or the Internet to make drug cards for the following.

a. Carbamide peroxide (Debrox)

b. Cortisporin otic

c. Pilocarpine ophthalmic

d. Betoptic

e. Diamox

f. Acular

g. Livostin

h. Tobrex

i. Bleph-10

j. Timoptic

MEDICAL RECORD ACTIVITIES

1. A patient comes to the office complaining of pain and swelling in the left eye. While obtaining the history, Amy, the medical assistant, finds that the patient may have wood chips in her eye. The physician orders an eye irrigation. Amy administers 100 cc of sterile saline into the patient's left eye. Document the case and the procedure using the SOAPE format.

   S: ____

   O: ____

Copyright © 2011, 2007, 2003 by Saunders, an imprint of Elsevier Inc. All rights reserved.

Refer to the charts in the following figure to answer the next group of questions.

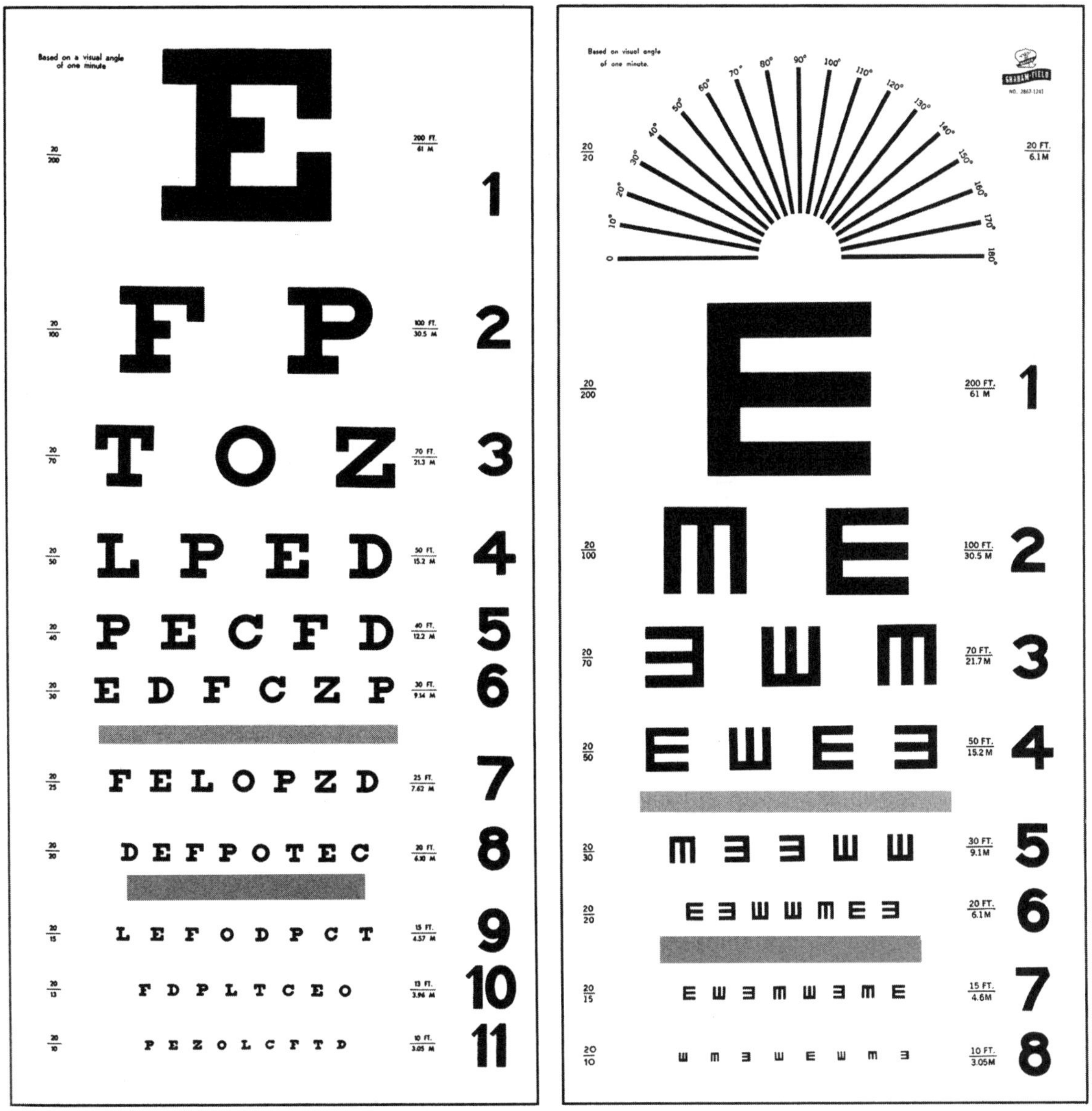

2. Your patient can read line number 8 with the right eye, number 9 with the left eye, and number 8 with both eyes on the Snellen chart. Document your findings. Use appropriate abbreviations. Be sure to include the date and your signature.

____

____

____

____

Copyright © 2011, 2007, 2003 by Saunders, an imprint of Elsevier Inc. All rights reserved.

3. Your patient cannot read English. He indicates that he can see line number 6 with the right eye, number 5 with the left eye, and number 6 with both eyes on the E chart. How will you have your patient respond so that you know your findings are accurate? Document your findings below.

____

____

____

____

4. You are ordered to perform a bilateral ear irrigation on a 72-year-old patient with impacted cerumen. In the right ear, a large amount of dark brown cerumen completely covers the tympanic membrane; in the left ear, a moderate amount of golden brown cerumen covers the side of the tympanic membrane. After the procedure, both membranes are visible. The patient had no complaints of discomfort. Document the procedure below.

____

____

____

____

Copyright © 2011, 2007, 2003 by Saunders, an imprint of Elsevier Inc. All rights reserved.

38 Assisting in Dermatology

VOCABULARY REVIEW

Define the following terms.

1. alopecia

____

2. cryosurgery

____

3. debridement

____

4. ecchymosis

____

5. electrodesiccation

____

6. exacerbation

____

7. hyperplasia

____

8. jaundice

____

9. keratin

____

10. leukoderma

____

11. opaque

____

12. remission

____

Copyright © 2011, 2007, 2003 by Saunders, an imprint of Elsevier Inc. All rights reserved.

Fill in the blanks with the correct terms.

13. Sebaceous glands release ________________, an oily substance that lubricates the skin.
14. The epidermis is the thin uppermost layer, and the ________________ is the thicker layer beneath.
15. A variety of microorganisms, called normal or resident ________________, are found on the skin and may increase the risk of integumentary system infections.
16. ________________ is a common, contagious, superficial infection caused by streptococci or *Staphylococcus aureus*.
17. ________________ is a disorder of the hair follicle and sebaceous gland unit.
18. ________________ is characterized by a vesicular, pruritic rash on the face, neck, elbows, and posterior knees and behind the ears.
19. Individuals with ________________, an inherited recessive trait, are unable to produce melanin, so they have white hair and skin and lack pigment in the iris.
20. Cancer cells are undifferentiated and ________________ in nature.
21. Jaundice is caused by deposits of ________________ in the tissues, which creates an orange discoloration of the skin.
22. A patient with an extremely pruritic skin rash may scratch so much that the area becomes ________________.
23. A(n) ________________ is a raised, firm scar caused by overgrowth of collagen at the site of a skin injury.
24. A patient who is given an antipruritic cream for an itchy skin lesion is receiving ________________ treatment.
25. Small purple hemorrhages under the skin that may resemble a rash are called ________________.
26. Accutane is an extremely dangerous ________________ that is contraindicated in women of childbearing age.
27. A(n) ________________ disorder is one that has no known cause.
28. Ischemia of the extremities that results in cyanosis and pain is called ________________.
29. SLE is a(n) ________________ disorder that results when the immune system attacks the body's connective tissue.

SKILLS AND CONCEPTS

1. Describe the major functions of the skin.

____

____

____

Copyright © 2011, 2007, 2003 by Saunders, an imprint of Elsevier Inc. All rights reserved.

2. Label the three layers of the skin in the following drawing.

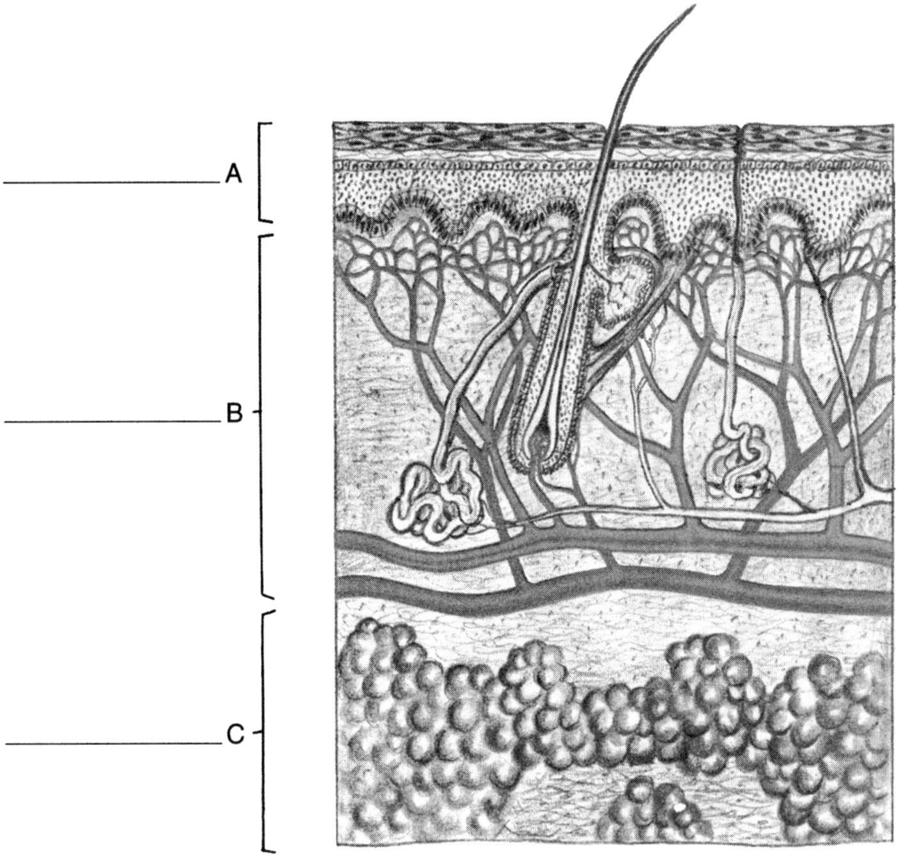

Define and give an example of the following.

3. Macule

____

____

4. Papule

____

____

5. Plaque

____

____

6. Fissure

____

____

7. Pustule

____

____

Copyright © 2011, 2007, 2003 by Saunders, an imprint of Elsevier Inc. All rights reserved.

8. Vesicle

____

____

9. Bulla

____

____

10. Cyst

____

____

11. Ulcer

____

____

12. Wheal

____

____

13. List and describe four types of inflammatory skin disorders.

a. _______________

b. _______________

c. _______________

d. _______________

14. List and describe two types of autoimmune disorders.

a. _______________

b. _______________

15. List and describe the three different types of burns.

a. _______________

b. _______________

c. _______________

16. Complete the following table.

Characteristic	**Benign Tumor**	**Malignant Tumor**
Cellular structure		
Type of growth		
Rate of growth		
Destruction of localized tissue		

17. Explain the seven warning signs of cancer.

a. C _______________

b. A _______________

c. U _______________

 Copyright © 2011, 2007, 2003 by Saunders, an imprint of Elsevier Inc. All rights reserved.

d. T ______

e. I ______

f. O ______

g. N ______

18. Describe the early warning signs of malignant melanoma.

a. ______

b. ______

c. ______

d. ______

e. ______

19. List and describe three ways to perform allergy testing.

a. ______

b. ______

c. ______

20. Explain three procedures for appearance modification.

a. ______

b. ______

c. ______

21. Explain the connection between chickenpox and herpes zoster and describe the typical signs and symptoms of shingles. Name the two vaccines used to prevent shingles. Who should receive them?

22. Explain the difference between basal and squamous cell carcinoma.

23. Describe how to perform a wound culture procedure. Include in your description the difference between aerobic and anaerobic microorganisms.

Copyright © 2011, 2007, 2003 by Saunders, an imprint of Elsevier Inc. All rights reserved.

CASE STUDIES

1. Alicia Ramsey, 16 years old, is being seen today for complaints of acne breakouts. What are the typical causes of acne vulgaris and how is it treated? Would the physician prescribe Accutane for this patient? Why?
2. Mrs. Rosa Philippe complains of frequent flushing across the nose, forehead, cheeks, and chin with pustule formation. The physician diagnosis is rosacea. What happens as the condition progresses? Explain to Mrs. Philippe the signs and symptoms of the condition and the treatment prescribed by the physician.
3. A patient calls and states that she has redness on her upper arm. What questions do you need to ask before scheduling the appointment? What vital signs should be obtained for the patient? Why? With a partner, role-play the case and document your findings.
4. A 6-year-old patient comes to the office today with a red, raised area around the mouth and nose. As Melissa, the medical assistant, examines the area, she notices that it is moist, inflamed, and crusted. What type of infection do these symptoms represent? With your knowledge of this infection, what patient education can you provide the patient and parents for stopping the spread of the infection? What types of medications are used to treat this infection? Document the case.
5. A 15-year-old patient comes to the office today with several boils forming on his anterior forearm. The physician is concerned about the development of cellulitis in the area. The patient's mother doesn't understand what the physician told her about her son's problem. Explain cellulitis to the mother, including the primary concerns of the infection, and the physician's prescribed treatment.

WORKPLACE APPLICATIONS

1. Patient education is an important part of Melissa's job as a medical assistant. Often patients are not aware of the medical terms used for common infections. Examine the following list of mycotic infections and provide the common name for each.
   a. Tinea pedis
   b. Tinea cruris
   c. Tinea corporis
   d. Tinea unguium

   What type of medication is used to treat mycotic infections?
2. Scabies (itch mite) and pediculosis (lice) are the two most common parasites that infest people. Dr. Lee has asked Melissa to develop a patient education handout on how to prevent the spread of these infestations. Include common medications used for treatment and how they are taken. What can patients do around the house to eliminate mites or lice? Who should be treated?
3. One of Melissa's duties is to assist the physician during tissue biopsies. What types of things should she do to prepare for such procedures?
4. Understanding the processes of staging and grading of tumors is an important part of patient care for patients diagnosed with a malignancy. Define the two terms and explain how they are performed.

INTERNET ACTIVITIES

1. Search the Internet for a list of sun safety recommendations. How can you reduce the risk of skin cancer? Create a list of ideas and compare it with those of your classmates.
2. Locate an article online on the treatment and management of different types of burns. Summarize the article and be prepared to share your findings in class.
3. Investigate the National Cancer Institute's recommendations for the prevention of skin cancer. Develop a patient education brochure on this topic.

MEDICAL RECORD ACTIVITIES

1. A patient complains of a red, flat rash with intense itching. What types of questions should you ask this patient? Use the correct medical terminology to chart your findings. Use appropriate abbreviations. Be sure to include the date and your signature.

Copyright © 2011, 2007, 2003 by Saunders, an imprint of Elsevier Inc. All rights reserved.

2. A patient comes to the office with a red, raised rash with small blisters. What type of questions should you ask this patient? Use the correct medical terminology to chart your findings. Use appropriate abbreviations.

3. Constance Oliver, a 23-year-old patient, has repeated herpes simplex infections. She does not understand why she keeps getting the cold sores. Perform patient education about the disorder and include in your discussion the typical medications used for treatment. Document your discussion with the patient.

4. Alonzo Racine calls the office because he is concerned about his 10-year-old son, Jayce. Jayce had been outside sledding and came in complaining of burning, tingling, and numbness in his cheeks, fingers, and toes, which are a grayish color. Dr. Lee believes the child may have a mild to moderate case of frostbite. What would Dr. Lee suggest that the father do? Should the patient be seen today? Document your interaction in the patient's medical record.

Copyright © 2011, 2007, 2003 by Saunders, an imprint of Elsevier Inc. All rights reserved.

39 Assisting in Gastroenterology

VOCABULARY REVIEW

Provide the correct term for each definition.

1. _______ The surgical joining together of two normally distinct organs
2. _______ A hard, impacted mass of feces in the colon
3. _______ Narrow slits or clefts in the abdominal wall
4. _______ Gas expelled through the anus
5. _______ Abnormal enlargement of the liver
6. _______ The valve guarding the opening between the ileum and cecum
7. _______ The surgical formation of an opening of the ileum on the surface of the abdomen through which fecal material is emptied
8. _______ Black, tarry stool containing digested blood; usually caused by bleeding in the upper gastrointestinal tract
9. _______ Tumors on stems frequently found in the mucosal lining of the colon
10. _______ Physicians who specialize in diseases and disorders of the stomach, small intestine, large intestine (colon), and appendix and the accessory organs of the liver, gallbladder, and pancreas

Define the following terms.

11. peritoneum

____

12. mesentery

____

13. omentum

____

14. adhesions

____

15. ascites

____

16. carcinogens

____

17. sclerotherapy

____

18. endemic disease

____

Copyright © 2011, 2007, 2003 by Saunders, an imprint of Elsevier Inc. All rights reserved.

19. portal hypertension

____

20. lithotripsy

____

21. esophageal varices

____

22. hematemesis

____

23. peristalsis

____

24. Valsalva's maneuver

____

SKILLS AND CONCEPTS

1. Describe the three primary functions of the digestive system.

   a. _______________

   b. _______________

   c. _______________

2. Label the structures of the upper abdominal cavity on the following figure.

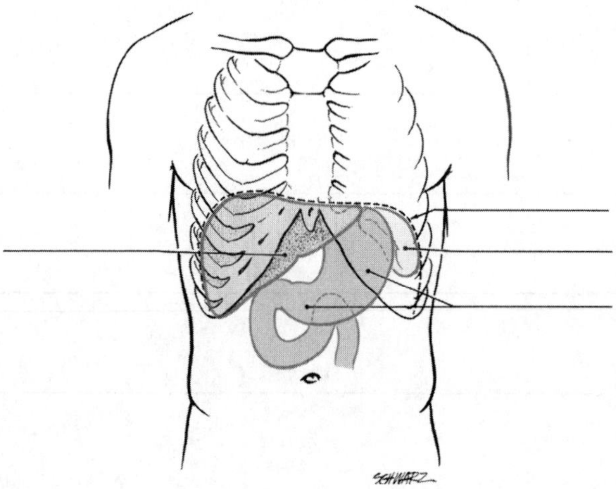

Copyright © 2011, 2007, 2003 by Saunders, an imprint of Elsevier Inc. All rights reserved.

Abdominal Regions

1. List the nine regions of the abdomen in the grid below.

Fill in the blanks.

2. The gallbladder is located in the ______ ______ quadrant of the abdomen.
3. The appendix is located in the ______ ______ quadrant of the abdomen.
4. The stomach is located in the ______ ______ quadrant of the abdomen.
5. The liver is located in the ______ ______ quadrant of the abdomen.
6. The pancreas is located in the ______ ______ quadrant of the abdomen.
7. List the seven parts of the large intestine in order, starting with the proximal end.
   a. ______
   b. ______
   c. ______
   d. ______
   e. ______
   f. ______
   g. ______

Complete the following sentences.

8. The ______ delivers bile from the liver to the duodenum where digestion is completed.
9. The ______ intestine is made up of the duodenum, jejunum, and ileum.
10. The small intestine is lined with transverse folds of tissue called ______.
11. Describe three disorders of the esophagus and stomach.
    a. ______
    b. ______
    c. ______
12. Describe 10 disorders of the intestines.
    a. ______
    b. ______
    c. ______
    d. ______
    e. ______
    f. ______
    g. ______
    h. ______
    i. ______
    j. ______

Copyright © 2011, 2007, 2003 by Saunders, an imprint of Elsevier Inc. All rights reserved.

13. Identify and explain two disorders of the liver and gallbladder.

a. ____

____

b. ____

____

14. Complete the following table.

Test	Description and Purpose	Patient Preparation
Barium swallow		
UGI		
Barium enema		
HIDA scan		
Ultrasonography of the liver, gallbladder, biliary system, pancreas		
Sigmoidoscopy		
Colonoscopy		
Endoscopy		

15. Complete the following chart.

Hepatitis Type	Mode of Transmission	Individuals at Risk
A (infectious hepatitis)		
B (serum hepatitis)		
C (non-A, non-B)		
D (delta virus)		
E		
G		

16. Explain the causes of the following GI system cancers.

Tumor	Cause or Contributing Factors
Oral tumors	
Esophageal cancer	
Gastric cancer	
Liver cancer	
Pancreatic cancer	
Colorectal cancer	

Copyright © 2011, 2007, 2003 by Saunders, an imprint of Elsevier Inc. All rights reserved.

CASE STUDIES

1. Dr. Sahani has ordered a screening hemoccult kit for a patient. Explain the test to the patient and why it is necessary. What collection instructions should Joan, the medical assistant, provide the patient?

2. While you are answering the telephone, a patient calls complaining of right upper quadrant pain. She is concerned about her appendix. Using your knowledge of acute appendicitis, what are the common signs? What questions should you ask the patient? What instructions should you provide the patient? Include the documentation for the patient's chart. What tests can be done to confirm the diagnosis?

3. Charles is scheduled for a barium swallow tomorrow. Explain the purpose of the procedure and any patient preparation involved.

4. Anna will have a colonoscopy next week. She calls the office and asks Joan whether she will be able to drive herself home after the test. What is Joan's response? Anna is also confused about the patient preparation for the test. What preparation should Joan explain to Anna with regard to the test?

5. A patient is suspected of having cholelithiasis. The patient is at 24 weeks' gestation. What test should be ordered for this patient? Why?

WORKPLACE APPLICATIONS

1. Many of Joan's patients are unsure of the risk factors for developing certain types of GI system cancers. List and describe some of the most common risk factors.

2. Dr. Sahani has asked Joan to create a patient education handout describing the definition, cause, signs, symptoms, diagnosis, and treatment options for GERD. Be sure to use terminology patients will understand.

3. You are expected to be able to ask questions designed to gather detailed information from patients about a variety of GI system complaints. List three questions you might ask a patient suffering from each of the problems listed below.

   a. nausea and vomiting

   ___

   ___

   ___

   b. diarrhea

   ___

   ___

   ___

   c. constipation

   ___

   ___

   ___

   d. abdominal pain

   ___

   ___

   ___

Copyright © 2011, 2007, 2003 by Saunders, an imprint of Elsevier Inc. All rights reserved.

4. Food poisoning is a disorder that results from the ingestion of food containing bacteria or toxic material. Create a chart for Joan to use as a resource when identifying the common sources, signs, and symptoms of different microorganisms.

Microorganism	Source	Signs and Symptoms
Staphylococcus aureus		
Escherichia coli		
Salmonella sp.		
Campylobacter jejuni		
Clostridium botulinum		

INTERNET ACTIVITIES

1. Investigate the Roux-en-Y weight loss surgery online. What criteria do patients have to meet to qualify for the surgery? What health conditions will improve with the weight loss that occurs after the procedure? How much does it cost? Does the procedure have any complications?

2. Use a drug reference book or the Internet to make drug cards for the following medications. Include drug classification, generic name, usual dose for an adult, and drug form.

   a. Imodium

   b. Lomotil

   c. Phenergan

   d. Tigan

   e. Anzemet

   f. Zofran

   g. Biaxin

   h. Bentyl

   i. Levsin

   j. Axid

   k. Prevacid

   l. Prilosec

   m. Tagamet

   n. Zantac

   o. Nexium

   p. Protonix

Copyright © 2011, 2007, 2003 by Saunders, an imprint of Elsevier Inc. All rights reserved.

MEDICAL RECORD ACTIVITIES

1. Joan's first patient of the day complains of pain in the RUQ. What kinds of questions should Joan ask the patient? In what position should the patient be placed? How should the patient be gowned and/or draped? What type of vital signs should Joan measure? Document the case.

2. Rita recently was diagnosed with a hiatal hernia. Dr. Sahani has prescribed Prilosec 20 mg once daily for the patient and has asked Joan to provide education on the drug (using the PDR), as well as any dietary modifications. Document the case.

3. Study the following case. Then rewrite the case using medical terminology and the proper abbreviations.

   Ms. Pullman comes to the office today complaining of pain in the upper right area of her abdomen. Her symptoms include a lack of appetite, profuse sweating, and a yellowish hue to her skin. On examination, Dr. Sahani finds an abnormal enlargement of the liver. The blood tests reveal a decrease in the volume percentage of red blood cells in the whole blood.

   ____

   ____

   ____

   ____

   ____

Copyright © 2011, 2007, 2003 by Saunders, an imprint of Elsevier Inc. All rights reserved.

40 Assisting in Urology and Male Reproduction

VOCABULARY REVIEW

Define the following terms.

1. albuminuria

2. azotemia

3. casts

4. copulation

5. erythropoietin

6. urgency

7. urology

Supply the terms for the following four types of urinary tract infections.

8. Inflammation of the urethra

9. Infection of the urinary bladder

10. Inflammation of the renal pelvis and kidney

11. Degenerative inflammation of the glomeruli

Define the following term and acronyms.

12. creatinine

13. BUN

Copyright © 2011, 2007, 2003 by Saunders, an imprint of Elsevier Inc. All rights reserved.

14. UA

____

15. PSA

____

16. DRE

____

Match the following terms with their definitions.

_______ 17. A long, coiled tube that rests on the top and lateral side of each testis	a. Epididymis
_______ 18. Bed wetting	b. Balanitis
_______ 19. Kidney stones	c. Impotence
_______ 20. A condition in which the signs and symptoms include urinary urgency and frequency, difficulty starting urination, hematuria, and repeated UTIs	d. Prostatitis
_______ 21. Undescended testicles	e. BPH
_______ 22. Inflammation of the prostate	f. Cryptorchidism
_______ 23. Inflammation of the glans penis	g. Hydrocele
_______ 24. A form of erectile dysfunction	h. Enuresis
_______ 25. A sac of clear fluid in the scrotum	i. Renal calculi

Skills and Concepts

1. Describe the five functions of the renal system.

   a. ____

   b. ____

   c. ____

   d. ____

   e. ____

2. List and describe the three processes of urine formation.

   a. ____

   b. ____

   c. ____

Copyright © 2011, 2007, 2003 by Saunders, an imprint of Elsevier Inc. All rights reserved.

3. Label the following diagrams to outline urine formation from the glomerulus to excretion through the urethra.

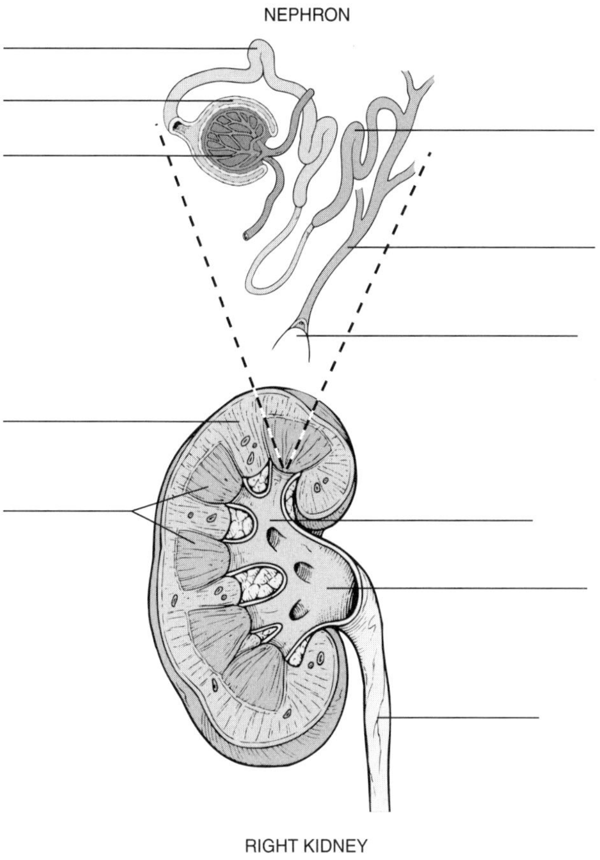

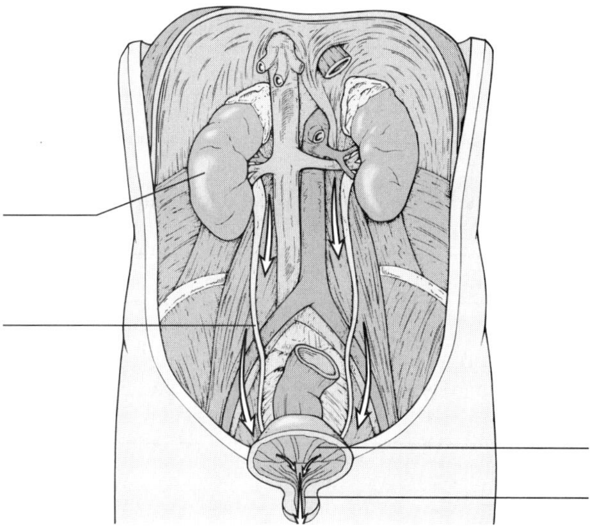

4. Explain stress incontinence in women and the exercise recommended for treatment.

____

____

____

5. List the general signs and symptoms of a urinary tract infection.

a. ____

b. ____

c. ____

d. ____

6. Explain the difference between acute glomerulonephritis and chronic glomerulonephritis. How is each treated?

____

____

____

____

Copyright © 2011, 2007, 2003 by Saunders, an imprint of Elsevier Inc. All rights reserved.

7. Explain polycystic kidney disease. What is happening to the kidneys? How can a patient develop it? How is it treated?

___

___

___

8. What is Wilms' tumor? What age group is at risk for this health problem?

___

___

9. Cryptorchidism can cause serious problems for developing boys. Describe this disorder, summarize the health issues that can occur if it is not corrected, and explain the procedure that is done to correct the problem.

___

___

___

10. Label the structures of the scrotum on the following figure.

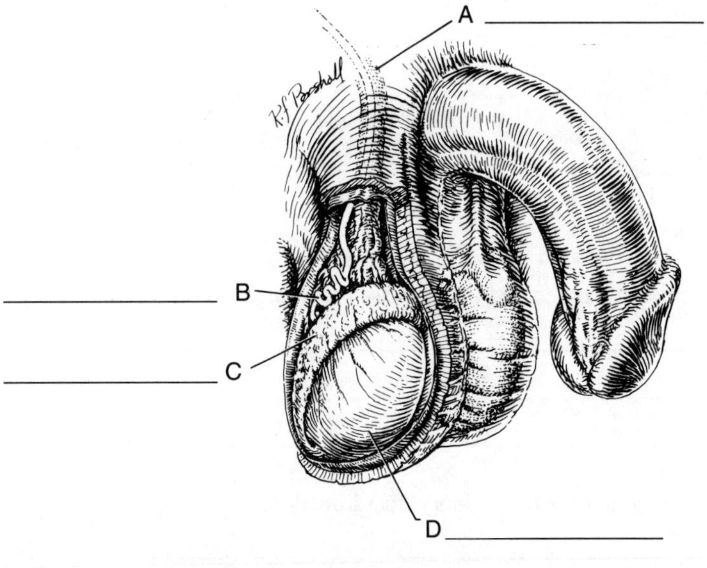

11. Summarize the important details you learned from your textbook about PSA tests.

___

___

___

___

12. Describe the treatments for prostate cancer.

a. ___

b. ___

c. ___

Copyright © 2011, 2007, 2003 by Saunders, an imprint of Elsevier Inc. All rights reserved.

13. Summarize the details of the three bacterial STDs and their treatment.

____

____

____

____

____

14. Explain the difference between HIV and AIDS. Describe three different diagnostic tests that can be used to diagnose HIV. Summarize the opportunistic infections that are commonly seen in patients with AIDS.

____

____

____

____

____

15. Discuss HIPAA applications for patients with HIV or AIDS.

____

____

____

16. Understanding renal system diagnostic tests and the required patient preparation for each is an important part of the medical assistant's responsibilities. Complete the following table.

Test	Description	Patient Preparation
Kidney-ureter-bladder (KUB) x-ray	Flat plate films of the abdomen; shows the size, shape, location, malformations of kidneys and bladder; used to visualize calculi	
Renal scanning		Patient should void before the procedure; no sedation or fasting is required; patient should drink two or three glasses of water before scanning; contraindicated in pregnancy
Cystography and voiding	X-ray evaluation with contrast dye to study bladder structure or function	
Intravenous pyelography (IVP); may be called intravenous urography (IUG)		Contraindicated in pregnancy and iodine allergies; laxative given the evening before; liquid diet 8 hours before; adequate fluids after; may have enema morning of the study
Arteriography (angiography)	Injection of dye into the renal artery; computerized fluoroscopy permits visualization of the blood flow of the kidneys, and serial x-ray films are taken; used to diagnose stenosis of the renal artery and highly vascular renal cancers	

Continued

Copyright © 2011, 2007, 2003 by Saunders, an imprint of Elsevier Inc. All rights reserved.

Renal computed tomography (CT)	Can be done with or without contrast dye; transverse views of the kidney are taken by CT to detect tumors, abscesses, cysts, and hydronephrosis	
Renal ultrasonography		No food or fluid restrictions; noninvasive and painless
Cystoscopy		Enemas to clear bowel; force fluids before procedure if local anesthesia is used; for general anesthesia, NPO after midnight; preprocedure sedative to reduce bladder spasms; aftercare: monitor urinary output for 24 hours
Retrograde pyelography	Dye injected into the bladder, ureters, and kidneys through a cystoscope to detect stones and other obstructions; can replace an IVP for patients with renal failure, obstructions, or allergies to IV dye	

CASE STUDIES

1. A patient comes to the office today complaining of severe lumbar pain and dysuria. The patient has a history of kidney stones. What diagnostic procedures might the physician order? Why? What type of patient preparation will Sara, the medical assistant, need to provide for the patient? If the patient had allergies to dye, what test would then be recommended?

___

___

___

2. Joe Hackett is a 68-year-old patient recently diagnosed with cancer of the bladder. What are the treatment options for this type of cancer? What might have caused the tumor to form? What diagnostic tool will the physician use to check for recurrences of the tumor?

___

___

___

3. Amir Wood, 7 years old, is being seen today because of chronic enuresis. What are some reasons this problem might occur? What diagnostic studies might the physician order to determine the cause of the problem? How is it treated?

___

___

___

Copyright © 2011, 2007, 2003 by Saunders, an imprint of Elsevier Inc. All rights reserved.

WORKPLACE APPLICATIONS

1. Sara, the medical assistant, deals with many patients with renal failure. She must be proficient in explaining the differences between peritoneal dialysis and hemodialysis. What are the advantages and disadvantages of each?

2. Design a handout explaining the details and instructions for a testicular self-examination.
   a. What is the importance of this exam? How often should it be done? Who should be performing it?
   b. What are the different approaches Sara could take to educate her male patients about testicular self-examinations? What types of resources could she provide?

3. The numbers of patients being seen with genital herpes and genital warts are on the rise. You are responsible for reinforcing patient education, so you need to know the problems these two viral STDs can cause and how they are treated. Summarize the information below.

   ____

   ____

   ____

   ____

INTERNET ACTIVITIES

1. Use a drug reference book or the Internet to make drug cards for the following medications. Include the drug classification, generic name, usual dose, and drug form.
   a. Keflex
   b. Bactrim
   c. Viagra
   d. Flomax
   e. Cardura
   f. Detrol
   g. Ditropan
   h. Xylocaine
   i. Cialis
   j. Interferon
   k. Proscar
   l. Zithromax
   m. Retrovir
   n. Rescriptor
   o. Valtrex

2. Use the Internet to search for conferences and training sessions in your area that would aid your continuing education.
   a. Why is it important to attend these conferences?
   b. Do the conferences you found offer continuing education units?
   c. Share your findings with the rest of the class.

3. Advances in HIV diagnosis and treatment are constantly occurring. Search the CDC's Web site *(www.cdc.gov)* for the most recent diagnostic tests and medications for treatment of HIV.

Copyright © 2011, 2007, 2003 by Saunders, an imprint of Elsevier Inc. All rights reserved.

MEDICAL RECORD ACTIVITIES

1. A 29-year-old male patient comes to the office complaining of discharge of pus, an itching sensation at the opening of the urethra, and burning on urination. What type of questions should Sara, the medical assistant, ask the patient? How should the patient disrobe and be positioned? What tests might the physician order to diagnosis the problem? What type of patient education should Sara provide? Document the case.

2. You collected a clean-catch urine specimen from a male patient. The urine is dark orange but clear. The amount of urine was 460 cc. The patient appeared to be comfortable during the procedure. Document your findings. Use appropriate abbreviations. Be sure to include the date and your signature.

3. Sally Lange, a 23-year-old patient with a history of UTIs, is seen today because of complaints of burning on urination, bladder spasms, urinary urgency, and urine that is dark and foul smelling. She had a Pyridium prescription at home and has already taken several doses. What would you expect her urine to look like? What will the physician order to determine whether Sally has a UTI? Sally is diagnosed with a repeat UTI and is prescribed Bactrim for 14 days. What patient education should she receive? Document the case study in the medical record.

Copyright © 2011, 2007, 2003 by Saunders, an imprint of Elsevier Inc. All rights reserved.

41 Assisting in Obstetrics and Gynecology

VOCABULARY REVIEW

Define the following terms.

1. rectocele

____

2. uterine prolapse

____

3. cystocele

____

4. PID

____

5. endometriosis

____

6. dilation and curettage

____

7. abruptio placentae

____

8. placenta previa

____

9. hysterectomy

____

10. ultrasonography

____

11. chorionic villus sampling

____

12. amniocentesis

____

13. alpha-fetoprotein (AFP)

____

14. mammography

____

15. colposcopy

____

16. cryosurgery

____

Copyright © 2011, 2007, 2003 by Saunders, an imprint of Elsevier Inc. All rights reserved.

Fill in the blanks with the correct terms.

17. Term pertaining to women who have had two or more pregnancies

___

18. Thin, yellow, milky fluid secreted by the mammary glands a few days before and after delivery

___

19. An x-ray procedure to guide the insertion of a needle into a specific area of the breast

___

20. Spotting or bleeding between menstrual cycles

___

21. Excessive menstrual blood loss, such as a menses lasting longer than 7 days

___

22. Absence of menstruation for a minimum of 6 months

___

23. Absence of menstruation for 35 days to 6 months

___

24. A hormone secreted by the placenta that is found in the urine of pregnant females

___

25. Thinning of the cervix during labor, measured in percentages from 0% to 100%

___

26. Abnormal cellular development that is diagnosed from a Pap smear

___

27. Congenital anomalies of the brain and spinal column that occur during embryonic development

___

28. A disease or condition that has no known cause

___

29. Toxic substances that cause severe fetal deformities or death

___

30. A test that uses a combination of fetal monitoring, maternal reports of fetal movement, and the fetal heart rate to determine the health of the baby in utero

___

Copyright © 2011, 2007, 2003 by Saunders, an imprint of Elsevier Inc. All rights reserved.

SKILLS AND CONCEPTS

1. Label the structures in the following figure.

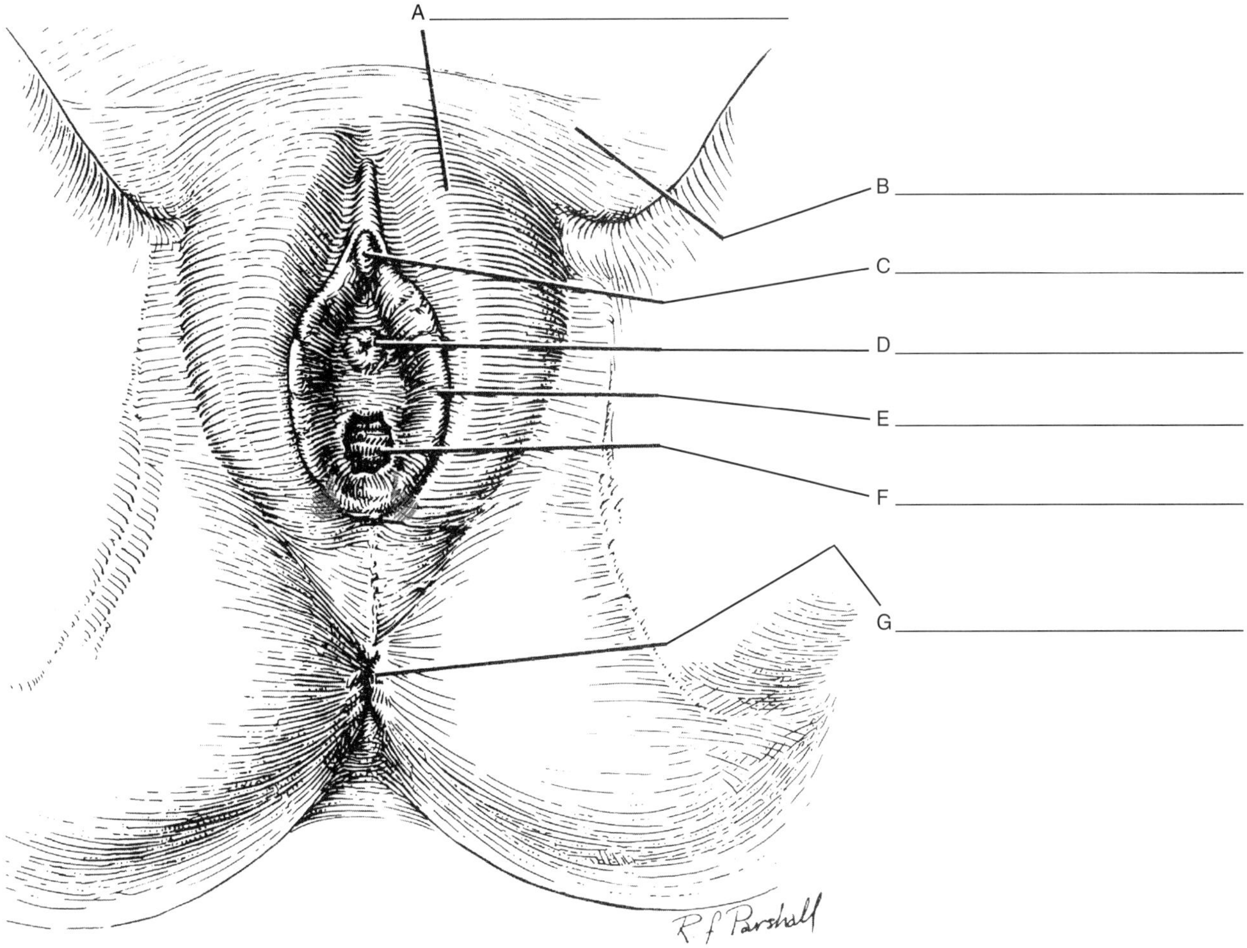

2. List and describe the three phases of menstruation.

   a. ______________________________

   b. ______________________________

   c. ______________________________

Copyright © 2011, 2007, 2003 by Saunders, an imprint of Elsevier Inc. All rights reserved.

3. Medical assistants should have a basic understanding of STDs, their typical signs and symptoms, and their treatment. Provide the missing information about STDs in the following table.

Disease (Causative Organism)	Signs and Symptoms	Treatment
Chlamydia *(Chlamydia trachomatis)*		Curable with antibiotic therapy; azithromycin (Zithromax), tetracycline, or Vibramycin
Genital herpes simplex virus (HSV-2)	Painful genital vesicles and ulcers; erythema and pruritus; tingling or shooting pain 1-2 days before outbreak; cycle through episodes. Viral shedding may occur during asymptomatic periods. Newborns can be infected by active lesions in vagina at birth.	
Genital warts (HPV)		Goal of treatment is to remove symptomatic warts; cryotherapy to lesions; podofilox solution or imiquimod cream to lesions
Gonorrhea *(Neisseria gonorrhoeae)*—bacteria	Dysuria; urinary frequency; abdominal pain; increased or decreased vaginal discharge. May cause endometritis, PID, and urethritis.	
Syphilis *(Treponema pallidum)*—spirochete bacteria		Penicillin G (Wycillin); if allergic to penicillin, doxycycline or tetracycline
Trichomoniasis *(T. vaginalis)*—protozoa		Metronidazole (Flagyl); need to treat partner

4. Describe three benign gynecologic tumors.

a. ______________________________

b. ______________________________

c. ______________________________

5. List and describe four gynecologic cancers.

a. ______________________________

____

b. ______________________________

____

c. ______________________________

____

d. ______________________________

____

Copyright © 2011, 2007, 2003 by Saunders, an imprint of Elsevier Inc. All rights reserved.

6. List and define five types of naturally occurring abortions.

a. ______________________________

b. ______________________________

c. ______________________________

d. ______________________________

e. ______________________________

7. List and describe two different types of placental abnormalities.

a. ______________________________

____

b. ______________________________

____

8. Labor is the physiologic process by which the uterus expels the fetus and the placenta. It is divided into three stages. Define each stage of labor.

Stage I ______________________________

____

Stage II ______________________________

____

Stage III ______________________________

____

9. Explain the difference between perimenopause and menopause. What are the typical discomforts reported by women at this time? How are they treated?

____

____

____

10. Your patient is trying to decide whether to breast-feed or bottle-feed. What are some benefits of breast-feeding you could explain through patient education?

____

____

____

____

Copyright © 2011, 2007, 2003 by Saunders, an imprint of Elsevier Inc. All rights reserved.

CASE STUDIES

1. A 20-year-old patient arrives today for her annual Pap smear. She has questions about the different types of birth control available. What are some of the factors involved in choosing a type of contraception? Using the following chart, create a patient education resource for the different types of contraception.

Type	Failure Rate	Characteristics	Contraindications	Side Effects
Condom (barrier method)				
Diaphragm or cervical cap (barrier method)				
Intrauterine device (IUD)				
Depo-Provera (DMPA)				
Oral contraceptives (OCPs)				
Hormonal patch				
Vaginal ring				

2. You receive a telephone call from a female patient who is experiencing side effects from oral contraceptives. What symptoms will you ask about?

A ______________________________

C ______________________________

H ______________________________

E ______________________________

S ______________________________

3. Carly comes to the office today for a prenatal checkup. She states that she has been experiencing some pelvic pain and burning on urination for 5 days. She also has recently stopped taking her prenatal vitamins, which she says make her nauseated. This is her first pregnancy, and she is very nervous about the examination. How can Betsy, the medical assistant, calm her fears? What test results and information should be gathered before the physician's examination? What patient education might be helpful? After Betsy has finished measuring the necessary vital signs and gathering the laboratory specimens, how should Carly be robed and draped? Once the physician begins the internal examination, how should she be positioned?

4. Dr. Beck has asked you to prepare a patient for a bimanual examination. How should the patient be robed and draped? How should you position the patient? What type of supplies will Dr. Beck need to complete the examination?

5. Mary has been instructed to have a baseline mammogram. What patient preparation should Betsy provide for Mary before her examination?

WORKPLACE APPLICATIONS

1. Dr. Beck has asked Betsy to create a patient education handout for patients with fibrocystic breast disease. Include the disease definition, possible causes, and signs and symptoms. Are any dietary restrictions required?

2. One of Betsy's duties includes instructing patients in the performance of breast self-examination. With a partner, explain the steps of this procedure. When should it be performed? For what should the patient be feeling? Why is breast self-examination important?

3. Betsy has been instructed to gather a health history on a patient. What type of questions should she ask? Include both open-ended and closed-ended questions. Practice your interviewing technique with a partner. What did you find most difficult about the interview?

Copyright © 2011, 2007, 2003 by Saunders, an imprint of Elsevier Inc. All rights reserved.

INTERNET ACTIVITIES

1. Use a drug reference book or the Internet to make drug cards for the following medication. Include the drug classification, generic name, usual dose, and drug form.

   a. Tamoxifen

   b. Premarin

   c. Prempro

   d. Methotrexate (for use in ectopic pregnancies)

   e. Evista

   f. Effexor

   g. Lupron

   h. Diflucan

   i. Flagyl

   j. Rocephin

   k. Boniva

2. Osteoporosis is a loss of bone tissue and a decrease in bone density. However, osteoporosis may be prevented and/or controlled with proper calcium intake. Search the Internet for public health programs or patient education programs available in your area that deal with osteoporosis prevention. How are the programs constructed? How do they increase awareness of this disease? How are the programs monitored? Is there a cost? Which program would you most recommend to someone you know? Share your research with your classmates.

3. Search the Internet for resources for pregnant and breast-feeding women. Develop a resource guide for these patients in an obstetric practice.

MEDICAL RECORD ACTIVITIES

1. Role-play with your partner the following case: Ashley Thomassio, 22 years old, is a new patient in the practice. You are responsible for gathering a gynecologic history, taking vital signs, and preparing the patient for a pelvic examination. Using the gynecologic history guidelines from your textbook, document this information in the medical record.

2. Carla Gomez, 48 years old, is being seen today because she discovered a hard mass on the outside of her left breast. What questions would you ask Mrs. Gomez about this problem? Role-play this case with a partner and document your results. How should the patient be gowned for the physician's examination? What diagnostic tests might the physician order?

3. Monica Anderson, 17 years old, is being seen today for follow-up of an endometriosis diagnosis. What symptoms would you expect Monica to describe? What are the possible treatments for endometriosis? Document your patient interaction in the medical record.

Copyright © 2011, 2007, 2003 by Saunders, an imprint of Elsevier Inc. All rights reserved.

42 Assisting in Pediatrics

VOCABULARY REVIEW

Match the following terms with their definitions.

1. ________ Weakened or changed virulence of a pathogenic microorganism
2. ________ Enlargement of the cranium caused by abnormal accumulation of cerebrospinal fluid within the cerebral system
3. ________ Visual examination of the voice box area through an endoscope equipped with a light and mirrors for illumination
4. ________ Small head size in relation to the rest of the body
5. ________ A continuous, dry rattling in the throat or bronchial tube caused by partial obstruction
6. ________ A thin, watery, serumlike drainage
7. ________ A shrill, harsh respiratory sound heard during inhalation with a laryngeal obstruction
8. ________ The formation and/or discharge of pus

a. Microcephaly
b. Serous
c. Hydrocephaly
d. Stridor
e. Rhonchi
f. Attenuated
g. Suppurative
h. Laryngoscopy

1. Explain the difference between growth and development.

____

____

____

____

SKILLS AND CONCEPTS

The Denver II Developmental Screening Test, a standardized tool, is given to children between 1 month and 6 years of age to screen healthy infants for developmental delays, to validate concerns about an infant's development, or to monitor high-risk children for the development of problems.

1. When should the test be administered?

____

2. The assessment focuses on the following four areas. Describe the following types of skills and provide examples of each.

   a. Gross motor skills

   ____

   ____

Copyright © 2011, 2007, 2003 by Saunders, an imprint of Elsevier Inc. All rights reserved.

b. Language skills

____

____

c. Fine-motor adaptive skills

____

____

d. Personal skills

____

____

3. The following chart describes different growth and development theories. Fill in the missing theories to complete the chart.

Age Group	Freud (1856–1939) Psychosexual Theory	Piaget (1896–1980) Cognitive Theory	Erikson (1902–1994) Psychosocial Theory	Kohlberg (1927–1987) Moral Reasoning
Infant	Oral stage; child operates with the pleasure principle, and the id develops.		Building basic trust versus mistrust; learning drive and hope.	
Toddler	Passes through oral aggressive stage to anal stage; elimination is used to control and inhibit.			Avoids punishment and the power of authority figures
Preschool to early school years		Intuitive-preoperational; preschoolers are egocentric and have magical thinking. Early school-aged children begin to develop understanding of cause and effect. Child functions symbolically using language; develops understanding of life events and relationships.	Preschool processing initiative versus guilt and attempting to develop direction and purpose. Children mimic others and are more purposeful in establishing goals.	

Continued

Copyright © 2011, 2007, 2003 by Saunders, an imprint of Elsevier Inc. All rights reserved.

School age		Concrete operations: uses mental reasoning to solve problems; attempts to reach logical solutions; tests beliefs to establish values.		Conventional morality; doing what is expected is important. Children need to be good in their own eyes as well as doing what they perceive others expect of them; they want to please others.
Adolescence	Genital stage		Identity versus role confusion; developing self-identity that will determine devotion and fidelity in future relationships.	

4. Using the growth charts, plot the measurements and answer the following questions.
   a. Simon Blackstone, 18 months: head circumference, 14¼ inches; 85 cm long; 14 kg. What are his height and weight percentiles?
   b. Carla Toomis, 9 years old: 50 inches tall and weighs 88 pounds. What are her stature and weight percentiles? What is her BMI?

5. Based on what you have learned about therapeutic approaches for the pediatric patient, what would be the best way to deal with the following patient situations?
   a. A crying 2-month-old scheduled for the first round of vaccinations

   ____

   ____

   b. A 3-year-old who is diagnosed with croup

   ____

   ____

   c. An 8-year-old who has to have his blood glucose checked with a glucometer

   ____

   ____

   d. A 13-year-old who has to receive a penicillin injection in the dorsogluteal site

   ____

   ____

6. Summarize five factors that are important safeguards for keeping vaccines safe during handling and storage.
   a. ____
   b. ____
   c. ____
   d. ____
   e. ____

Copyright © 2011, 2007, 2003 by Saunders, an imprint of Elsevier Inc. All rights reserved.

7. What are three common characteristics of children with autism?

a. ______________________________

b. ______________________________

c. ______________________________

Fill in the blanks in the following statements.

8. Infection or inflammation of the middle ear is called ______________.

9. ______________ is a viral inflammation of the larynx and the trachea that causes edema and spasm of the vocal cords.

10. During a(n) ______________, the bronchial tubes begin to spasm, reducing the amount of air that can pass through them; at the same time, the tissue lining the bronchioles becomes edematous and secretes mucus.

11. ______________ is a viral infection of the small bronchi and bronchioles that usually affects children under 3 years of age. The infection varies in severity and is seen in children with a family history of asthma and children exposed to cigarette smoke.

12. Common treatments for ______________ include zanamivir (Relenza), which is inhaled every 12 hours, and oseltamivir (Tamiflu), which is available in pill form.

13. ______________ can be caused by a bacterial or viral infection that produces a white or yellowish pus that may cause the eyelids to stick shut in the morning.

14. ______________, or "slapped cheek disease," is an infection caused by parvovirus B19.

15. ______________ is caused by a member of the herpes virus group and is transmitted by direct or indirect droplets from the respiratory tract of an infected person. The incubation period is 14 to 21 days.

16. ______________ is an inflammation of the membranes that cover the brain and spinal cord.

17. ______________ is the best prevention for Reye's syndrome.

18. ______________ is caused by the coxsackievirus. The symptoms include fever; sore throat; painful red blisters on the tongue, mouth, palms of the hands, and soles of the feet; headache; anorexia, and irritability.

19. ______________ is an inherited disorder that causes pulmonary obstruction and malabsorption problems.

20. ______________ is caused by a faulty gene that is passed from mothers to sons.

21. List eight details that must be documented when a vaccination is given.

a. ______________________________

b. ______________________________

c. ______________________________

d. ______________________________

e. ______________________________

f. ______________________________

g. ______________________________

h. ______________________________

22. List and discuss the five stages of Reye's syndrome.

a. ______________________________

____

b. ______________________________

____

Copyright © 2011, 2007, 2003 by Saunders, an imprint of Elsevier Inc. All rights reserved.

c. ______________________________

____

d. ______________________________

____

e. ______________________________

____

23. List 10 safety guidelines for parents with small children.

a. ______________________________

b. ______________________________

c. ______________________________

d. ______________________________

e. ______________________________

f. ______________________________

g. ______________________________

h. ______________________________

i. ______________________________

j. ______________________________

24. Complete the following table.

Vaccine and Disease	Route of Administration	Contraindications (Mild Illness Is not a Contraindication)	Side Effects
DtaP Diphtheria, tetanus, pertussis (whooping cough)		Moderate or severe acute illness, neurologic problem, complication such as fever or convulsion after previous dose	
HAV Hepatitis A (can use either Havrix or Vaqta brands)			Localized injection site reaction, fever, headache
HBV Hepatitis B (can use either Energix B or Recombivax HB brands)		Moderate or severe acute illness, yeast allergy, severe cardiovascular disease	
Hib *Haemophilus influenzae* serotype B meningitis			Minimal
HPV Human papilloma virus (Gardasil)		Hypersensitivity to the ingredients; pregnancy	Relatively few; mild headache and GI upset
Influenza Either trivalent inactivated influenza vaccine for 6 months; at 2 years use live, attenuated influenza vaccine			Uncommon; fever, local irritation at injection site, general malaise

Continued

Copyright © 2011, 2007, 2003 by Saunders, an imprint of Elsevier Inc. All rights reserved.

IPV Inactive poliovirus for polio			Uncommon
MMR Measles, mumps, rubella			Fever
Pneumococcal Pneumococcal pneumonia			
Rotavirus (Rota) RotaTeq for prevention of Rotavirus gastroenteritis			GI upset and blood disorders
Varicella Varicella (chickenpox)			

CASE STUDIES

1. Susie, a medical assistant, is concerned about approaching young children and how and when to involve the parents. Provide tips for approaching children in each of the following age groups.

   a. Infants (birth to 1 year)

   b. Toddlers and preschoolers (2 to 6 years)

   c. School-aged children (7 to 11 years)

   d. Adolescents (12 to 18 years)

2. A mother comes to the office complaining that her 4-week-old baby has had crying episodes lasting 3 to 4 hours four times during the past week. What type of questions should Susie ask the mother? Role-play this case with a partner and document your findings. The physician diagnoses the baby as having colic. What type of patient education should Susie provide to the mother?

3. The physician instructs a patient complaining of diarrhea to follow a "BRAT" diet. Define this dietary recommendation.

4. A patient recently was diagnosed with asthma. The physician has asked Susie to educate the patient and parents on the common triggers of asthma attacks. Document the conversation.

5. Susie is trying to obtain vital signs on a 4-year-old child who refuses to stand on the scale or cooperate while her temperature is taken. What can Susie do to try to obtain the child's cooperation? What is the best way to take this patient's temperature?

WORKPLACE APPLICATIONS

1. Childhood obesity is becoming an epidemic in the United States. The clinic for which you work is providing an in-service presentation to educate staff members about this growing problem. Susie and the other staff members are asked to create a list of possible reasons for this trend. List the possible causes and describe some solutions to be discussed during the in-service presentation.

2. At a recent office meeting, the staff concluded that a patient education handout on the common cold would benefit patients in the office. Susie has decided to take on this responsibility.

   a. Creatively design an informative handout for patients.

   b. Be sure to include the definition of the common cold.

   c. How is the infection spread to others? Describe ways to eliminate the spread of infection.

   d. What are the common signs and symptoms? When should the patient be seen in the office?

   e. What are some common OTC medications the physician would recommend?

   f. Include instructions for use of a bulb syringe.

Copyright © 2011, 2007, 2003 by Saunders, an imprint of Elsevier Inc. All rights reserved.

3. Susie is reorganizing the patient waiting room and wants to include some helpful and educational resources for the patients to view. Create a list of possible items Susie could place in the waiting room.

4. A father calls the office to report that his 4-year-old child is complaining of abdominal pain, occasional diarrhea, and a cough. Summarize five questions Susie should ask to gather more details about the problem.

INTERNET ACTIVITIES

1. Use a drug reference book or the Internet to make drug cards for the following medications. Include the drug classification, generic name, usual pediatric dose, and drug form.
   a. Amoxicillin
   b. Ceclor
   c. Cipro
   d. Augmentin
   e. EryPed
   f. Septra
   g. Singulair
   h. Albuterol
   i. Tamiflu
   j. Varivax
   k. Relenza
   l. Serevent
   m. Advair Diskus
   n. Zithromax
2. Search the CDC's Web site *(www.cdc.gov)* for VIS (vaccination information sheets). Print a copy for each of the immunizations recommended in the immunization schedule. Why is using these educational handouts in the office important?
3. Flu vaccinations are recommended for children over 6 months of age. Search the CDC's Web site *(www.cdc.gov)* for dosage instructions. Describe dosage instructions for children who have not previously been vaccinated and for those who have. When should a patient *not* receive the flu vaccine?

MEDICAL RECORD ACTIVITIES

1. Drew Cassandra, 3 months old, is being seen today for a well-baby checkup and her first round of immunizations, including her second Hep B immunization. What vaccinations will be given today? What is their route of administration? Explain the criteria for VIS use in this case. Document the visit in the baby's medical record.
2. Tommy Lango, a 2-year-old patient, is being seen today because of complaints of earache; a harsh, barking cough; and a fever. What are the medical assistant's responsibilities in this case? What questions should be asked to gather more details? Document the information in the patient's medical record.
3. Alisha Johnson, 10 years old, is being seen today for diarrhea that has lasted 3 days, abdominal cramping, and occasional blood in the stool. What are the medical assistant's responsibilities in this case? What questions should be asked to gather more details? Document the information in the patient's medical record.

Copyright © 2011, 2007, 2003 by Saunders, an imprint of Elsevier Inc. All rights reserved.

43 Assisting in Orthopedic Medicine

VOCABULARY REVIEW

Define the following terms.

1. kyphosis

2. lordosis

3. luxation

4. subluxation

5. thoracic

6. tendon

7. ligament

8. atrophy

9. bursae

10. periosteum

11. reduction

12. goniometer

13. crepitation

14. periosteum

15. epiphyseal plate

16. medullary cavity

Copyright © 2011, 2007, 2003 by Saunders, an imprint of Elsevier Inc. All rights reserved.

SKILLS AND CONCEPTS

1. List five general functions of the musculoskeletal system.

   a. ______________________________

   b. ______________________________

   c. ______________________________

   d. ______________________________

   e. ______________________________

2. In the figure below, label the bones of the extremities.

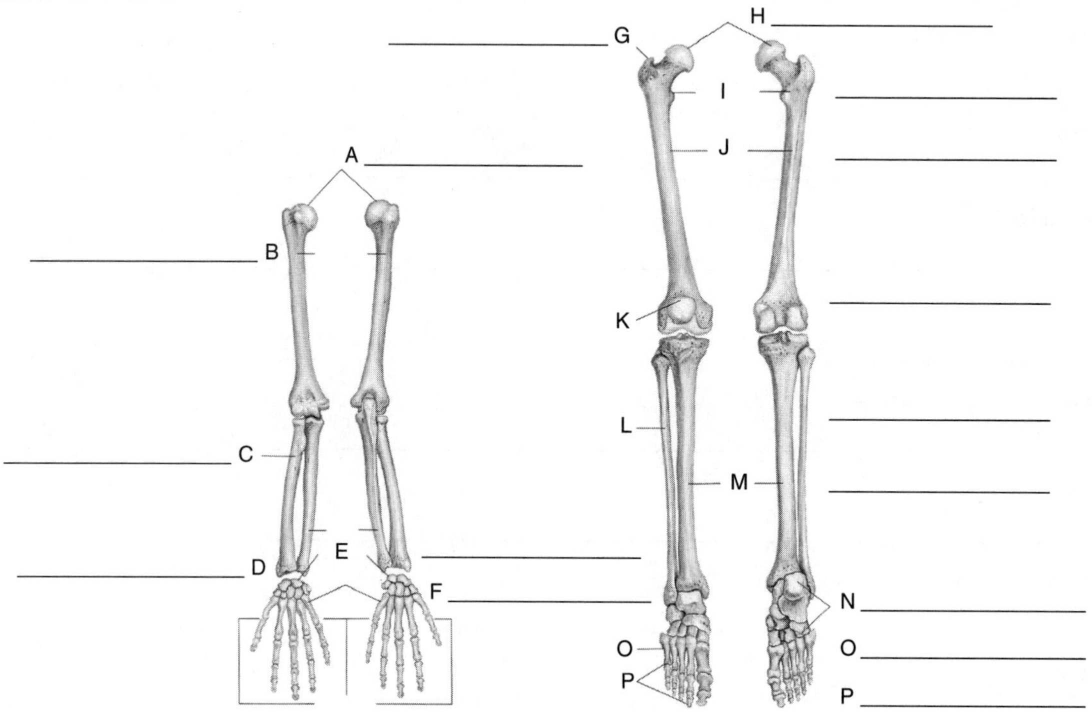

3. Label the following drawing with muscle, tendons, insertion, and origin.

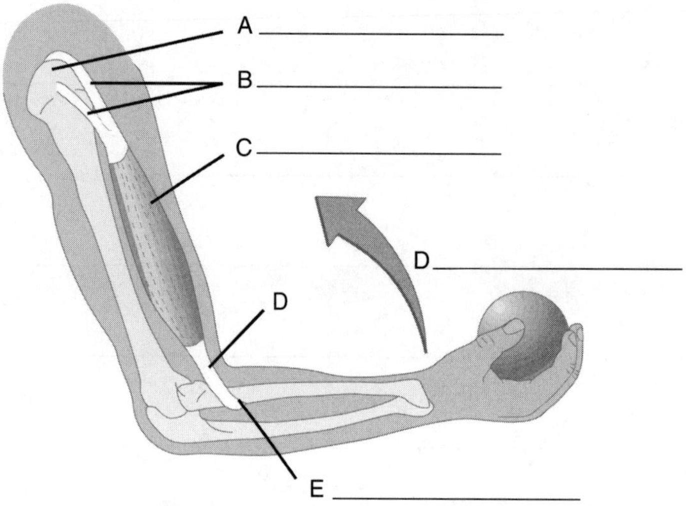

Copyright © 2011, 2007, 2003 by Saunders, an imprint of Elsevier Inc. All rights reserved.

4. Label the three types of muscles shown in the following figure.

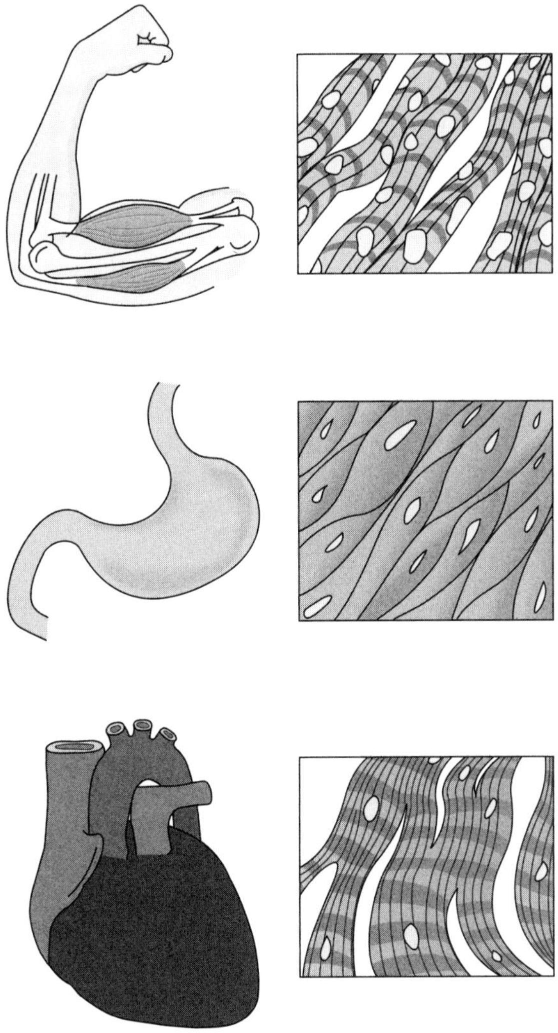

Identify the correct types of joints in the following descriptions.

5. ________________ permit the skull to grow with the child but have very limited flexibility.

6. ________________ allow for the greatest range of motion by permitting the joint to rotate in a complete circle.

7. The ________________ joints of the elbow and knee allow for movement in one plane, such as bending up and down.

Indicate which statements are true (T) and which are false (F).

8. ________ The tibia is distal to the femur.

9. ________ The patella is superior to the metacarpals.

10. ________ The radius is lateral to the ulna.

11. ________ The tibia is medial to the fibula.

12. ________ The metatarsals are inferior to the tarsals.

Copyright © 2011, 2007, 2003 by Saunders, an imprint of Elsevier Inc. All rights reserved.

13. Label each type of range of motion shown in the following figure.

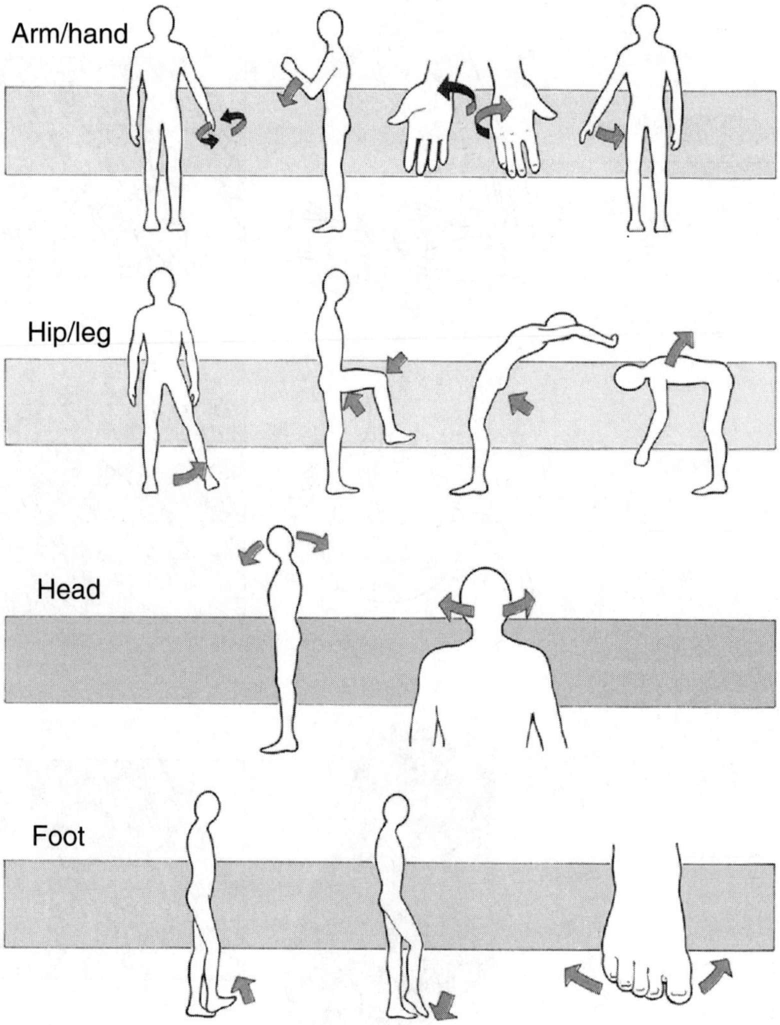

Copyright © 2011, 2007, 2003 by Saunders, an imprint of Elsevier Inc. All rights reserved.

Define the following.

14. Gout

15. Osteoarthritis

16. Rheumatoid arthritis

17. Myasthenia gravis

18. Osteomalacia

19. Herniated disk

20. SLE

21. Lyme disease

22. Compare and contrast hot and cold therapeutic modalities.

23. Explain the difference between therapeutic ultrasound and a TENS treatment.

Copyright © 2011, 2007, 2003 by Saunders, an imprint of Elsevier Inc. All rights reserved.

24. Review the fractures shown in the following figure. Match the name of the fracture with the letter corresponding to the illustration of the fracture in the figure in the list.

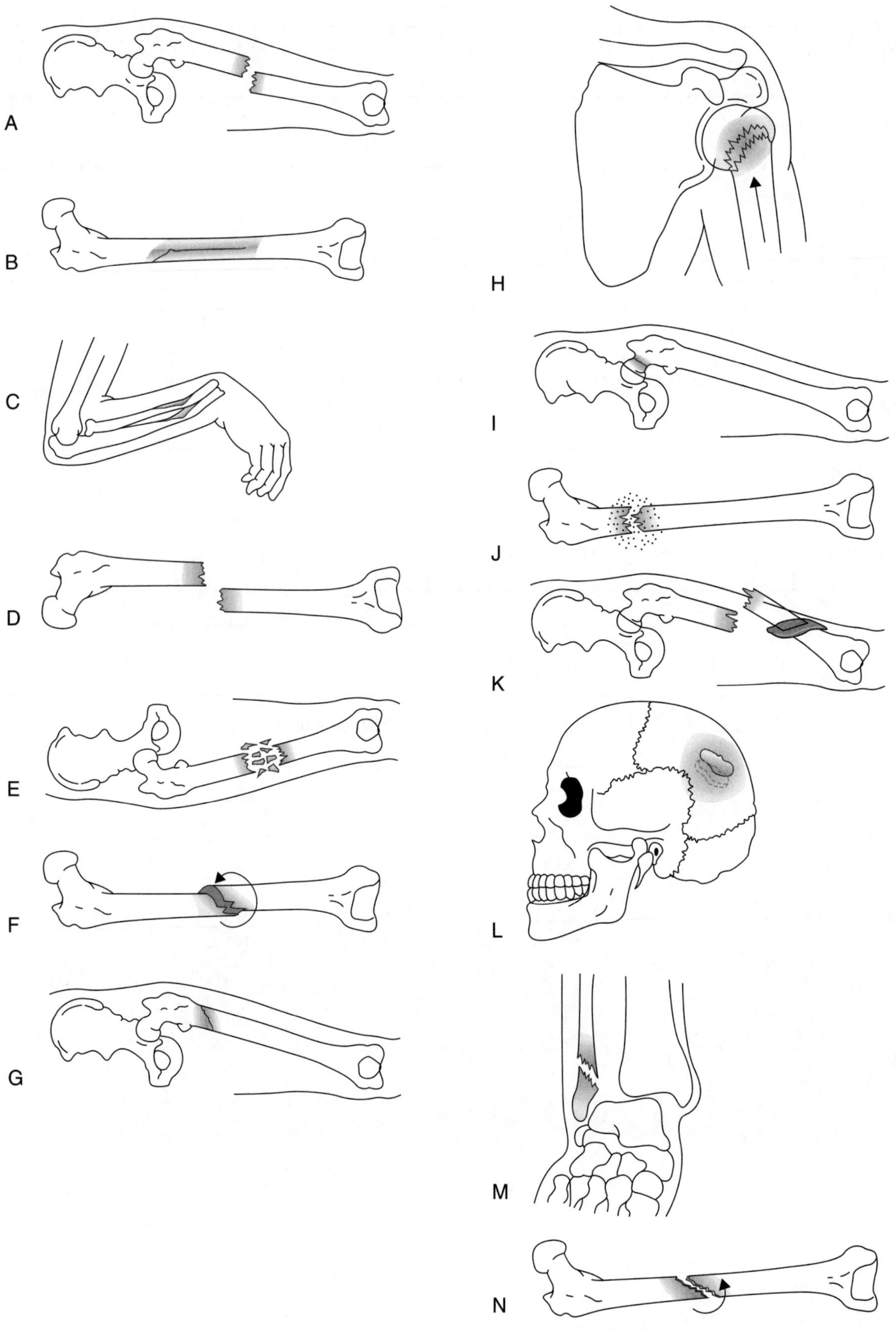

Copyright © 2011, 2007, 2003 by Saunders, an imprint of Elsevier Inc. All rights reserved.

_______ 1. Transverse
_______ 2. Spiral
_______ 3. Simple
_______ 4. Pathologic
_______ 5. Oblique
_______ 6. Longitudinal
_______ 7. Intracapsular
_______ 8. Impacted
_______ 9. Greenstick
_______ 10. Extracapsular
_______ 11. Fracture/dislocation
_______ 12. Depressed
_______ 13. Compound
_______ 14. Comminuted

25. Compare and contrast sprains, strains, and spasms.

Explain the purpose of each of the following diagnostic procedures. Indicate when each procedure would be used.

26. ROM testing

27. Muscle strength evaluation

28. X-ray studies

29. CT scans

30. MRI

Copyright © 2011, 2007, 2003 by Saunders, an imprint of Elsevier Inc. All rights reserved.

31. Arthrograms

32. EMG/NCS

33. DEXA scan

CASE STUDIES

1. A patient comes to the office with pain, tenderness, and deformity of the fingers. What questions should you ask? What medications will you ask about? Document the case.

2. A patient calls the office asking about fibromyalgia. She heard about the disease on a TV commercial and would like some information about the disorder. What can you tell her about the signs, symptoms, associated disorders, diagnosis, and treatment?

3. A patient on crutches comes to the office for a recheck of an ankle sprain. The medical assistant should be aware of what when obtaining the patient's weight, height, and vital signs? How should the patient be prepared for the examination?

4. The physician has ordered crutches for a patient with a knee injury. Kaiwan, the medical assistant, is responsible for fitting the patient properly. How should Kaiwan fit the patient? What patient education should Kaiwan provide?

WORKPLACE APPLICATIONS

1. The office manager has asked you to develop an osteoporosis awareness prevention program for the office staff. Together with a partner, brainstorm ideas for the development of this program.
   a. Many of the staff are young women. Why should they be concerned with osteoporosis?
   b. What are common risk factors for osteoporosis?
   c. What can individuals do to reduce their risk?
   d. What are common treatments?
   e. Using your knowledge of the disease, what type of activities can you implement in this program?

2. The office manager asks you to reinforce the correct method for using a walker with an elderly patient in the practice. What guidelines should you include?

Copyright © 2011, 2007, 2003 by Saunders, an imprint of Elsevier Inc. All rights reserved.

INTERNET ACTIVITIES

1. Use a drug reference book or the Internet to make drug cards for the following medications. Include the drug classification, generic name, usual adult dose, and drug form.
   a. Remicade
   b. Ridaura
   c. Prednisone
   d. Zyloprim
   e. Colchicine
   f. Anaprox
   g. Cataflam
   h. Relafen
   i. Toradol
   j. Voltaren
   k. Naprosyn
   l. Orudis
   m. Celebrex
   n. Acetaminophen
   o. Ambien
   p. Lyrica
   q. Fosamax
   r. Actonel
   s. Evista
   t. Miacalcin
   u. Soma
   v. Flexeril
   w. Benemid
   x. Plaquenil
   y. Imuran
   z. Cytoxan

2. Search the Internet for information describing proper lifting and patient transfer techniques. Why are proper mechanics important? Make notes on the different techniques and demonstrate your findings to the class.

Copyright © 2011, 2007, 2003 by Saunders, an imprint of Elsevier Inc. All rights reserved.

MEDICAL RECORD ACTIVITIES

1. A patient calls the office and requests the results of her recent MRI study. After finding the patient's medical record, you notice that the physician has not yet reviewed the results. The impression states: HNP of L3 and L4. What should you tell the patient? Why? Document a message in the patient's medical record.

2. A patient calls the office explaining that he has just fallen and twisted his ankle. What questions should you ask about the injury? What instructions should you give about applying ice to the ankle? Document the information in the patient's medical record.

3. Mrs. Alonzo Smith is being seen today for possible Lyme disease. How is Lyme disease transmitted? The physician asks you to reinforce teaching on how to prevent Lyme disease. Include in your documentation the patient education criteria for this health issue.

Copyright © 2011, 2007, 2003 by Saunders, an imprint of Elsevier Inc. All rights reserved.

44 Assisting in Neurology and Mental Health

VOCABULARY REVIEW

Define the following terms.

1. anomalies

   ____

2. ataxia

   ____

3. atrophy

   ____

4. coma

   ____

5. diplopia

   ____

6. gait

   ____

7. aura

   ____

8. contralateral

   ____

9. paresthesia

   ____

10. syncope

    ____

11. blood-brain barrier

    ____

12. exacerbation

    ____

13. ipsilateral

    ____

Copyright © 2011, 2007, 2003 by Saunders, an imprint of Elsevier Inc. All rights reserved.

14. papilledema

____

15. myelin sheath

____

Define the following procedures.

16. MRI

____

____

17. CT

____

____

18. EEG

____

____

19. Lumbar puncture

____

____

SKILLS AND CONCEPTS

1. Label the functional structures and lobes of the brain on the following figure.

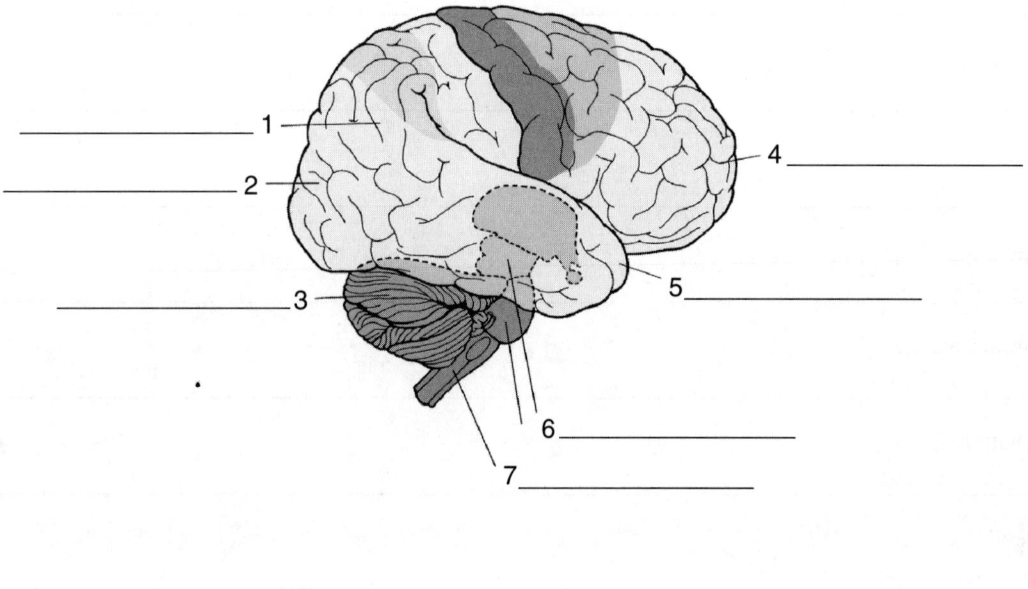

 Copyright © 2011, 2007, 2003 by Saunders, an imprint of Elsevier Inc. All rights reserved.

Describe the functions of each of the following.

2. CSF

____

____

3. Brainstem

____

____

4. Hypothalamus

____

____

5. Cerebrum

____

____

6. Spinal nerves

____

____

7. Cranial nerves

____

____

8. Autonomic nerves

____

____

9. Cerebellum

____

____

Copyright © 2011, 2007, 2003 by Saunders, an imprint of Elsevier Inc. All rights reserved.

10. Label the cranial nerves on the following figure.

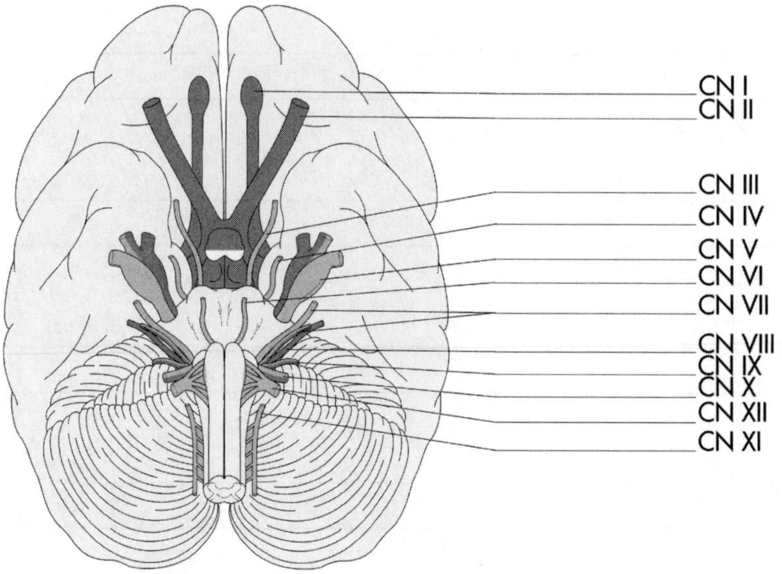

CN I ______________________________

CN II ______________________________

CN III ______________________________

CN IV ______________________________

CN V ______________________________

CN VI ______________________________

CN VII ______________________________

CN VIII ______________________________

CN IX ______________________________

CN X ______________________________

CN XI ______________________________

CN XII ______________________________

Copyright © 2011, 2007, 2003 by Saunders, an imprint of Elsevier Inc. All rights reserved.

11. Differentiate between a thrombus and an embolus.

____

____

____

12. Compare the afferent and efferent nervous pathways.

____

____

____

13. Label the parts of the neuron in the following picture.

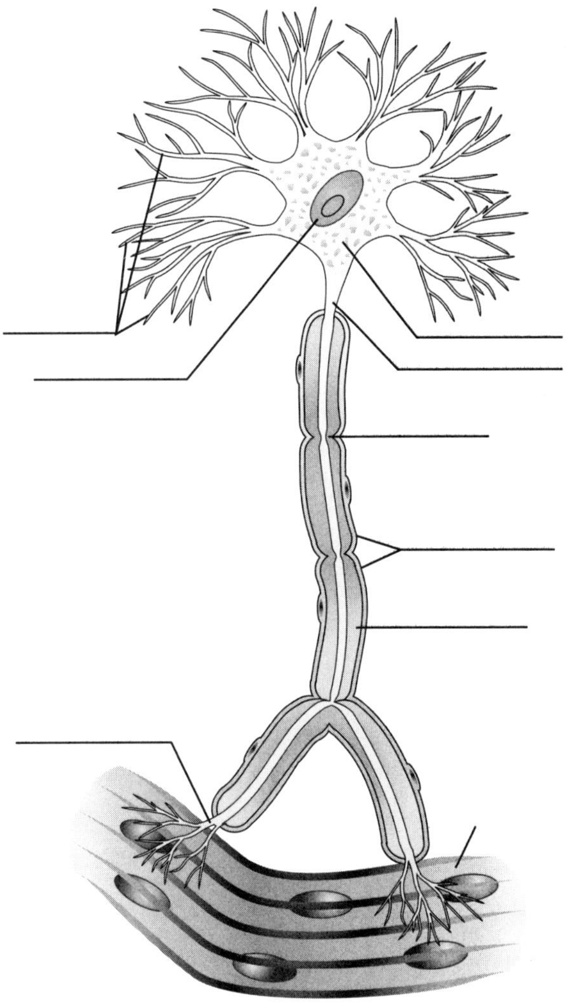

Copyright © 2011, 2007, 2003 by Saunders, an imprint of Elsevier Inc. All rights reserved.

14. Describe the three layers of the meninges and the spaces between each.

____

____

____

____

____

15. Explain the three different types of CVAs.

____

____

____

____

____

Fill in the blanks.

16. A(n) ______________ occurs when the blood supply to a particular part of the brain is inadequate for a limited period.

17. CVA is commonly referred to as ______________ or brain attack.

18. This ______________ often consists of some form of visual disturbance, such as dark lines across or spots within the visual field.

19. Absence or ______________ seizures are a less serious form of seizure consisting of momentary clouding of consciousness and loss of contact with reality.

20. The typical presentation of ______________ includes muscular rigidity, unilateral pill-rolling tremor of the hand, a high-pitched monotone voice, and a(n) ______________-like facial expression. The patient has a bent-forward posture with the head bowed. Muscular tremors and ______________ increase.

21. ______________ results from progressive inflammation and deterioration of the myelin sheaths, which leaves the nerve fibers uncovered.

22. ______________, or Lou Gehrig's disease, is a progressive, destructive neurologic disease that results in muscle atrophy.

23. ______________ affects the seventh cranial nerve in the face. It occurs suddenly and usually subsides spontaneously over several weeks to several months.

24. Carpal tunnel syndrome results from a compression or entrapment of the ______________ nerve as it courses past the carpal bones of the hand.

25. List nine signs and symptoms that suggest possible neurologic problems.

    a. ____
    b. ____
    c. ____
    d. ____
    e. ____
    f. ____
    g. ____
    h. ____
    i. ____

Copyright © 2011, 2007, 2003 by Saunders, an imprint of Elsevier Inc. All rights reserved.

26. Describe Brudzinski's sign. How is it performed and what does it demonstrate?

27. Compare and contrast encephalitis and meningitis.

28. Explain the difference between an epidural and a subdural hematoma.

29. Explain the difference between spinal transection and paraplegia and quadriplegia spinal cord injuries.

30. Describe the treatment recommendations for depression and the typical medications prescribed.

31. Summarize four risk factors for suicide.

a.

b.

c.

d.

32. Discuss the possible treatments for schizophrenia.

Copyright © 2011, 2007, 2003 by Saunders, an imprint of Elsevier Inc. All rights reserved.

CASE STUDIES

1. A patient comes to the office complaining of numbness in the left side of the face and difficulty walking. The patient is having difficulty with speech and is easily confused. With a partner, role-play this case. Measure vital signs. What questions should you ask the patient? What appears to be the preliminary diagnosis?

2. A mother calls and states that her son suffered a head injury at school today while playing football. She is concerned about the possibility of a concussion. What questions should the medical assistant ask the mother? Explain to the mother the signs and symptoms that might occur immediately after the injury, as well as those that could develop in a few days.

3. A patient comes to the office to discuss depression. She is crying and upset while you take her vital signs. What communication skills should you remember to use? What questions should you ask the patient? Describe some of the common signs and symptoms of depression.

WORKPLACE APPLICATIONS

1. The office has been asked to discuss depression at a community health seminar. What can you tell the audience about depression? What are some of the symptoms of depression?

2. Your office manager has asked you to create a patient education guide describing the common risk factors for CVA. What should be included?

3. Patients on warfarin (Coumadin) must constantly be monitored. Blood work is ordered regularly. How might an office ensure that patients are following orders and getting their laboratory work done on a timely basis? Why is this close monitoring necessary?

INTERNET ACTIVITIES

1. Use a drug reference book or the Internet to make drug cards for the following medications. Include the drug classification, generic name, usual adult dose, and drug form.

   a. Coumadin
   b. Plavix
   c. Imitrex
   d. Heparin
   e. Maxalt
   f. Sumatriptan succinate
   g. Effexor
   h. Dilantin
   i. Phenobarbital
   j. Valproic acid
   k. Prozac
   l. Zomig
   m. Topamax
   n. Neurontin
   o. Klonopin
   p. Lamictal
   q. Risperdal
   r. Zyprexa
   s. Xanax
   t. BuSpar

Copyright © 2011, 2007, 2003 by Saunders, an imprint of Elsevier Inc. All rights reserved.

u. Zoloft

v. Celexa

w. Rilutek

x. Avonex

y. Mirapex

z. Requip

2. Neurologic diseases and disorders can have an overwhelming impact on family members. Research online the support groups and area resources available for patients with the following conditions:

   a. Alzheimer's disease

   b. Parkinson's disease

   c. ALS

   d. Schizophrenia

   e. MS

   f. Epilepsy

   g. Spinal cord injuries

MEDICAL RECORD ACTIVITIES

1. On discharge from the hospital, a patient is prescribed Coumadin. Inform the patient about the drug's actions, side effects, and precautions for taking the medication. Document your patient education session.

2. Mary O'Reilly, age 37, has just been diagnosed with multiple sclerosis. The physician asks you to reinforce patient education about the cause of the disease, recommended treatment, and the remission/relapse cycle that typically occurs. Document your patient interaction.

3. Carl Westover calls today and wants a refill on his Xanax prescription. Carl is an Army veteran who suffers from posttraumatic stress disorder. Document your interaction with the patient.

Copyright © 2011, 2007, 2003 by Saunders, an imprint of Elsevier Inc. All rights reserved.

45 Assisting in Endocrinology

VOCABULARY REVIEW

Match the following terms with their definitions.

1. _______ A hormone produced by the alpha cells of the pancreatic islets that stimulates the liver to convert glycogen into glucose
2. _______ The abnormal presence of glucose in the urine
3. _______ The sugar (starch) formed from glucose and stored mainly in the liver

A. Glycosuria

B. Glycogen

C. Glucagon

Fill in the blanks.

4. Excessive thirst is called ________________.
5. ________________ is a hormone that stimulates the production and secretion of glucocorticoids; it is released by the anterior pituitary gland.
6. ________________ is a hormone secreted by the beta cells of the pancreatic islets in response to increased levels of glucose in the blood.
7. ________________ is the abnormal production of ketone bodies in the blood and tissue as a result of fat catabolism in cells. Ketones accumulate in large quantities when fat instead of glucose is used as fuel for energy in cells.
8. ________________ is a hormone secreted by the anterior lobe of the pituitary gland that stimulates the secretion of hormones produced by the thyroid gland.
9. ________________ means increased appetite.
10. ________________ is a hormone secreted by the posterior pituitary gland; it encourages fluid resorption in the renal tubules of the kidneys and a possible elevation in blood pressure. It is also known as *vasopressin.*
11. ________________ is excessive urine production.
12. ________________ is an anabolic action in the liver that forms glucose out of proteins and fats.
13. ________________, also called *somatotropic hormone,* is responsible for stimulating the epiphyseal plates of the long bones to create new tissue.
14. ________________ is produced by the anterior pituitary and stimulates the development of breast tissue.

SKILLS AND CONCEPTS

1. Identify the gland that produces the following hormones and the purpose of each hormone.

   a. Melatonin ____

   ____

   b. TSH ____

   ____

   c. Adrenaline____

   ____

Copyright © 2011, 2007, 2003 by Saunders, an imprint of Elsevier Inc. All rights reserved.

d. Insulin ______________________________

____

e. Glucagon ______________________________

____

2. Explain the difference between an exocrine gland and an endocrine gland.

____

____

____

3. Define negative feedback and give an example of how it works in the body.

____

____

____

4. Describe the hormones released by the anterior pituitary gland.

a. ______________________________

b. ______________________________

c. ______________________________

d. ______________________________

e. ______________________________

f. ______________________________

5. Define the three conditions related to alterations in growth hormone.

a. ______________________________

b. ______________________________

c. ______________________________

6. Define the following.

a. Diabetes insipidus

____

b. Addison's disease

____

c. Cushing's syndrome

____

7. You are interviewing two different patients who have a provisional diagnosis of hypothyroidism and hyperthyroidism. What signs and symptoms would you expect for each condition?

Hypothyroidism ______________________________

____

Hyperthyroidism ______________________________

____

Copyright © 2011, 2007, 2003 by Saunders, an imprint of Elsevier Inc. All rights reserved.

8. Explain prediabetes and how it is diagnosed.

____

____

____

9. Differentiate between diabetes mellitus type 1 and type 2.

____

____

____

10. Differentiate between diabetic coma and insulin shock.

____

____

____

11. Name and define the three "poly" conditions of diabetes mellitus.

a. ____

b. ____

c. ____

12. Medical assistants must be familiar with the different types of insulin that may be prescribed. Complete the following table.

Insulin Type	Onset of Action	Peak Action	Effective Duration	Appearance	Comments
Rapid acting					
		1–2 hr	2–5 hr	Clear	
Short acting					
Regular (Novolin R, Humulin R)		2-4 hr	3-5 hr	Clear	Take 30 min before meal
Intermediate acting					
	2–4 hr	4–10 hr			Take at bedtime to minimize nighttime hypoglycemia
Lente		4-12 hr	12-18 hr	Clear	
Long acting					
	6-10 hr	Minimal peak		Clear	
Glargine	4-6 hr	Peakless	24 hr	Clear	
Pre-mixed					
	30-60 min	2-10 hr	10-16 hr		

Copyright © 2011, 2007, 2003 by Saunders, an imprint of Elsevier Inc. All rights reserved.

13. Treatment for diabetes mellitus type 2 can involve a complicated combination of oral hypoglycemics, diet, and exercise. Provide the missing information about the most prescribed hypoglycemics.

Medication	**Action**
Micronase, Glucotrol, Amaryl	Increase insulin release from the pancreas
	Reduce hepatic glucose production; slightly increase muscle glucose uptake
Avandia	
Precose, Glyset	
Glucovance (Micronase and Glucophage)	
Avandamet (Avandia and Glucophage)	

14. You are responsible for drawing blood and following through with diagnostic orders for patients suspected of having diabetes mellitus. Identify the diagnostic criteria for DM.

____

____

____

15. Describe each of the following laboratory tests.

a. Thyroid-stimulating hormone (TSH)

____

____

____

b. OGGT

____

____

____

c. FBS

____

____

____

d. NFBS

____

____

____

e. Glycohemoglobin or hemoglobin A_{1c}

____

____

____

Copyright © 2011, 2007, 2003 by Saunders, an imprint of Elsevier Inc. All rights reserved.

CASE STUDIES

1. A patient at the clinic recently was diagnosed with diabetes insipidus. The physician asked you to educate the patient on the common signs and symptoms. What information do you want to be sure to include?

2. A patient comes to the office today complaining of fatigue, hair loss, muscle cramps, menorrhagia, and thick, dry, puffy skin. Her vital signs show a pulse of 56/minute, a temperature of 97.7° F, and a weight gain of 25 pounds over the past 3 months. What condition do these signs and symptoms suggest? What laboratory work will the physician most likely order?

3. A patient calls the office today stating that she is 20 weeks pregnant and is concerned about her risk for gestational diabetes. What questions would you ask her? How would you educate the patient on the risk factors of gestational diabetes.

4. Miguel, a medical assistant, has been assisting with diabetes nutritional education for Jerry for more than 6 months now. Unfortunately, the effort seems to be unsuccessful. Jerry explains that he feels good and does not see why he should change his eating habits. How would Miguel explain to Jerry the different types of long-term complications related to poorly controlled diabetes? Should Miguel provide any additional patient education? Why or why not? Are any community resources available that might prove useful for this patient?

WORKPLACE APPLICATIONS

1. Medical assistants must have a knowledge of the different medications prescribed for patients with endocrine abnormalities. Use the PDR to identify the indications for the following drugs:
   a. Synthroid
   b. Prednisone
   c. Byetta
   d. DiaBeta
   e. Glucophage
   f. Prandin
   g. Micronase
   h. Glucovance
   i. Avandia
   j. Actos
   k. Symlin
   l. Florinef
   m. Levoxyl
   n. Desmopressin

2. Create a handout that explains the difference between hypoglycemic and hyperglycemic episodes.

3. Carrie has been using her glucometer for the past 4 months and states that she does not feel the routine controls need to be done. How would you explain to Carrie the importance of the routine controls and when they should be performed?

4. Mr. Carlos Mantea has long-term diabetes type 2 and is complaining about numbness and tingling in his toes. What types of questions could you ask Mr. Mantea to gather comprehensive information about his condition for documentation?

Copyright © 2011, 2007, 2003 by Saunders, an imprint of Elsevier Inc. All rights reserved.

INTERNET ACTIVITIES

1. Go to the Web site *www.diabetes.org*. Locate the diabetes risk assessment tool and take the test. Are you surprised at the results? What lifestyle changes can you make to reduce your risk for diabetes?

2. Patients on a diabetic meal plan often feel that they are limited in the different foods they are allowed to eat. Search the Internet for different recipes and their nutritional exchanges for diabetics. Create a small collection of recipes you can share with your patients. Be sure your selections include a variety of foods so that your list appeals to a large population.

MEDICAL RECORD ACTIVITIES

1. Samantha Carson, a 16-year-old patient with diabetes type 1, is experiencing frequent episodes of hypoglycemia. The physician asks you to reinforce with her the Rule of 15 if she experiences hypoglycemic symptoms. Summarize the guidelines and document your interaction with the patient.

2. Scott Anderson has been newly diagnosed with diabetes type 2. Scott does not understand the complexities of his care, and you are responsible for reinforcing the physician's patient education. Summarize a patient education approach for a patient newly diagnosed with diabetes and document your interaction in the patient's medical record.

3. A patient with diabetes has come to your office because of a sore on his right great toe. He states that he was trimming a corn a week ago, and the area has become painful. You notice that the area is red and warm to the touch. The patient is wearing beach sandals. The patient's fasting blood sugar (FBS) is 348 mg/dL. His oral temperature is 100.9° F; blood pressure is 182/110 mm Hg; and pulse is 88/minute. Should you provide patient education on diabetic foot care? What should you include? Document the case.

Copyright © 2011, 2007, 2003 by Saunders, an imprint of Elsevier Inc. All rights reserved.

46 Assisting in Pulmonary Medicine

VOCABULARY REVIEW

Define the following terms.

1. apnea

___

2. atelectasis

___

3. dyspnea

___

4. empyema

___

5. hemoptysis

___

6. hemothorax

___

7. hypercapnia

___

8. hyperpnea

___

9. hypoxemia

___

10. orthopnea

___

11. pleurisy

___

12. pneumothorax

___

13. pyothorax

___

14. rhinoplasty

___

Copyright © 2011, 2007, 2003 by Saunders, an imprint of Elsevier Inc. All rights reserved.

15. rhinorrhea

____

16. tachypnea

____

17. thoracotomy

____

SKILLS AND CONCEPTS

1. _______________ is the abnormal dilation of the bronchi and bronchioles that may lead to COPD.
2. The _______________ are tiny, hair-like projections lining the respiratory tract that trap particles and move these unwanted substances up and out of the system.
3. Chronic tissue hypoxia can lead to an abnormal enlargement of the ends of the fingers called _______________.
4. Explain the process of ventilation. Include the action of the diaphragm and the intercostal muscles.

____

____

____

5. Label the following drawing with these anatomic landmarks: anterior, posterior, and midaxillary lines.

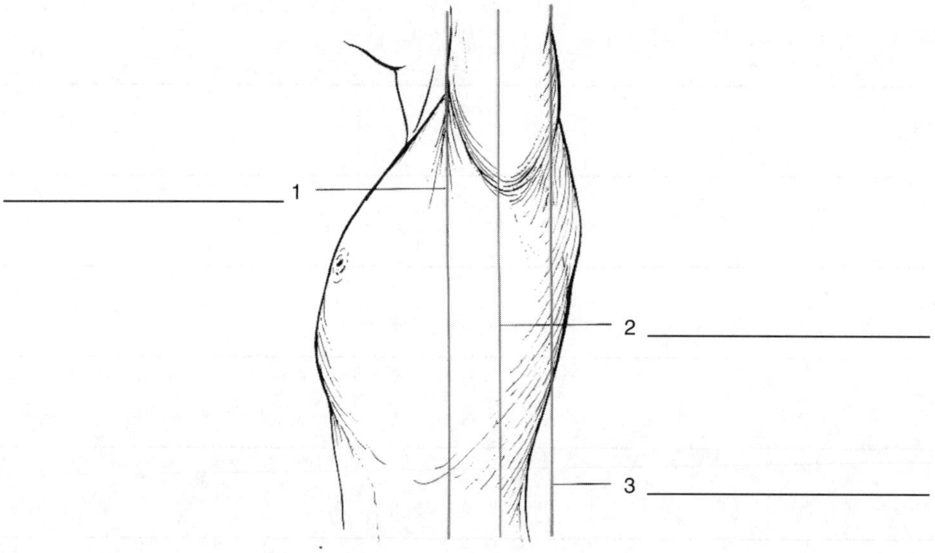

Copyright © 2011, 2007, 2003 by Saunders, an imprint of Elsevier Inc. All rights reserved.

6. On the following figure, label the structures of the respiratory system, head, and chest.

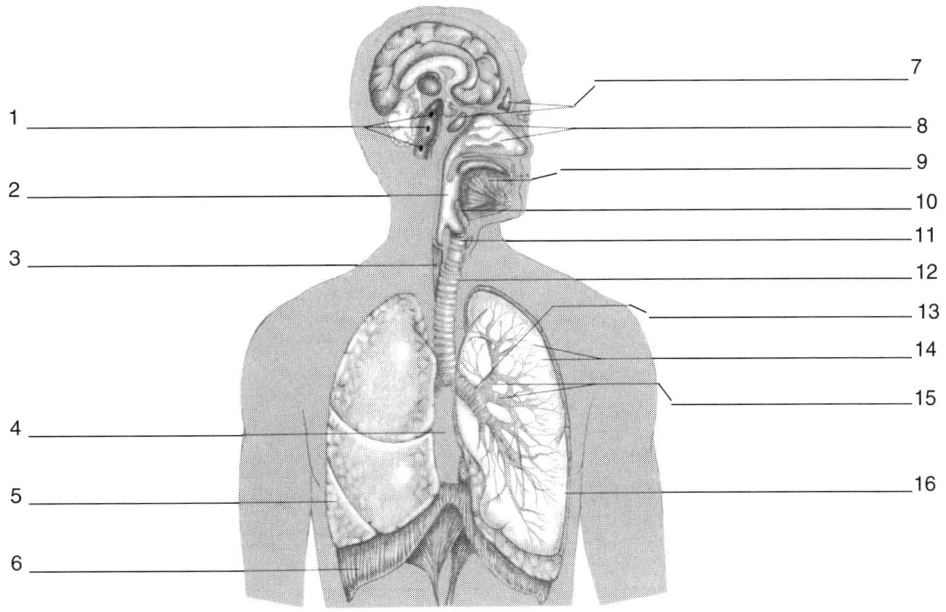

7. Label the lobes of the lungs on the following figure.

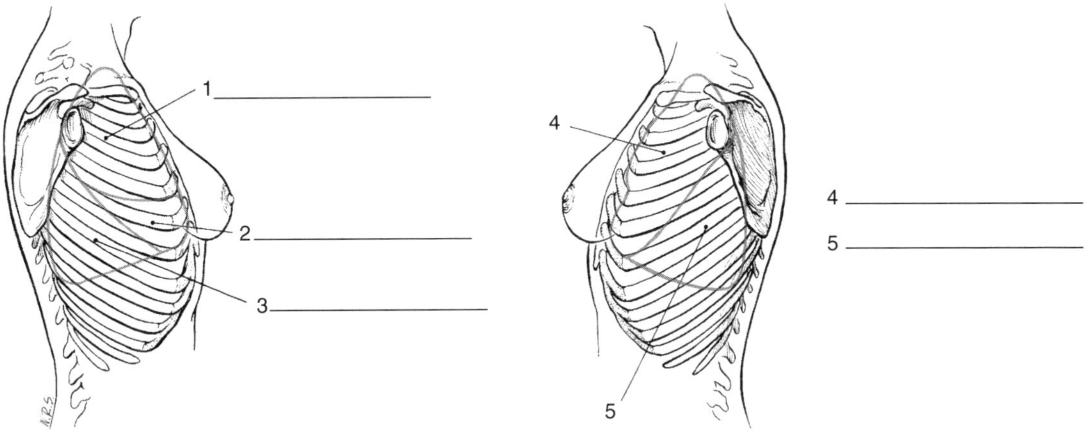

8. The signs and symptoms of sinusitis include:

____

____

9. Identify the medications that are used to treat allergic rhinitis.

____

____

Copyright © 2011, 2007, 2003 by Saunders, an imprint of Elsevier Inc. All rights reserved.

Fill in the blanks.

10. ________________ cancer is the leading cause of cancer-related deaths for both men and women in the United States.

11. A positive ________________ reaction indicates the possibility of active or dormant tuberculosis or exposure to the disease.

12. ________________ is a noninvasive method of evaluating the oxygen saturation of hemoglobin in arterial blood, as well as the pulse rate.

Match the following occupations with the associated lung diseases.

13. ________ Stone cutting or sand blasting
14. ________ Insulation and ship building
15. ________ Coal mining

a. Anthracosis
b. Silicosis
c. Asbestosis

16. Define the four tests used to diagnose TB.

a. ____
b. ____
c. ____
d. ____

17. Discuss the difference between latent and active tuberculosis.

____
____
____
____

18. Discuss how tuberculosis is treated.

____
____
____
____

19. Explain what happens during an asthma attack and how the patient should be treated.

____
____
____

20. You are responsible for teaching a patient how to use an inhaler. Explain the procedure below.

____
____
____
____

Copyright © 2011, 2007, 2003 by Saunders, an imprint of Elsevier Inc. All rights reserved.

21. List six signs and symptoms of obstructive sleep apnea.

a. ______________________________

b. ______________________________

c. ______________________________

d. ______________________________

e. ______________________________

f. ______________________________

22. Carcinoma of the ________________ is pathologically linked to smoking and chronic alcohol consumption.

CASE STUDIES

1. Dr. Samuelson orders a nebulizer treatment for a patient having an acute asthma attack. How should Michael prepare for this procedure? Describe the steps for administering a nebulizer treatment to a patient. What information should you provide for the patient? What should Michael watch for while the patient is undergoing the treatment?

2. A patient calls the office and requests an antibiotic for chest congestion. The patient is busy working today and refuses an appointment. What should the medical assistant do in this situation? Why?

3. A patient arrives today complaining of high fever, chills, dyspnea, chest pain during inspiration, and general malaise. The patient is a smoker. Dr. Samuelson suspects pneumonia. What tests are done to confirm the diagnosis? How may the physician determine whether the pneumonia is viral or bacterial? What is the treatment for bacterial pneumonia? What is the treatment plan for viral pneumonia?

WORKPLACE APPLICATIONS

1. Create a handout outlining a spirometry procedure including the lung function studies that are assessed during the procedure.

2. Michael is getting ready to obtain a sputum sample. What universal precautions should Michael follow? What equipment will he need to use? Why?

3. What instruction should the medical assistant provide a patient while scheduling a bronchoscopy?

INTERNET ACTIVITIES

1. One of the duties of a medical assistant is to serve as a resource for patients. Search the Internet for pulmonologists and respiratory durable medical equipment providers in your area. Create either a circular file or an address book with the names, addresses, phone numbers, and fax numbers for each resource. Include any additional information your patients may need (e.g., accepted insurance plans, services provided, hospital contacts).

2. The medical assistant must have knowledge of the different medications prescribed for patients with respiratory system abnormalities. Use the PDR to identify the indications for the following drugs:

   a. Allegra

   b. Flonase

   c. Singulair

   d. Alupent

   e. Advair

Copyright © 2011, 2007, 2003 by Saunders, an imprint of Elsevier Inc. All rights reserved.

f. Nasalcrom

g. Isoniazid (INH)

h. Rifampin

i. Accolate

j. Flovent Diskus

MEDICAL RECORD ACTIVITIES

1. Maura, a 10-year-old patient, has recently been diagnosed with asthma. To help her better understand how to recognize her symptoms, Dr. Samuelson has asked Michael to teach Maura how to use a peak flow meter. Role-play with a partner and document the case.

2. Juan Garcia, a 42-year-old patient, has just been diagnosed with active TB. What symptoms would you expect Mr. Garcia to exhibit? How would you protect yourself from exposure? What patient education will Mr. Garcia need to protect his family and co-workers from the disease? Document the case in the medical record.

3. Document the following case. Use correct medical terminology for respiratory system terms.

   Mabel Bishop, a 73-year-old patient of Dr. Samuelson's, has been a long-time smoker with a history of a collapsed right lung, difficulty breathing, and the only position she finds comfortable for breathing is sitting upright. She has come to the office today complaining of blood when she coughs; stabbing pain when she breathes, especially on the right side; and excessive nasal drainage. Dr. Samuelson listens to her lungs and can hear both a popping and rumbling sound in the right and left lower lobes.

Copyright © 2011, 2007, 2003 by Saunders, an imprint of Elsevier Inc. All rights reserved.

47 Assisting in Cardiology

VOCABULARY REVIEW

Fill in the blanks.

1. An abnormal sound or murmur heard on auscultation of an organ, vessel, or gland is a(n) ________________.
2. Recurring cramping in the calves caused by poor circulation of blood to the muscles of the lower leg is called ________________ claudication.
3. ________________ is an autoimmune disorder that affects the blood vessels and connective tissue, causing fibrous degeneration of the major organs.
4. The heart is enclosed in a double-membrane sac called the ________________.
5. The middle layer of the heart is the ________________, which is the muscle layer.
6. The medical term for heart attack is ________________.
7. Patients with ________________ have an inherited predisposition for the development of aneurysms.
8. The inner layer of the heart is the ________________, which includes the valves of the heart.
9. Describe the action of depolarization and repolarization.

____

____

____

10. Define essential and secondary hypertension.

____

____

____

SKILLS AND CONCEPTS

1. Describe the conduction system of the heart.

____

____

____

Copyright © 2011, 2007, 2003 by Saunders, an imprint of Elsevier Inc. All rights reserved.

2. Label the parts of the heart and describe the blood flow through the heart in the following figure.

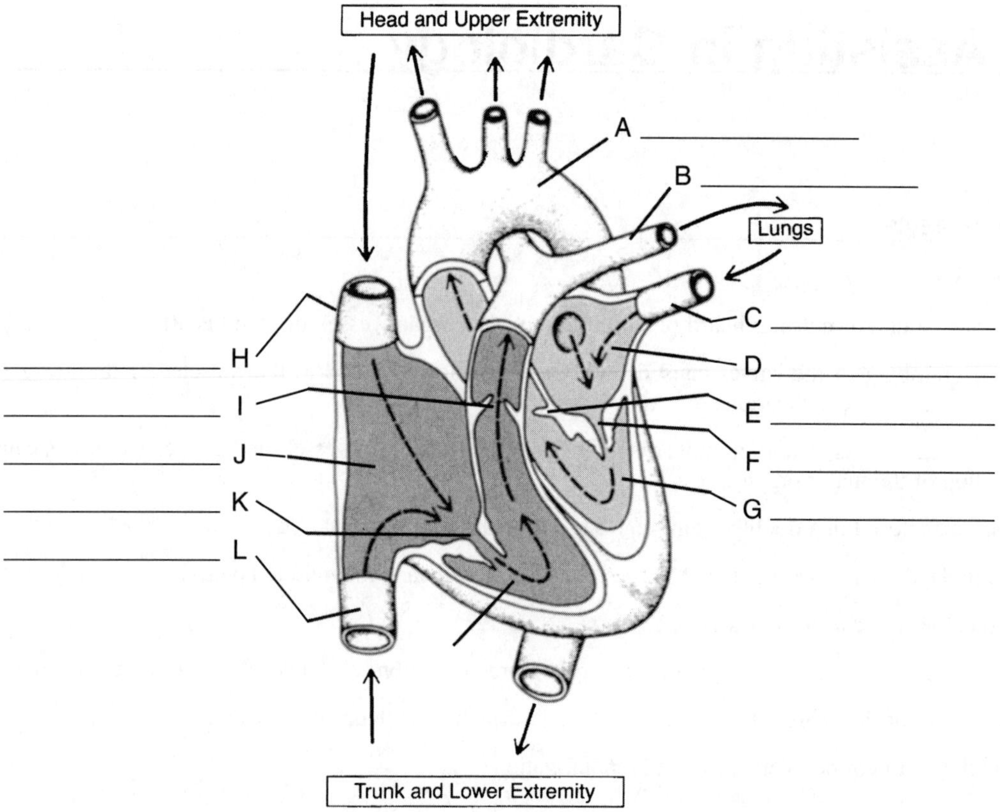

3. List three risk factors for heart disease that cannot be changed.

a. ______

b. ______

c. ______

4. Summarize six lifestyle factors that put a patient at risk for heart disease.

a. ______

b. ______

c. ______

d. ______

e. ______

f. ______

5. Explain the process of atheroma formation in a patient with hypercholesterolemia.

______

______

______

Copyright © 2011, 2007, 2003 by Saunders, an imprint of Elsevier Inc. All rights reserved.

6. Summarize the signs and symptoms typically seen in male and female patients experiencing an MI.

Male ____

____

Female____

____

7. Explain the use of blood tests in diagnosing an MI.

CK levels ____

____

Troponin levels ____

____

8. _______________, such as _______________, are administered intravenously to dissolve coronary artery blockage and prevent permanent myocardial damage. However, to be most effective, this treatment must be started within _______________ of the episode.

9. Explain the difference between a CABG procedure and a coronary angioplasty.

____

____

____

10. Complete the following table, which summarizes the various stages of hypertension and how they are treated.

Blood Pressure	**Treatment**
Prehypertension	Lifestyle modification
	Drug therapy in patients with:
Stage 1	Consider coexisting conditions
	Medication
Stage 2	Consider coexisting conditions
	Medication

11. List five conditions that can result from hypertension.

a. ____

b. ____

c. ____

d. ____

e. ____

Copyright © 2011, 2007, 2003 by Saunders, an imprint of Elsevier Inc. All rights reserved.

12. Complete the following table, which presents medications used to treat hypertension.

Classification/Name	Action	Treatment Protocol
Thiazide diuretics (Hydrodiuril, Lasix, Lozol, Aldactone)		First drugs of choice for treatment of hypertension; enhance the action of other BP medications; used in patients with diabetes and chronic kidney disease who have prehypertension.
Beta blockers (Tenormin, Lopressor, Ziac, Inderal)		May be used with a diuretic for stage 1 or stage 2 hypertension
Angiotensin-converting enzyme (ACE) inhibitors (Lotensin, Capoten, Vasotec, Monopril, Prinivil, Zestril)		May be used with a diuretic for stage 1 or stage 2 hypertension; also for hypertension in patients with coronary artery disease, heart failure, or kidney failure
Angiotensin II receptor blockers (Cozaar, Atacand, Diovan)		May be used with a diuretic for stage 1 or stage 2 hypertension; also for hypertension in patients with coronary artery disease, heart failure or kidney failure
Calcium channel blockers (Norvasc, Lotrel, Cardizem, Procardia, Vascor)		May be used with a diuretic for stage 1 or stage 2 hypertension; also used to treat angina and/or some arrhythmias

13. Identify the causes of the various types of shock.

Type of Shock	Causes
Cardiogenic	
Hypovolemic	
Neurogenic	
Anaphylactic	
Septic	

Fill in the blanks.

14. ________________ is diagnosed if the patient experiences a drop in blood pressure when standing.

15. Damage and scar formation on the heart's valves are often seen in patients with ________________.

16. ________________ carries oxygenated blood away from the heart.

17. ________________ is an incompetence in the mitral valve resulting from a congenital defect or vegetation from endocarditis.

18. Dilated, tortuous, superficial veins in the legs are called ________________.

19. A cardiac pacemaker is most often used for treatment of ________________.

20. A(n) ________________ is used for patients experiencing frequent episodes of ventricular fibrillation.

CASE STUDIES

1. A patient is prescribed Tenormin 25 mg once daily. Prepare a prescription for the physician's signature on the following form. Order enough medication for a 3-month supply with two refills. Explain to the patient the effects of Tenormin on the body.

Copyright © 2011, 2007, 2003 by Saunders, an imprint of Elsevier Inc. All rights reserved.

DEA#: 8543201 John Jones, M.D. Tel: 544-8976
108 N. Main St.
City, State

Patient ______________________ DATE ___________

ADDRESS ___________________________________

Rx:

Disp:

Sig:

Refill _____ Times
Please label ☑ ______________________________

2. Adam, a medical assistant, is taking vital signs on a patient and records a blood pressure in the right arm of 168/98 mm Hg. What steps should Adam take next?

3. A patient has been diagnosed with prehypertension. Adam should educate the patient to make what type of lifestyle modifications?

4. A patient complains of calf pain and swelling in the left leg. The leg is warm to the touch. What questions should the medical assistant ask this patient? If a DVT is suspected, what tests can be done to confirm the diagnosis? What is the common treatment for DVT? What precautions should the medical assistant take when performing venipuncture on a patient taking warfarin (Coumadin)?

WORKPLACE APPLICATIONS

1. You are updating the policy and procedures manual. The new version will include telephone screening templates, which will guide other medical assistants in the proper handling of situations. Create a list of circumstances in which the medical assistant should activate emergency medical services for a patient with chest pain.

2. Corina visits the office and states that she would like the results of her neighbor's heart catheterization. Corina states that her neighbor had a difficult time understanding the results when the physician called her, so Corina thought she might be better able to relay any messages. Can Adam give Corina the requested information? What steps should Adam take to make sure the patient correctly understands the physician's message?

3. An elderly patient, Miss Kate Glasgow, is being seen in the office today for complaints of vertigo and syncope when she stands. The physician suspects orthostatic hypotension. Explain how you would check Miss Glasgow's BP for this condition.

INTERNET ACTIVITIES

1. As discussed in the text, many risk factors are involved in the development of heart disease. Visit the Web site *www.americanheartassociation.com* and use the risk assessment tool to determine your risk for heart disease. Did any of the results surprise you? What type of modifications can you make to reduce your risk for heart disease?

Copyright © 2011, 2007, 2003 by Saunders, an imprint of Elsevier Inc. All rights reserved.

2. The medical assistant must be knowledgeable about the different medications prescribed for patients with respiratory system abnormalities. Use the PDR to identify the indications for the following drugs:
   a. Activase
   b. Retavase
   c. Tenormin
   d. Lopressor
   e. Inderal
   f. Lipitor
   g. Mevacor
   h. Zocor
   i. Hydrodiuril
   j. Lasix
   k. Lozol
   l. Aldactone
   m. Lopressor
   n. Ziac
   o. Inderal
   p. Lotensin
   q. Capoten
   r. Vasotec
   s. Monopril
   t. Prinivil
   u. Zestril
   v. Norvasc
   w. Lotrel
   x. Cardizem
   y. Procardia
   z. Vascor

MEDICAL RECORD ACTIVITIES

1. Lucille Kring, a 48-year-old patient, has been diagnosed with metabolic syndrome. What signs and symptoms would you expect to see in this patient? The physician has asked you to reinforce her patient education about risk factors for cardiac disease. What would you include in this information? Document the patient education intervention and the vital signs you would expect to gather in this patient.
2. A 52-year-old male patient calls the office complaining of jaw and neck pain that seems to radiate to both arms. For the past 2 hours, he has been increasingly short of breath, has had pressure in his chest, and has been sweating. What do you suspect the problem may be? What advice would you give this patient? Document the case.
3. Simon Jacobson is scheduled for a transesophageal echocardiogram as a follow up for a congenital mitral valve prolapse. He has never had this particular procedure before, and is quite concerned about how it will be done and whether he will experience any pain. Explain the procedure to Mr. Jacobson and document your teaching intervention in the patient's medical record.

Copyright © 2011, 2007, 2003 by Saunders, an imprint of Elsevier Inc. All rights reserved.

48 Assisting in Geriatrics

VOCABULARY REVIEW

Match the following terms with their definitions.

1. _______ The secretion or discharge of tears
2. _______ A sore or ulcer over a bony prominence caused by ischemia from prolonged pressure; a bedsore
3. _______ Age-related farsightedness that makes focusing on near objects difficult
4. _______ Protein that forms the inelastic fibers of tendons, ligaments, and fascia
5. _______ Pertaining to the ribs
6. _______ A decreased ability to hear high frequencies and to discriminate sounds; age-related hearing loss
7. _______ An essential part of elastic connective tissue that is flexible and elastic when moist
8. _______ Waxy, greasy papules on the skin that vary from tan to dark brown; also called *age spots*

a. Collagen
b. Costal
c. Decubitus ulcer
d. Elastin
e. Lacrimation
f. Seborrheic keratoses
g. Presbyopia
h. Presbycusis

SKILLS AND CONCEPTS

1. List five myths and stereotypes about aging.
   a. ____
   b. ____
   c. ____
   d. ____
   e. ____

2. Describe the effects of aging on the cardiovascular system.
____
____
____
____

3. What can aging patients do to reduce their risk of cardiovascular disease? ____
____
____
____
____

Copyright © 2011, 2007, 2003 by Saunders, an imprint of Elsevier Inc. All rights reserved.

4. List six risk factors for cognitive decline.

a. ______________________________

b. ______________________________

c. ______________________________

d. ______________________________

e. ______________________________

f. ______________________________

g. ______________________________

5. Explain the purpose of the Mini-Mental Status Examination. What abilities does it assess, and how is it performed?

____

____

____

____

6. Describe the stages of Alzheimer's disease.

First stage ______________________________

____

Second stage ______________________________

____

Terminal stage ______________________________

____

7. List six suggestions for helping elderly individuals prevent and treat dry skin.

a. ______________________________

b. ______________________________

c. ______________________________

d. ______________________________

e. ______________________________

f. ______________________________

8. Explain the changes that occur in the pulmonary system with aging.

____

____

____

____

Copyright © 2011, 2007, 2003 by Saunders, an imprint of Elsevier Inc. All rights reserved.

9. List six suggestions for helping an older adult with mobility, dexterity, and balance.

a. ______________________________

b. ______________________________

c. ______________________________

d. ______________________________

e. ______________________________

f. ______________________________

10. Summarize the medical assistant's role in caring for elderly patients.

____

____

____

CASE STUDIES

1. A patient is having difficulty staying steady on his feet and must use a walker to remain mobile. How can the medical assistant aid the patient? What approach should the medical assistant take in preparing the patient for the physician's examination?

2. A patient recently stopped complying with her diabetes treatment plan. What factors should Bill, the medical assistant, be aware of that may affect the patient's diabetes management? How can Bill help the patient deal with these factors?

3. Mary is concerned about her risk for osteoporosis. What can Bill tell Mary about common risk factors for the development of osteoporosis? Can she do anything to prevent the decrease in bone density? What tests are done to diagnosis osteoporosis? Describe methods for preventing and treating osteoporosis.

4. Mr. Carlos Rozera, age 82, has both hearing and vision impairments because of age-related changes. What suggestions can you give Bill to help him communicate with Mr. Rozera?

5. Mr. Herbert Sampson's daughter brings him to the office today because of concerns about his increasing difficulty with memory and confusion. A number of conditions can cause cognitive changes in aging individuals. What risk factors may be contributing to Mr. Sampson's memory loss and confusion? What methods might the family use to improve Mr. Sampson's cognitive ability?

WORKPLACE APPLICATIONS

1. You are asked to speak at a local community center about the prevention of injuries in aging people. What suggestions can you make for preventing falls in this age group?

2. Your office sees many geriatric patients daily. What are some common barriers for aging patient's when they come into the office? What changes can you make to provide a safe and welcoming environment?

3. One of the duties of the medical assistant is to inform patients about advance directives. What information should the medical assistant provide to the patient? Why is it important for a patient to have an advance directive?

4. Patient education is vital to helping patients understand various disease processes and health maintenance. Describe some guidelines for effective patient education with older adults.

Copyright © 2011, 2007, 2003 by Saunders, an imprint of Elsevier Inc. All rights reserved.

5. You are interviewing an aging patient and begin to suspect that the patient may be suffering from abuse. What are the indications of elder abuse? How are elder abuse cases handled in your state?

INTERNET ACTIVITIES

1. Aging individuals frequently need assistance to be able to remain in their homes and maintain independence. The medical assistant should be prepared to provide details on community resources that could be useful to older patients and their families. Conduct a search online for resources that could provide assistance to aging people and develop a resource guide that could be used as a referral source in the ambulatory care setting.

2. One reason patients do not comply with medication orders is the lack of prescription coverage. Search the Internet for programs that provide patient assistance for medications. What are the criteria for enrollment? Be prepared to discuss your findings in class.

3. The medical assistant must be knowledgeable about the different medications prescribed for patients with respiratory system abnormalities. Use the PDR to identify the indications for the following drugs:

   a. Fosamax

   b. Actonel

   c. Evista

   d. Calcimar

   e. Miacalcin

   f. Aricept

   g. Exelon

   h. Reminyl

   i. Namenda

   j. Ambien

   k. Restoril

   l. Sonata

   m. Lunesta

   n. Reclast

MEDICAL RECORD ACTIVITIES

1. A patient comes to the office today for a follow-up appointment because of orthostatic hypotension. What questions should Bill ask the patient? How should Bill measure the patient's vital signs? Document the case.

2. While Bill is taking Mrs. Simoni's health history, she complains of chronic constipation. What questions should Bill ask her? What are the possible causes of constipation in elderly individuals? What dietary measures may help provide relief? Document the case.

3. Dr. Kennedy is concerned that Mrs. Isabel Carmassi may be suffering from a nutritional deficiency. What factors could be contributing to her poor dietary choices? What questions should the medical assistant ask to obtain detailed information about her dietary habits? Document the case.

Copyright © 2011, 2007, 2003 by Saunders, an imprint of Elsevier Inc. All rights reserved.

49 Principles of Electrocardiography

VOCABULARY REVIEW

Match the following terms with their definitions.

1. ________ Bradycardia
2. ________ Bundle of His
3. ________ Cardiac arrest
4. ________ Cardioversion
5. ________ Defibrillator
6. ________ Dyspnea
7. ________ Hypertension
8. ________ Infarction
9. ________ Ischemic
10. ________ Myocardial
11. ________ Arrhythmia
12. ________ Orthopnea
13. ________ Sinoatrial (SA) node
14. ________ Tachycardia

a. Complete cessation of cardiac contractions
b. Use of electroshock to convert an abnormal cardiac rhythm to a normal one
c. An irregular heart rhythm
d. A heart rate less than 60 beats per minute
e. Fibers that conduct electrical impulses from the AV node to the ventricular myocardium
f. A heart rate greater than 100 beats per minute
g. An area of tissue that has died because of lack of blood supply
h. A temporary interruption in blood supply to a tissue or organ
i. Pertaining to the heart muscle
j. Difficulty breathing when in the supine position
k. The pacemaker of the heart, located in the right atrium
l. A machine used to deliver an electroshock to the heart through electrodes placed on the chest wall
m. Difficulty breathing
n. High blood pressure in which the diastolic pressure is greater than 90mm Hg

SKILLS AND CONCEPTS

1. Describe diastole and systole.

____

____

____

____

Copyright © 2011, 2007, 2003 by Saunders, an imprint of Elsevier Inc. All rights reserved.

2. Label each structure on the following figure.

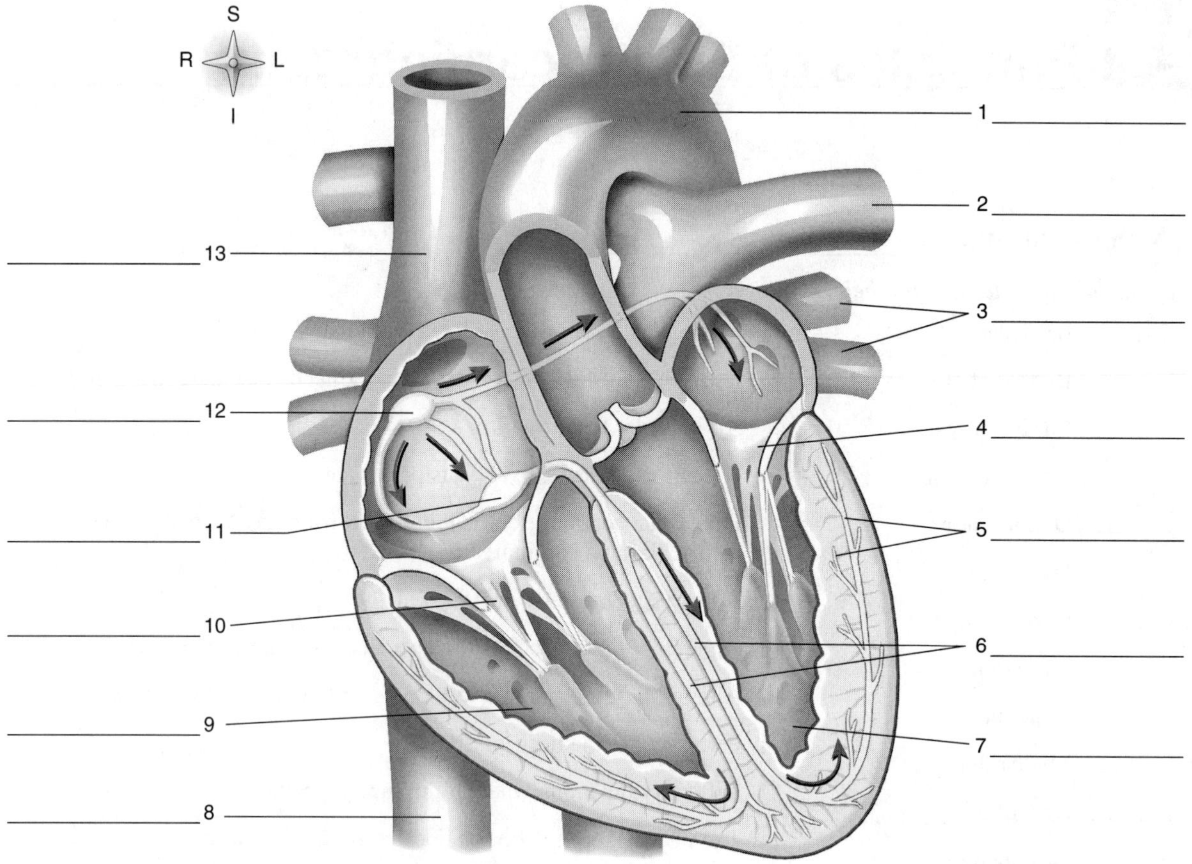

3. Describe the conduction pathways of the heart.

____

____

____

____

4. Label the precordial leads on the following drawing.

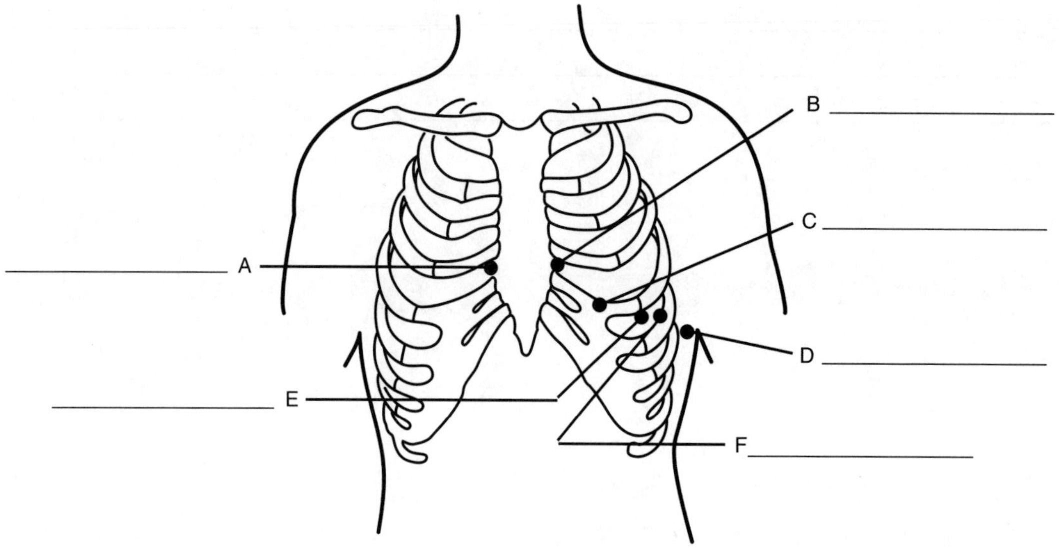

Copyright © 2011, 2007, 2003 by Saunders, an imprint of Elsevier Inc. All rights reserved.

5. Name the rhythm shown in the following illustration.

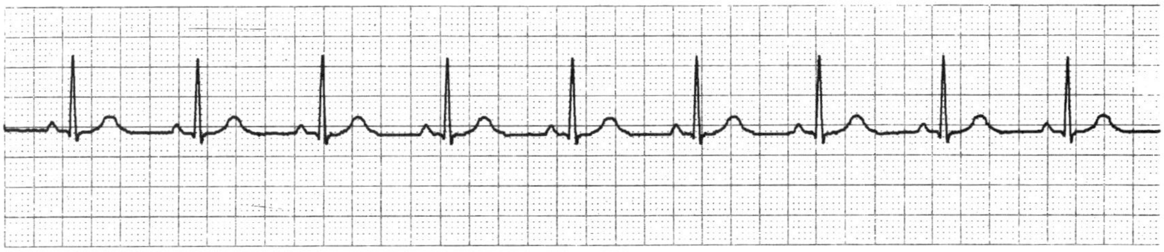

____

6. Name the rhythm shown in the following illustration.

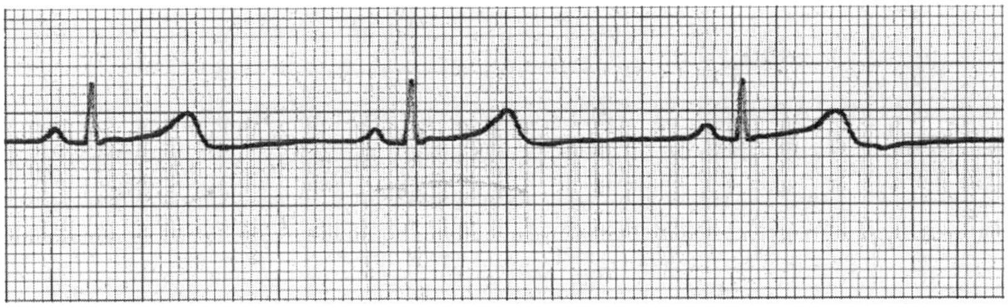

____

7. Name the rhythm shown in the following illustration.

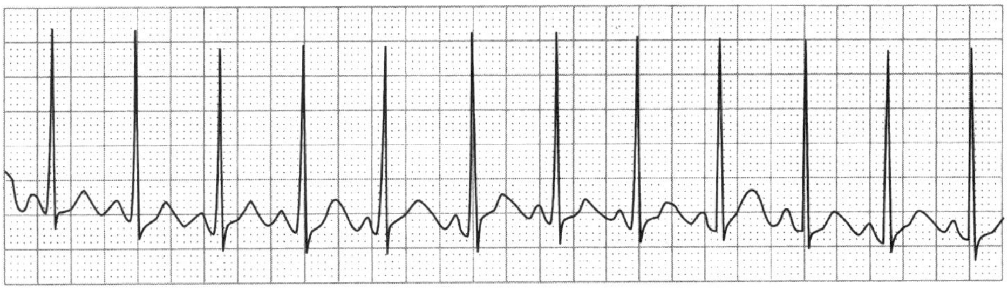

____

8. Name the rhythm shown in the following illustration.

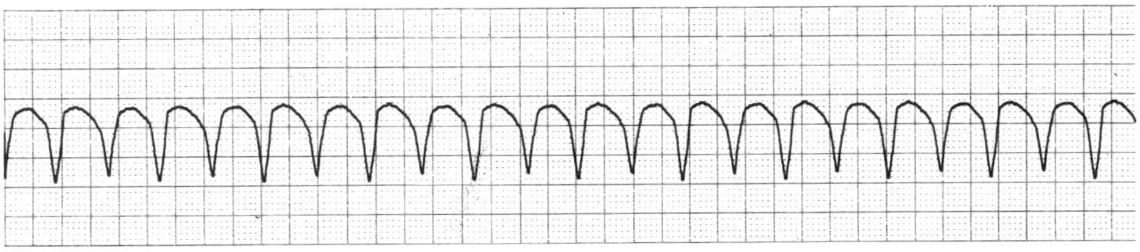

____

9. Name the rhythm shown in the following illustration.

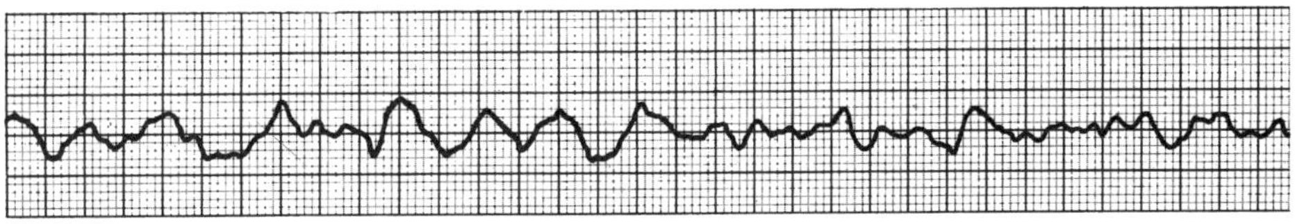

____

Copyright © 2011, 2007, 2003 by Saunders, an imprint of Elsevier Inc. All rights reserved.

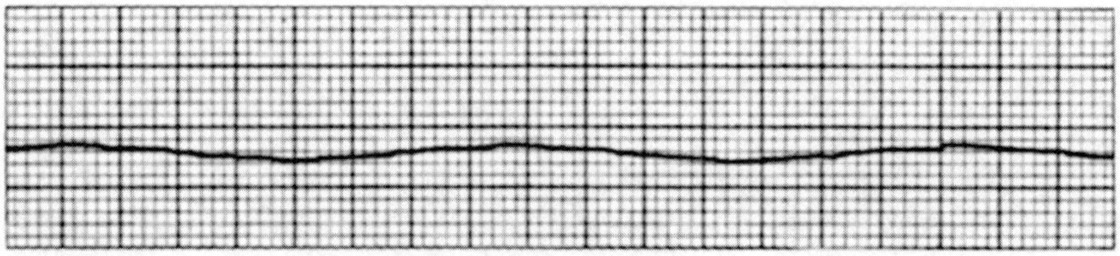

10. Name the rhythm shown in the following illustration.

11. Describe the procedure shown in the following illustration.

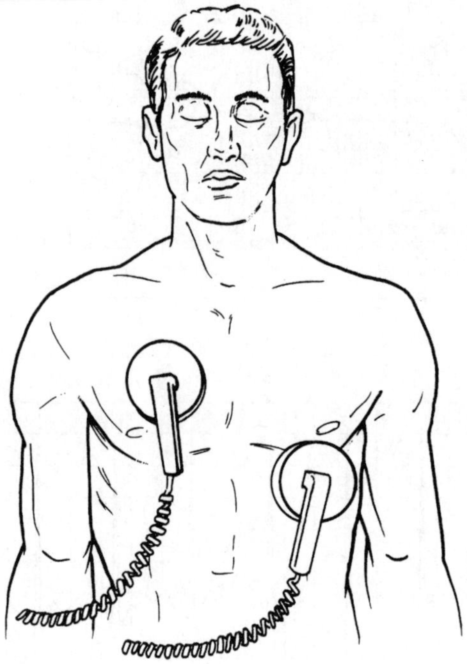

Fill in the blanks.

12. The ________________ wave occurs during the contraction of the atria and shows the beginning of cardiac depolarization.
13. The ________________ complex shows the contraction of both ventricles and also reflects the completion of cardiac depolarization.
14. The ________________ interval is the time from the beginning of atrial contraction to the beginning of ventricular contraction.
15. The T wave indicates ventricular recovery, or ________________ of the ventricles.
16. ECG paper has horizontal and vertical lines at ________________-mm intervals.
17. When running at normal speed, one small, 1-mm square passes the stylus every ________________ seconds.
18. One large, 5-mm square passes the stylus every ________________ seconds.
19. Lead I records the electrical activity between the ________________ arm and the ________________ arm.

 Copyright © 2011, 2007, 2003 by Saunders, an imprint of Elsevier Inc. All rights reserved.

20. Lead ________________ records the electrical activity between the right arm and the left leg.

21. Lead III records the electrical activity between the ________________ arm and the left leg.

22. ________________ records the activity from midway between the left leg and the left arm to the right arm.

23. ________________ records the activity from midway between the right arm and the left leg to the left arm.

24. ________________ records the activity from midway between the right arm and the left arm to the left leg.

25. With the ________________ baseline, the stylus gradually shifts away from the center of the paper.

26. ________________ shows up on the recording as jagged peaks of irregular height and spacing and a shifting baseline.

27. ________________ occurs when the electric connection has been interrupted.

28. ________________ interference appears as a series of uniform small spikes on the paper.

29. Cardiac ________________ testing is conducted to observe and record the patient's cardiovascular response to measured exercise challenges.

30. A(n) ________________ monitor is a portable system for recording the cardiac activity of a patient over a 24-hour period or longer.

31. The stylus should deflect exactly ________________ when the standardization button is depressed.

32. The standard speed for an ECG recording is ________________.

33. A(n) ________________ monitors the heart rhythm and delivers a shock to the heart if it detects a dangerous tachycardia or fibrillation.

34. What information should be analyzed when an ECG strip is read?

 a. ____

 b. ____

 c. ____

 d. ____

 e. ____

35. Summarize the classic changes that occur in the ECG when a patient experiences an MI.

____

36. List three reasons cardiac stress tests are performed.

 a. ____

 b. ____

 c. ____

37. ________________ is a screening tool that allows physicians to see the amount of plaque in the coronary arteries by showing the presence of calcium deposits.

CASE STUDIES

1. You have been instructed to perform an ECG on a 51-year-old man. As you start to prepare the patient for the examination, you notice a large amount of body hair on his chest. Can the procedure still be performed? What should you do? Why?

2. Martha, the medical assistant, is performing electrocardiography on a patient who complains of orthopnea. In what position can the patient be placed?

Copyright © 2011, 2007, 2003 by Saunders, an imprint of Elsevier Inc. All rights reserved.

3. During the ECG recording, the patient coughs and starts talking. What type of artifacts would you expect to see?

4. The physician has reviewed a patient's ECG and has concluded that the patient has PACs. Explain to the patient what is happening to the heart during this time. What are some common causes of PACs?

5. The physician has just prescribed digoxin for a patient. What can Martha tell the patient about the effects of the drug? Refer to the PDR for important drug information.

WORKPLACE APPLICATIONS

1. Martha is showing a new employee around the office during orientation. The office has both a multichannel and a single-channel ECG machine. Describe the difference between these two machines. Which one is more convenient?

2. A new shipment of ECG paper and electrodes has just arrived at the office. What should Martha remember when storing the supplies? Why?

3. Martha is nervous that she will not remember the lead placement while performing electrocardiography. Describe the lead placement.

   RA ____________________

   RL ____________________

   LA ____________________

   LL ____________________

   V_1 ____________________

   V_2 ____________________

   V_3 ____________________

   V_4 ____________________

   V_5 ____________________

   V_6 ____________________

4. What can the medical assistant do to prevent AC interference on the ECG strip?

5. As you are preparing a patient for Holter monitor testing, he asks why a Holter monitor would be ordered instead of an ECG. How should you respond? The patient states that he is too busy to record the daily activities. Explain to the patient the importance of keeping a diary during Holter monitor testing.

6. You are hired to work in a cardiologist's practice and are concerned about understanding the immediate treatment for a patient who is suffering an MI. Summarize the typical treatment protocol for this cardiac emergency.

INTERNET ACTIVITY

The office is considering the purchase of a Holter monitor. You have been asked to research the different types of equipment available. Use the Internet to search for different suppliers of Holter monitors. Consider the usability, cost, and maintenance of the different products. Present your findings to the class. Which product would you recommend and why?

MEDICAL RECORD ACTIVITIES

1. You are responsible for explaining to a patient how to use an event monitor at home. Document your patient education intervention, including an explanation of the purpose of the monitor and directions on how to use it throughout the test period.

2. You have just performed an ECG on a patient. What type of information should be documented about the procedure?

Copyright © 2011, 2007, 2003 by Saunders, an imprint of Elsevier Inc. All rights reserved.

50 Assisting with Diagnostic Imaging

VOCABULARY REVIEW

Match the following terms with their definitions.

1. _______	distal	a. Forward or the front portion of the body or body part
2. _______	internal	b. Pertaining to the head; toward the head
3. _______	plantar	c. Away from the head; the opposite of cephalad
4. _______	medial or mesial	d. Away from the source or point of origin
5. _______	palmar	e. To the outside, at or near the surface of the body or a body part
6. _______	external	f. Below, farther from the head
7. _______	anterior	g. Deep, near the center of the body or a part; the opposite of external
8. _______	inferior	h. Referring to the side; away from the center to the left or right
9. _______	lateral	i. Toward the center of the body or of a body part; the opposite of lateral
10. _______	posterior	j. Referring to the palm (anterior surface) of the hand
11. _______	cephalic, cephalad	k. Referring to the sole of the foot
12. _______	caudal, caudad	l. Backward or the back portion of the body or body part; the opposite of anterior
13. _______	superior	m. Toward the source or point of origin; the opposite of distal
14. _______	proximal	n. Above, toward the head; the opposite of inferior

Fill in the blanks with the correct terms.

1. ________________ refers to the making of x-ray images called *radiographs*.
2. X-rays can penetrate most substances to some degree, but some substances, such as metal and bone, are more difficult to penetrate and are said to be ________________.
3. ________________ is a technique performed with special equipment that allows the radiologist to view x-ray images in motion.
4. The ________________ scanner consists of a movable table with remote control, a circular gantry structure that supports the x-ray tube and detectors, an operator console with a monitor, and the supporting computer system.
5. ________________ medicine scans do not provide clear images of anatomic structures. They are used to obtain information about the function of organs and tissues.
6. A(n) ________________ is the radioactive substance administered to patients for nuclear medicine imaging procedures.
7. The ________________ is the moving grid device that prevents scatter radiation from fogging x-ray film.
8. The ________________ is the part of the sonography machine in contact with the patient; it sends high-frequency sound waves and receives the sound echoes that return from the patient's body.
9. A(n) ________________ is a fluoroscopic examination of the soft tissue components of joints with direct injection of a contrast medium into the joint capsule.
10. Barium sulfate is an example of a(n) ________________.

Copyright © 2011, 2007, 2003 by Saunders, an imprint of Elsevier Inc. All rights reserved.

11. The ________________ is the part of the CT scan that surrounds the patient and gathers imaging data.

12. A(n) ________________ may be created on x-ray film if the patient wears clothing with heavy seams or buttons during an x-ray procedure.

Fill in the blanks by choosing the correct terms from the following list.

recumbent	supine
upright	dorsal recumbent
prone	ventral recumbent
lateral recumbent	

13. Lying face down is known as the ________________ position.

14. Lying down is referred to as the ________________ position.

15. Lying on the back with the knees bent and the feet flat on the table is called the ________________ position.

16. Lying on the side is the ________________ position.

17. Lying face down, prone, is called the ________________ position.

18. Lying face up is known as the ________________ position.

19. An x-ray examination performed while the patient is standing or seated would be called a(n) ________________ view.

SKILLS AND CONCEPTS

1. Name the directions and planes of the body shown in the following figure.

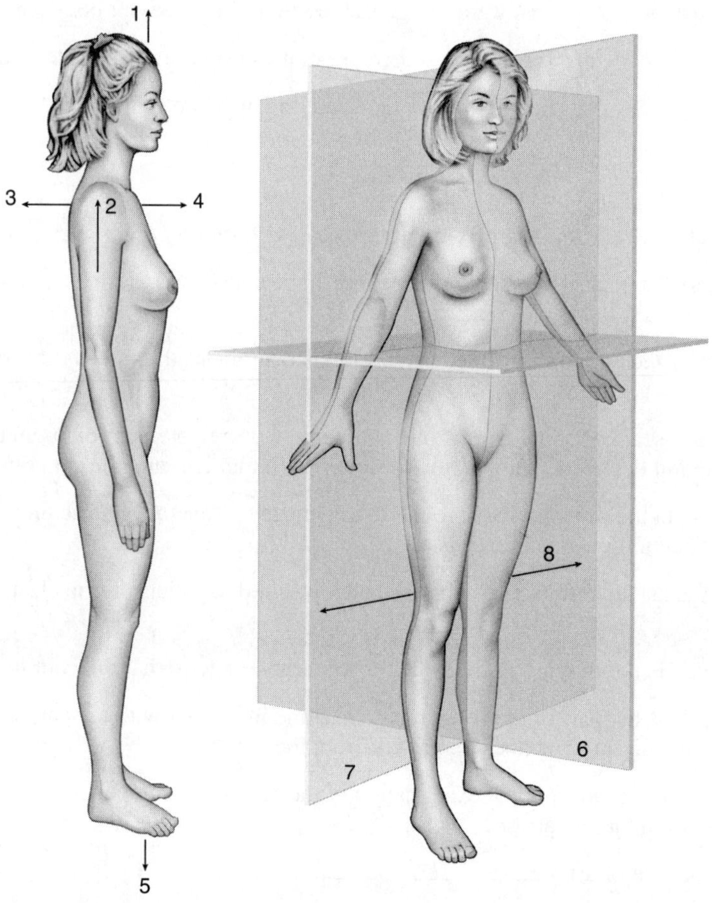

Copyright © 2011, 2007, 2003 by Saunders, an imprint of Elsevier Inc. All rights reserved.

1. ____
2. ____
3. ____
4. ____
5. ____
6. ____
7. ____
8. ____

2. List and describe the four prime factors of exposure.

a. ____
b. ____
c. ____
d. ____

Indicate which statements are true (T) and which are false (F).

3. ________ Patients with cardiac pacemakers cannot have MRI examinations.

4. ________ Radiation control regulations do not require that female patients of childbearing age be advised of potential radiation hazards before an x-ray examination.

5. ________ If the patient is supine facing the x-ray tube, the projection is said to be anteroposterior (AP).

6. ________ X-rays do not linger in the room after the exposure, and they are not capable of making the objects in the room radioactive.

Fill in the blanks.

7. The radiographer selects the correct cassette and places a(n) ________________ marker on it to identify the patient's right or left side.

8. The ________________ (R) is the conventional unit of radiation exposure that represents a measurement of radiation intensity and is determined by the interaction of the x-ray beam with air.

9. The conventional unit for measuring both therapeutic radiation doses and specific tissue doses received in diagnostic applications is the ________________, which stands for "radiation absorbed dose."

10. The dose-equivalent unit used to measure the occupational dose or other exposure that may involve more than one type of radiation is the ________________, which stands for "roentgen equivalent in man."

Copyright © 2011, 2007, 2003 by Saunders, an imprint of Elsevier Inc. All rights reserved.

11. Identify each type of radiographic projection in the following pictures.

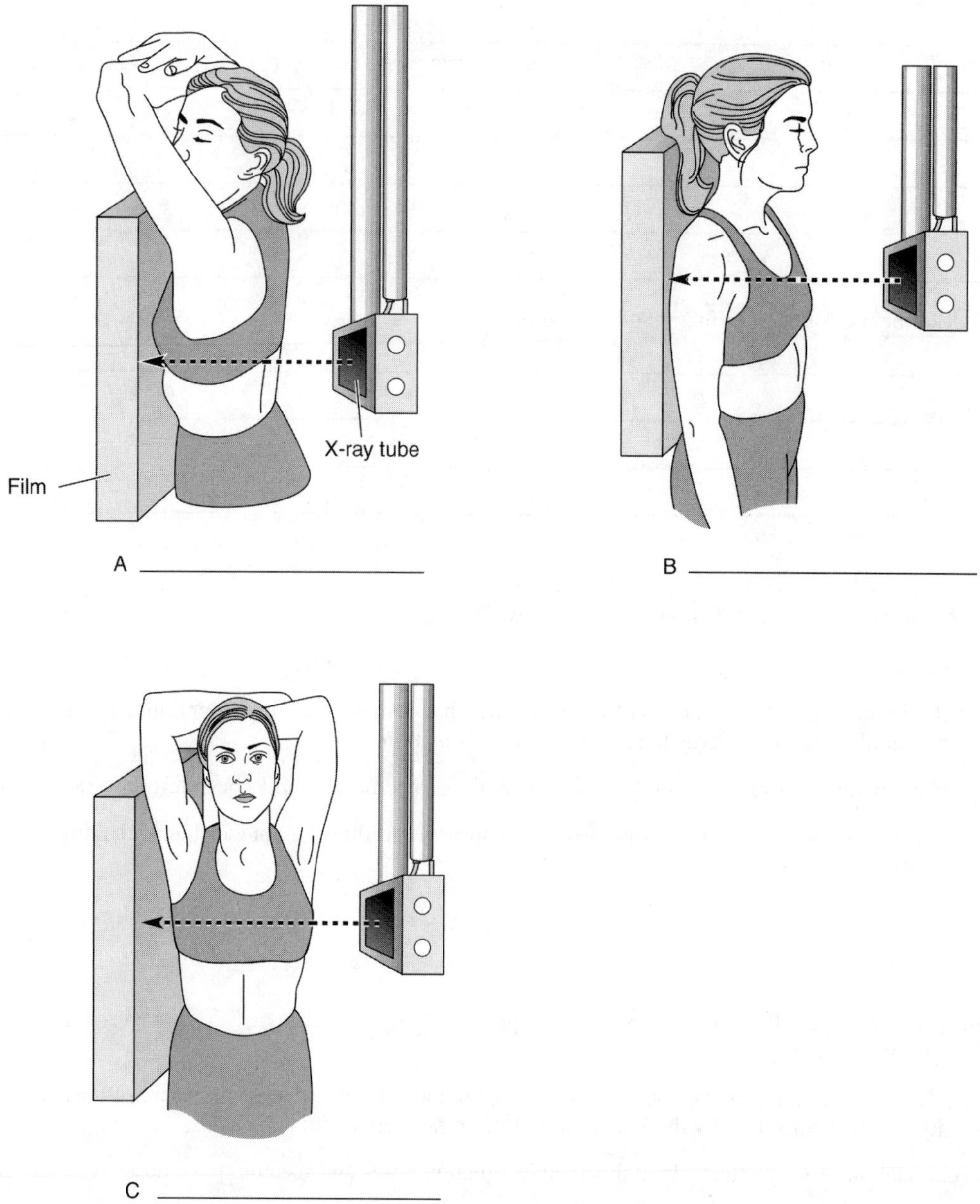

A ______________________

B ______________________

C ______________________

Copyright © 2011, 2007, 2003 by Saunders, an imprint of Elsevier Inc. All rights reserved.

12. Medical assistants must understand the purpose of diagnostic procedures and must be able to reinforce patient education on how to prepare for them. Complete the following table to demonstrate your knowledge of this topic.

Study	Diagnostic Purpose	Procedure	Patient Preparation
Arteriogram		Catheter is inserted into the femoral or brachial artery and advanced, under fluoroscopy, to the target site. Dye is injected, and x-ray images are taken.	
Arthrogram		Fluoroscopic and radiographic examination of a joint after injection of air or contrast dye.	
Barium enema		Fluoroscopic and radiographic examination of the colon after a barium enema to detect internal structural abnormalities; takes approximately 1 hour.	
Barium swallow		Fluoroscopic and radiographic examination performed as barium is swallowed to detect abnormalities of the pharynx, esophagus, and stomach; takes about 15 minutes.	
Bone scan	To detect bone cancer; bone infection; osteoarthritis; and osteomyelitis		
Computed tomography (CT)	To obtain detailed, cross-sectional views of all types of tissue; one of the best tools for studying the chest and abdomen		
Intravenous urogram (IVU) or intravenous pyelogram (IVP)	To evaluate the structure and function of the kidneys, ureters, bladder		
Magnetic resonance imaging (MRI)	To aid diagnosis of intracranial and spinal lesions, aneurysms, heart defects, multiple sclerosis, and soft tissue abnormalities in the body		
Myelogram		Fluoroscopic and radiographic examination of the spinal column after injection of a contrast medium into the subarachnoid space; takes about 1 hour.	

Copyright © 2011, 2007, 2003 by Saunders, an imprint of Elsevier Inc. All rights reserved.

13. Nuclear medicine studies are difficult for patients to understand and can be frightening because of the potential exposure to radioactive materials. Complete the following table by providing the purpose of several nuclear medicine procedures.

Procedure	Purpose
Bone scan	
Brain scan	
Liver scan	
Lung scan	
PET scan	
Thallium stress test	
Thyroid scan	

CASE STUDIES

1. A patient with irritable bowel syndrome has been ordered to have a barium enema. What can Sara, the medical assistant, tell the patient about the examination? What patient preparation is involved?

2. Sara is providing instructions to a patient for whom a DEXA scan has been ordered to check for evidence of osteoporosis. Describe the procedure and the patient preparation.

3. Sara is assisting a patient during an x-ray examination. The patient asks, "What does the x-ray show? Is anything broken?" How should Sara respond?

WORKPLACE APPLICATIONS

1. Sara occasionally assists the radiology technician in preparing and positioning patients during x-ray procedures. Should she wear a dosimeter? Explain the purpose of a dosimeter and how the employer must manage these devices.

2. Sara is putting away a recent shipment of films. What factors should she remember when handling and storing films?

3. Describe the methods Sara can use to minimize unnecessary exposure of her patients to radiation.

4. You are responsible for scheduling a patient for several diagnostic procedures. Summarize the proper sequencing order for scheduling various types of diagnostic studies.

INTERNET ACTIVITY

Visit the Web site of the Radiological Society of North America. Become familiar with the site, especially the patient education section. Is the Web site something you could find useful in a healthcare setting? What are the different features of the site?

MEDICAL RECORD ACTIVITIES

1. You are responsible for explaining to a patient how to prepare for an LGI. Document your patient teaching intervention.

2. Tara Silverman, a 7-year-old patient, is scheduled for multiple x-ray films the next day. Her mother is quite concerned about Tara and whether she will be able to be with her during the procedures. Summarize the guidelines for pediatric x-ray examinations for Mrs. Silverman and document appropriately.

Copyright © 2011, 2007, 2003 by Saunders, an imprint of Elsevier Inc. All rights reserved.

51 Assisting in the Clinical Laboratory

VOCABULARY REVIEW

Write the correct term in the space provided.

1. ________ A term used to describe a blood sample in which the red blood cells have ruptured.
2. ________ A cylindric glass or plastic tube used to deliver fluids.
3. ________ The substance or chemical being analyzed or detected in a specimen.
4. ________ A sample of body fluid, waste product, or tissue collected for analysis.
5. ________ A substance known to cause cancer.
6. ________ The ability of the eye to distinguish two objects that are very close together; the sharpness of an image.
7. ________ A portion of a well-mixed sample removed for testing.
8. ________ A substance that burns or destroys tissue by chemical action.
9. ________ A liquid used to dilute a specimen or reagent.
10. ________ A chemical added to the blood after collection to prevent clotting.
11. ________ An order found on a laboratory requisition indicating that the test must be done immediately (from the Latin word *statin,* meaning "at once").
12. ________ A substance known to cause birth defects.
13. ________ Fluids with a high concentration of protein and cellular debris, which have escaped from the blood vessels and been deposited in tissues or on tissue surfaces.
14. ________ A sac filled with blood, possibly the result of trauma.
15. ________ Fluid within the subarachnoid space, the central canal of the spinal cord, and the four ventricles of the brain.
16. ________ Substances added to a specimen to prevent deterioration of cells or chemicals.
17. ________ Private or hospital-based laboratories that perform a wide variety of tests, many of them specialized. Physicians often send specimens collected in the office to one of these for testing.
18. ________ The study of cells using microscopic methods.

SKILLS AND CONCEPTS

1. Explain the concept of normal or reference ranges for laboratory specimens.

____

____

2. Convert the following from Greenwich time to military time or from military time to Greenwich time.

   a. 2:30 PM ________________________

   b. 12 PM ________________________

   c. 4:20 AM ________________________

Copyright © 2011, 2007, 2003 by Saunders, an imprint of Elsevier Inc. All rights reserved.

d. 1500 hours ______________________________

e. 1815 hours ______________________________

3. Label the parts of a microscope in the following figure and define each.

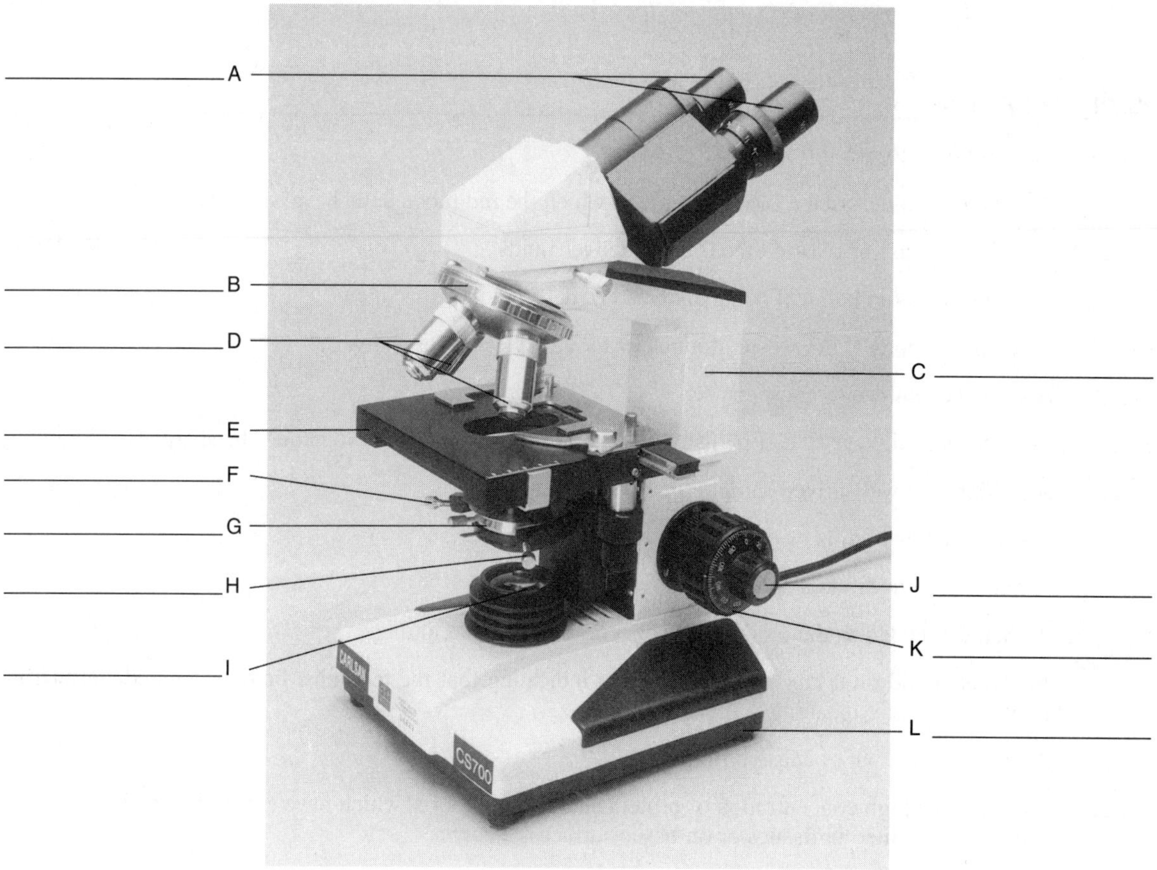

4. One blood glucose meter always reads 10% too high. Another meter reads anywhere from 5% to 9% too high. Which one is the more precise? Which one is the more accurate? How is accuracy different from precision?

____

____

____

____

5. List five occasions when it is absolutely necessary to wash your hands in the laboratory area.

a. ____

b. ____

c. ____

d. ____

e. ____

Copyright © 2011, 2007, 2003 by Saunders, an imprint of Elsevier Inc. All rights reserved.

6. Name three types of hazards in the laboratory setting.

a. ______________________________

b. ______________________________

c. ______________________________

7. Summarize methods for preventing physical hazards in the clinical laboratory.

____

____

____

____

8. Explain the hazard identification system developed by the National Fire Protection Association to provide information on the potential health, flammability, and chemical reactivity hazards of materials.

____

____

____

____

9. Differentiate between qualitative and quantitative results. Give an example of each.

____

____

____

____

10. Identify and explain the four major divisions of the clinical laboratory.

a. ______________________________

____

b. ______________________________

____

c. ______________________________

____

d. ______________________________

____

11. Label each of the following according to its clinical laboratory division.

Hemoglobin ______________________________

Urine specific gravity ______________________________

Urine culture ______________________________

Blood glucose ______________________________

Throat culture ______________________________

Copyright © 2011, 2007, 2003 by Saunders, an imprint of Elsevier Inc. All rights reserved.

White blood cell count ____________________

Cholesterol ____________________

Complete blood count ____________________

12. What is an MSDS? What type of information does it include?

____

____

____

13. What is the role of OSHA in the clinical laboratory?

____

____

____

14. What is CLIA, and what are the three different levels of laboratory testing?

____

____

____

____

15. Medical assistants are trained to perform CLIA-waived tests in the ambulatory healthcare setting. Complete the following table with the information medical assistants should know about these tests.

CLIA-Waived Test	Function
Dipstick or tablet reagent urinalysis (nonautomated) for bilirubin, glucose, hemoglobin, ketone, leukocytes, nitrite, pH, protein, specific gravity, urobilinogen	
Urine pregnancy tests: visual color comparison tests	
Urine chemistry analyzer; automated urine dipstick analysis	
Urine chemistry analyzer for microalbumin and creatinine	
Ovulation tests: visual color comparison tests for luteinizing hormone	
Fecal occult blood	
Erythrocyte sedimentation rate: nonautomated	
Hemoglobin-copper sulfate: nonautomated	
HemoCue hemoglobin system	
Blood glucose by glucose monitoring devices cleared by the FDA specifically for home use	
HemoCue B	

Continued

Copyright © 2011, 2007, 2003 by Saunders, an imprint of Elsevier Inc. All rights reserved.

Spun microhematocrit	
STAT-CRIT hematocrit	
Hemoglobin and hemoglobin A_{1c} by single analyte instruments with self-contained or component features to perform specimen-reagent interaction	
Cholestech LDX	
Blood mononucleosis antibodies	
Helicobacter pylori antibodies	
Borrelia burgdorferi antibodies	
Whole blood OraSure HIV-1 test	
Nasal influenza A and B	
Streptococcus A throat swab	

16. Describe the chain of custody. Why is it important? What steps must be followed?

____

____

____

____

17. Summarize the label information typically required when specimens are sent to a reference laboratory.

____

____

____

____

18. Explain the basic units of the metric system used in the clinical laboratory.

____

____

19. Which of the following statements is/are true about laboratory beakers?

_______ Beakers are wide, straight-sided cylindric vessels used for mixing or reagent preparation.

_______ Beakers are calibrated to hold an exact volume.

_______ Erlenmeyer flasks are used for reagent preparation and are calibrated for exact measurements.

20. Which of the following statements is/are true about pipets?

_______ A bulb or vacuum pump–type device is required to draw liquid into a pipet.

_______ A TD pipet delivers a specified volume by drawing the liquid up to the calibration mark and then allowing it to drain out vertically, unassisted.

_______ A serologic pipet has a large tip opening that delivers a fast flow of liquid with accuracy.

Copyright © 2011, 2007, 2003 by Saunders, an imprint of Elsevier Inc. All rights reserved.

21. How is a 1:10 dilution prepared in the medical laboratory?

____

____

____

22. Explain the functions of the following clinical laboratory equipment.

Incubator

____

____

____

Autoclave

____

____

____

CASE STUDIES

1. Marsha, the medical assistant, is preparing to draw blood from a patient. What Standard Precautions should she take when performing the procedure?

2. Marsha has been asked to develop a safety manual for the office. What information should be included?

3. Marsha is in charge of performing quality assurance in the office. Describe when QA testing should be done for the following tests:

   a. Urinalysis

   b. Pregnancy tests

   c. Glucometer test strips

   d. Automated chemistry analyses

   e. Temperature logs

Copyright © 2011, 2007, 2003 by Saunders, an imprint of Elsevier Inc. All rights reserved.

WORKPLACE APPLICATIONS

1. Marsha is preparing a requisition form for a collected specimen. What information must be included?

2. On the thermometer drawings provided, mark the range of common laboratory temperatures for the following:

   a. Body and incubator temperature

   b. Room temperature

   c. Freezer temperature

   d. Refrigerator temperature

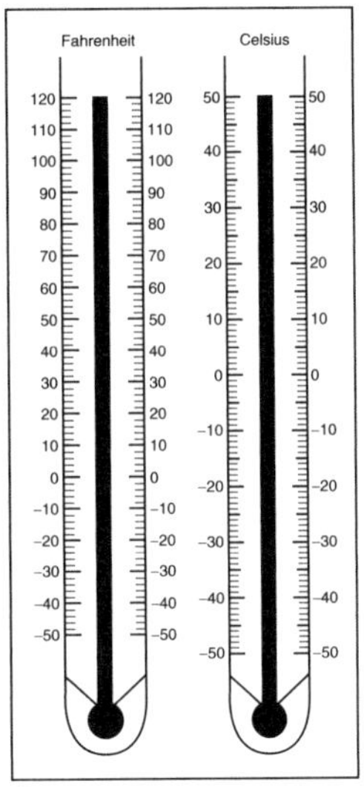

A

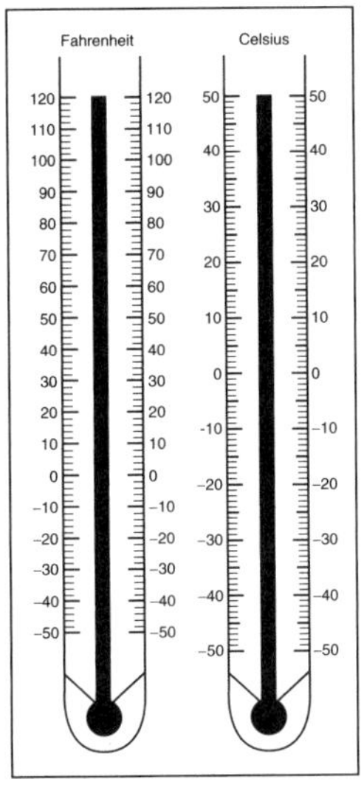

B

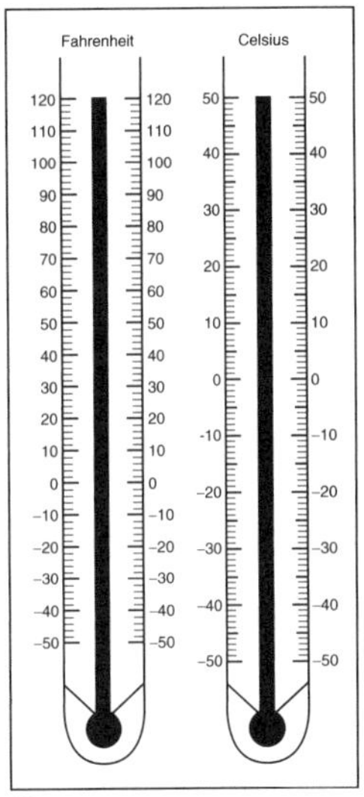

C

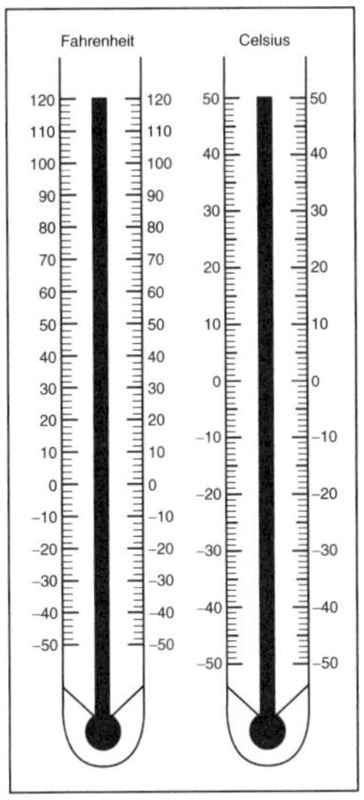

D

3. Your centrifuge starts to vibrate markedly while you are spinning a specimen. What should you check? What precautions should you take while operating a centrifuge?

Copyright © 2011, 2007, 2003 by Saunders, an imprint of Elsevier Inc. All rights reserved.

4. Record the volume in milliliters for the two cylinders pictured.

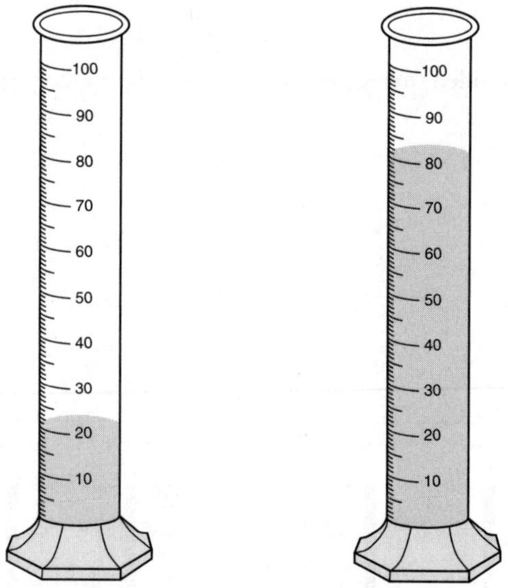

a. ______________ b. ______________

a. How much diluent is added to a 1 mL sample to make a 1:10 dilution? ________ mL

b. How much diluent is added to a 2 mL sample to make a 1:10 dilution? ________ mL

c. How much diluent is added to a 1 mL sample to make a 1:20 dilution? ________ mL

d. How much diluent is added to a 2 mL sample to make a 1:10 dilution? ________ mL

5. Marsha is evaluating the laboratory for the risk of fire. What type of equipment should be kept in the laboratory in case of an open flame emergency?

INTERNET ACTIVITY

Visit OSHA's Web site, www.osha.gov, and locate the list of Standard Precautions. What tools does the Web site offer healthcare workers?

MEDICAL RECORD ACTIVITIES

1. You are responsible for collecting a throat specimen and sending it to the reference laboratory for analysis. Document the procedure in the patient's medical record.

2. Marsha is conducting a quality control test on the urinalysis dipsticks used routinely in the clinic. Explain the significance of the QC check and discuss the documentation required for this procedure.

Copyright © 2011, 2007, 2003 by Saunders, an imprint of Elsevier Inc. All rights reserved.

52 Assisting in the Analysis of Urine

VOCABULARY REVIEW

Fill in the blanks with the correct vocabulary terms from this chapter.

1. _______ Abnormal presence of a hemoglobin-like chemical of muscle tissue in urine as the result of muscle deterioration.
2. _______ Essential amino acid found in milk, eggs, and other foods.
3. _______ Decreased blood flow to a body part or organ caused by constriction or plugging of the supplying artery.
4. _______ Chemical reaction controlled by an enzyme.
5. _______ White blood cells; leukocytes that have segmented nuclei; also known as *polymorphonuclear neutrophils* (PMNs) or *segmented neutrophils*.
6. _______ Presence of glucose in the urine.
7. _______ White blood cells; leukocytes that have unsegmented nuclei; monocytes and lymphocytes in particular.
8. _______ Causing light to refract, creating a sharp boundary or image.
9. _______ Level above which a substance cannot be reabsorbed by the renal tubules and therefore is excreted in the urine.
10. _______ Fluid that remains after a liquid is passed through a membranous filter.
11. _______ A sealed glass float with a calibrated paper scale in its stem. With a slight spinning motion, it is placed in a cylinder containing a urine sample, and the value is read at the meniscus of the urine.
12. _______ Strips used to test the specific gravity of urine.
13. _______ Device that measures the refraction of light through solids in a liquid.
14. _______ Glucose test on a reagent strip. A tablet is dropped into a test tube of urine, and the color of the tube's contents is compared with a chart.
15. _______ Reagent tablets used to test for fat metabolism byproducts.
16. _______ Substance detected by all pregnancy tests.
17. _______ Increases in the concentration of urine shortly before ovulation.
18. _______ Shape of urates or phosphates that settle out of unrefrigerated urine samples.
19. _______ Procedure performed in the microbiology laboratory in which a specimen is cultured on artificial media to detect bacterial or fungal growth, followed by appropriate screening for antibiotic sensitivity.
20. _______ Medical term for a urine sample with a persistent greenish yellow foam that may indicate the patient has viral hepatitis.
21. _______ Definitive diagnostic test to which all others are compared.
22. _______ Protein that has taken on the size and shape of the renal tubules that is washed into the urine.

Copyright © 2011, 2007, 2003 by Saunders, an imprint of Elsevier Inc. All rights reserved.

SKILLS AND CONCEPTS

1. Identify the structures of the urinary system shown in the following figure.

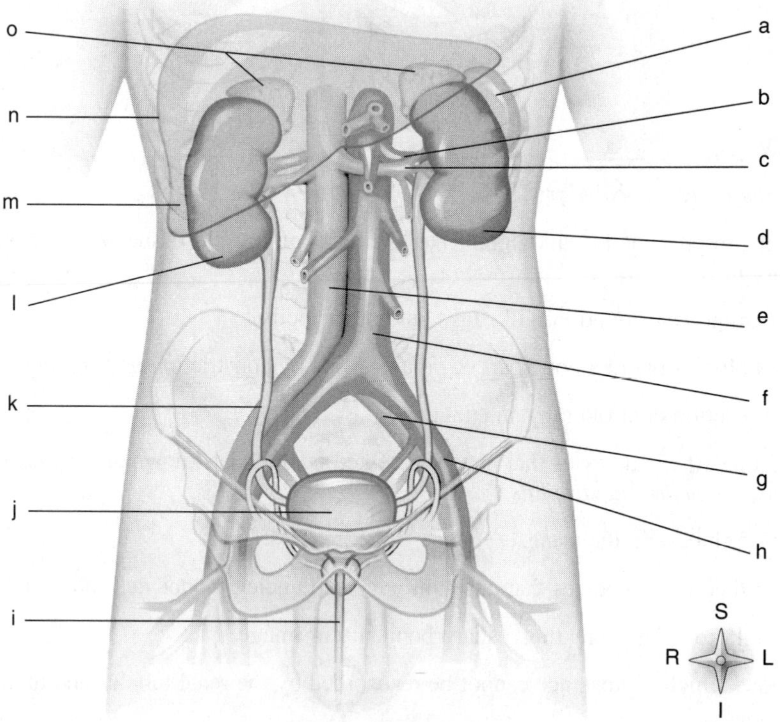

a. ______________________________

b. ______________________________

c. ______________________________

d. ______________________________

e. ______________________________

f. ______________________________

g. ______________________________

h. ______________________________

i. ______________________________

j. ______________________________

k. ______________________________

l. ______________________________

m. ______________________________

n. ______________________________

o. ______________________________

Copyright © 2011, 2007, 2003 by Saunders, an imprint of Elsevier Inc. All rights reserved.

2. Label the structures of the kidney shown in the following figure.

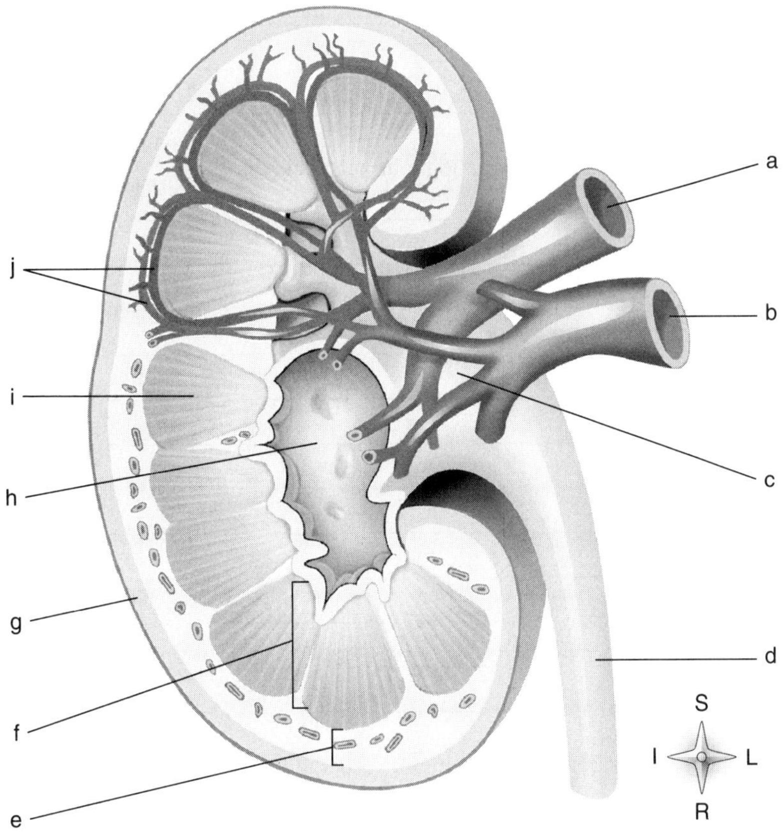

a. ______________________________

b. ______________________________

c. ______________________________

d. ______________________________

e. ______________________________

f. ______________________________

g. ______________________________

h. ______________________________

i. ______________________________

j. ______________________________

3. Urine is formed after three separate processes occur in the kidney. What are they, and in which anatomic structures of the kidney do they occur?

____

____

____

____

Copyright © 2011, 2007, 2003 by Saunders, an imprint of Elsevier Inc. All rights reserved.

4. Requesting a urine specimen make create an embarrassing moment for the patient. How can the medical assistant make this request without causing the patient undue discomfort?

____

____

____

5. List and describe six different methods of collecting a urine specimen.

a. _______________

____

b. _______________

____

c. _______________

____

d. _______________

____

e. _______________

____

f. _______________

____

6. Why must a sterile container be used if a urine culture is ordered?

____

7. Explain the five components of the physical examination of urine.

a. _______________

b. _______________

c. _______________

d. _______________

e. _______________

8. Explain the eight chemical components of urine.

a. _______________

b. _______________

c. _______________

d. _______________

e. _______________

f. _______________

g. _______________

h. _______________

Copyright © 2011, 2007, 2003 by Saunders, an imprint of Elsevier Inc. All rights reserved.

9. Explain how urine samples are used to screen for bladder cancer.

____

____

____

CASE STUDIES

1. A patient brings a urine sample to the office in an old "pill bottle." Should Rosa, the medical assistant, accept the urine sample for testing? Why or why not?

2. One of Rosa's duties is to perform urine drug testing in the office. How may urine be altered to affect the results of the drug test? What can Rosa do to prevent this from happening?

WORKPLACE APPLICATIONS

1. You are performing a microscopic examination of urine, and you notice the blood cells shown in the following figure. What type are they?

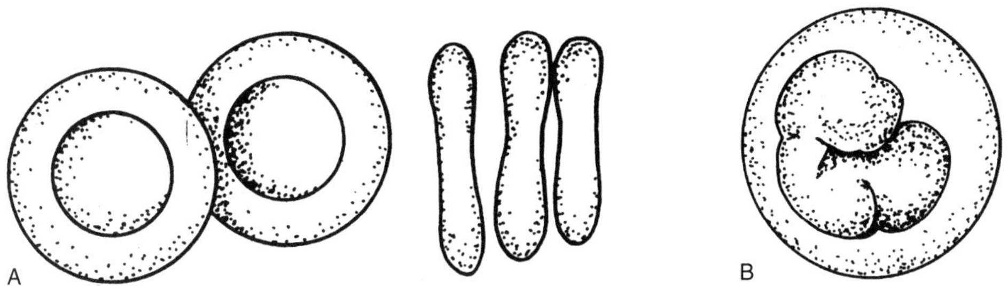

a. ____

b. ____

Copyright © 2011, 2007, 2003 by Saunders, an imprint of Elsevier Inc. All rights reserved.

2. You are performing a microscopic examination of urine, and you notice the pathogens shown in the following figure. What type are they?

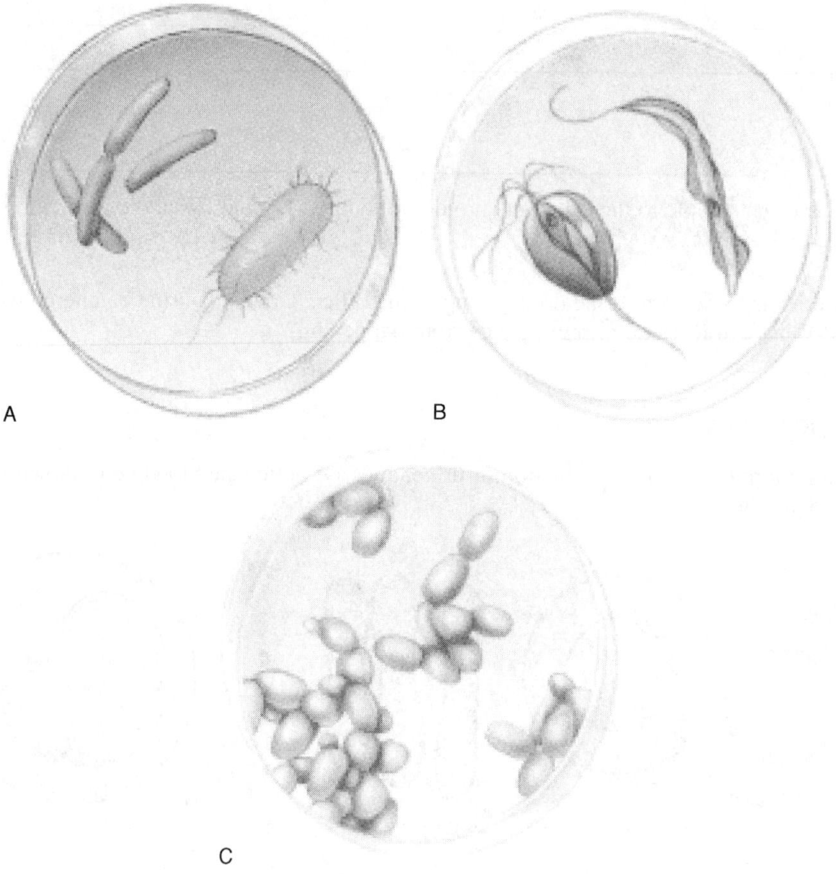

a. ______________________________

b. ______________________________

c. ______________________________

3. Dr. Hill has ordered both a UA and C&S. Which test should Rosa perform first? Why?

____

____

4. You are responsible for collecting urine samples from patients, handling them properly, and preparing them for transport to a reference laboratory. How should you perform these procedures?

____

____

____

5. Explain how to perform a specific gravity determination in the physician's office setting.

____

____

____

____

Copyright © 2011, 2007, 2003 by Saunders, an imprint of Elsevier Inc. All rights reserved.

INTERNET ACTIVITY

Search the Internet for different types of home pregnancy tests. How are they similar? How do they differ? How do these tests work, and what hormone are these tests detecting in the body? When should the patient seek a physician's advice when performing these tests? Prepare to discuss your findings in class.

MEDICAL RECORD ACTIVITIES

1. Dr. Hill has asked Rosa to obtain a clean-catch urine sample from a patient. What instructions should Rosa provide the patient? Document the case.

2. Dr. Hill has asked Rosa to instruct a patient on the collection of a 24-hour urine sample. What should Rosa include in the patient teaching intervention? Document the case.

Copyright © 2011, 2007, 2003 by Saunders, an imprint of Elsevier Inc. All rights reserved.

53 Assisting in Phlebotomy

VOCABULARY REVIEW

Fill in the blanks with the correct terms.

1. A blood draw that is ordered to be done immediately is a(n) ________________ order.
2. A laboratory paper used to collect a blood sample from newborns is a(n) ________________.
3. ________________ The liquid portion of whole blood that remains after the blood has clotted
4. ________________ The liquid portion of whole blood that contains active clotting agents
5. ________________ A situation in which the concentration of blood cells is increased in proportion to the plasma
6. ________________ Fainting
7. ________________ The destruction or dissolution of red blood cells, with subsequent release of hemoglobin
8. ________________ A material that appears to be a solid until subjected to a disturbance, such as centrifugation, at which point it becomes a liquid
9. ________________ An agent that inhibits bacterial growth and can be used on human tissue

SKILLS AND CONCEPTS

1. On the following figure, identify the parts of a Vacutainer (evacuated tube) system.

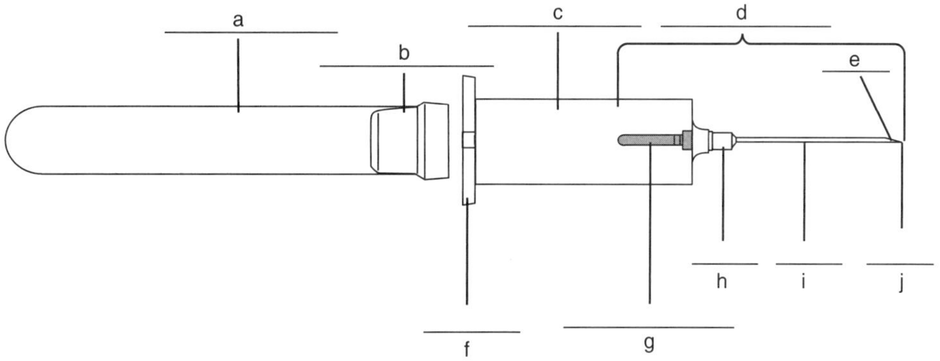

a. ________________________________ f. ________________________________

b. ________________________________ g. ________________________________

c. ________________________________ h. ________________________________

d. ________________________________ i. ________________________________

e. ________________________________ j. ________________________________

Copyright © 2011, 2007, 2003 by Saunders, an imprint of Elsevier Inc. All rights reserved.

2. On the following figure, label the veins used for venipuncture.

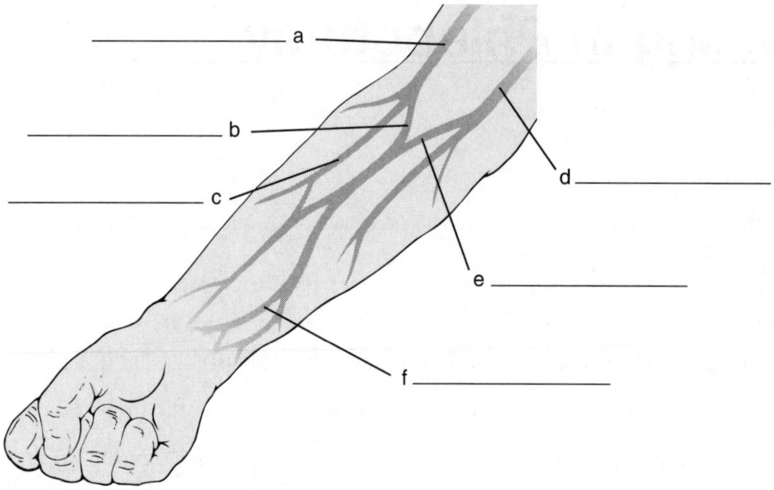

3. Capillary puncture may be warranted in:

a. ______

b. ______

c. ______

d. ______

e. ______

f. ______

g. ______

Fill in the blanks.

4. ______ tubes, also known as *microhematocrit tubes,* are small glass or plastic tubes, open at each end, that will hold a volume of 75 μL.

5. Microcollection, or ______, tubes hold up to 750 μL of blood and are available with a variety of anticoagulants and additives.

6. For children younger than 1 year, dermal puncture is performed on the medial and lateral surfaces of the ______ surface of the heel.

7. The most commonly used skin preparation is ______%, also known as *rubbing alcohol.*

8. If a blood culture is ordered, additional preparation is needed at the venipuncture site to eliminate contaminating bacteria. ______-iodine solution (______) is commonly used.

Which needle gauge should be used in the following situations?

9. A blood bank typically uses ______-gauge needles to prevent hemolysis.

10. ______ gauge needles are used to collect samples from fragile or small veins.

11. Routine adult venipuncture requires a(n) ______-gauge needle.

Copyright © 2011, 2007, 2003 by Saunders, an imprint of Elsevier Inc. All rights reserved.

12. List three causes of a hematoma.

a. ______________________________

b. ______________________________

c. ______________________________

13. Describe the steps involved in performing a venipuncture.

____

____

____

14. Performing phlebotomy procedures on children can be challenging. Complete the following table by providing parenteral actions that may make the procedure less traumatic.

Age	Typical Mental State	Suggested Parental Involvement
Newborns (0-12 months)	Trust that adults will respond to their needs	
Infants and toddlers (1-3 years)	Minimal fear of danger but fear of separation; limited language and understanding of procedure	
Preschoolers (3-6 years)	Fearful of injury to body; still dependent on parent	
School-aged children (7-12 years)	Less dependent on parent and more willing to cooperate	
Teenagers (13-18 years)	Fully engaged in the process; embarrassed to show fear and may exhibit hostility to cover emotions	

15. Hemolysis of a blood sample usually requires a repeat blood draw. Complete the following table by explaining how to prevent hemolysis when performing phlebotomy.

Cause of Hemolysis	Explanation	Prevention
Alcohol preparation	Transfer of alcohol into the specimen causes hemolysis.	
Incorrect needle size	A high-gauge needle causes the blood to be forced through a small lumen with great force, shearing the cell membranes; a very low-gauge needle allows a large amount of blood to suddenly enter the tube with great force, causing frothing.	
Loose connections on the vacuum tube assembly	If the connection between the needle holder and the double-pointed needle or the syringe and needle is loose, air can enter the sample and cause frothing.	
Removing the needle from the vein with the tube intact	The remaining vacuum in the tube can cause air to be drawn forcefully into the tube.	
Underfilled tubes	Underfilling tubes leads to an improper blood to additive ratio.	
Syringe collections	Pulling back forcibly on the plunger draws blood too quickly through the needle, shearing cell membranes; transferring blood into a vacuum tube further traumatizes red blood cells.	

Continued

Copyright © 2011, 2007, 2003 by Saunders, an imprint of Elsevier Inc. All rights reserved.

Cause of Hemolysis	Explanation	Prevention
Mixing tubes too vigorously	All tubes except the red-stoppered tube must be mixed.	
Temperature and transport problems	Trauma and temperature extremes can damage cells.	
Separation of plasma or serum from red cells	Removing the serum or plasma from the cells minimizes the risk of contaminating the specimen with red cell contents.	
Prolonged tourniquet time	While the tourniquet restricts blood flow, interstitial fluid can leak into the veins and hemolyze red cells.	
Poor collection; blood flowing too slowly into the tube	The lumen of the needle may be blocked.	

16. Complete the following table by providing strategies to prevent or manage possible complications from a phlebotomy procedure.

Possible Complication	Strategies
Burned area	
Convulsions	
Damaged or scarred veins or infected areas	
Edema	
Hematoma	
Intravenous (IV) therapy or blood transfusion sites	
Mastectomy	
Nausea	
No blood	
Petechiae	
Syncope	

Copyright © 2011, 2007, 2003 by Saunders, an imprint of Elsevier Inc. All rights reserved.

17. The medical assistant must know which tube top color to use when drawing blood samples. Complete the following table to identify additives and their functions and the laboratory uses for each type of tube.

Vacutainer Color	Additive and Its Function	Laboratory Use
Yellow		
Red		
Red-gray (marbled)		
Light blue		
Green		
Green-gray (marbled)		
Yellow-gray (marbled)		
Lavender		
Gray		
Royal blue		

CASE STUDIES

1. Leah, the medical assistant, is gathering supplies for venipuncture. Explain to the patient why a tourniquet is necessary. Describe the proper way to apply a tourniquet. List three consequences of improper application.

2. As Leah is demonstrating a capillary puncture, the patient states, "I'm not a good bleeder; it may not be wise to waste the first drop of blood." Explain to the patient why the first drop of blood is wiped away.

3. One of Leah's co-workers has just experienced a needle stick. What instruction should Leah provide about care of the exposure site?

4. Leah is preparing a requisition for a patient's laboratory work. What information should be included on the requisition?

5. While Leah is performing venipuncture, she notices that the patient is becoming pale, is sweating, and is not conversing. What steps should be taken for patients who faint during venipuncture?

Copyright © 2011, 2007, 2003 by Saunders, an imprint of Elsevier Inc. All rights reserved.

WORKPLACE APPLICATIONS

1. The medical assistant must be able to recognize equipment and supplies used for phlebotomy. Identify the venipuncture supplies shown in the figure.

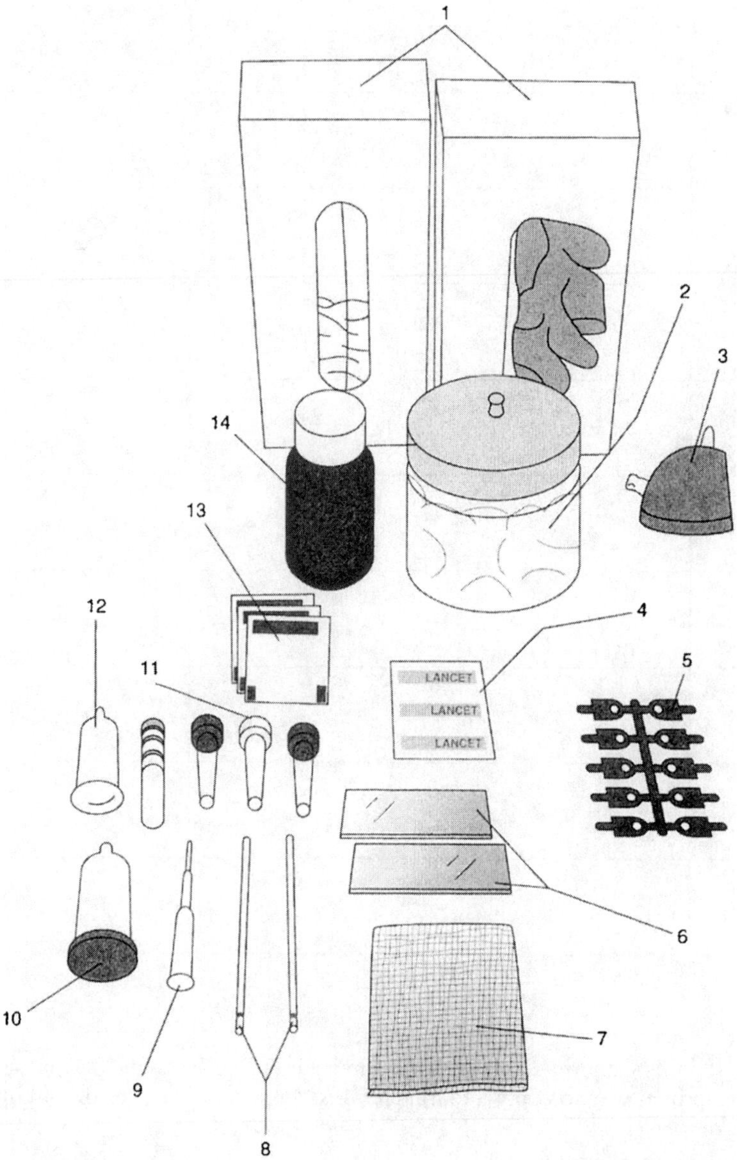

a. ______________________________

b. ______________________________

c. ______________________________

d. ______________________________

e. ______________________________

f. ______________________________

g. ______________________________

h. ______________________________

i. ______________________________

Copyright © 2011, 2007, 2003 by Saunders, an imprint of Elsevier Inc. All rights reserved.

j. ___

k. ___

l. ___

m. ___

n. ___

2. List seven reasons the laboratory may reject a specimen.

a. ___

b. ___

c. ___

d. ___

e. ___

f. ___

g. ___

The National Committee for Clinical Laboratory Standards has developed a set of standards outlining the order of draw for a multitube draw. The same order applies to the filling of tubes when the blood is collected in a syringe. A mnemonic device that is useful for remembering the order of the draw is STOP, RED LIGHT, GREEN LIGHT, READY, GO.

3. Use the mnemonic device and fill in the blanks.

a. ___ tubes are collected first, because they are sterile.

b. ___-topped tubes are collected second, because they have no additive and therefore nothing to transfer to another tube.

c. ___ blue-topped tubes are next, because other anticoagulants might contaminate the sample collected for coagulation studies.

d. ___-topped tubes are next, because heparin is less likely to interfere with EDTA than vice versa.

e. ___-topped tubes follow. EDTA binds with calcium, so this tube is drawn near the end.

f. ___-___ marble-topped tubes are next. They contain a clot activator that could interfere with specimens if passed into another tube.

g. The ___-topped tube is last because the contents can elevate electrolyte levels or damage cells if passed into another tube.

4. Leah is attending a conference on needle-stick prevention. List some of the ways accidental needle sticks can be prevented.

___

___

___

5. Develop an exposure control plan for the office to follow in case of accidental needle sticks. What should be included?

___

___

___

Copyright © 2011, 2007, 2003 by Saunders, an imprint of Elsevier Inc. All rights reserved.

6. Leah has just received a shipment of winged infusion sets (butterfly needles). When might Leah choose this equipment? When would Leah *not* want to choose a butterfly needle?

____

____

____

INTERNET ACTIVITY

Leah is in charge of replacing the old needles with the new safety needles. Search the Internet for the different types of safety needles. Print out some of the various examples and compare them. Which type do you like the best? Why is it so important to implement the use of safety needles?

Copyright © 2011, 2007, 2003 by Saunders, an imprint of Elsevier Inc. All rights reserved.

54 Assisting in the Analysis of Blood

VOCABULARY REVIEW

Match the following terms with their definitions.

1. _______ A condition marked by deficiency of red blood cells
2. _______ An apparatus consisting essentially of a compartment spun about a central axis to separate contained materials of different specific gravities or to separate colloidal particles suspended in a liquid
3. _______ Any of several complex proteins produced by cells that act as catalysts in specific biochemical reactions
4. _______ A substance, usually a peptide or steroid, produced by one tissue and conveyed by the bloodstream to another to effect physiologic activity, such as growth or metabolism
5. _______ A substance produced by metabolism
6. _______ An increase in the number of normal WBCs
7. _______ A condition marked by an abnormally large number of red blood cells in the circulatory system
8. _______ An abnormal condition of pregnancy characterized by hypertension, edema, and protein in the urine
9. _______ Tests performed to assess the compatibility of blood to be transfused
10. _______ The major nitrogenous end product of protein metabolism and the chief nitrogenous component of the urine
11. _______ An enzyme that catalyzes the hydrolysis of urea to form ammonium carbonate
12. _______ The layer of white cells or platelets found between the plasma and the packed RBCs after whole blood is centrifuged

a. Anemia
b. Enzyme
c. Urea
d. Hormone
e. Polycythemia vera
f. Toxemia
g. Metabolite
h. Leukocytosis
i. Centrifuge
j. Urease
k. Type and cross-match
l. Buffy coat

SKILLS AND CONCEPTS

1. List the three main functions of blood.

   a. ____

   b. ____

   c. ____

2. Describe the role of hematology in patient care.

   ____

   ____

   ____

Copyright © 2011, 2007, 2003 by Saunders, an imprint of Elsevier Inc. All rights reserved.

3. Identify the blood cells in the following illustration.

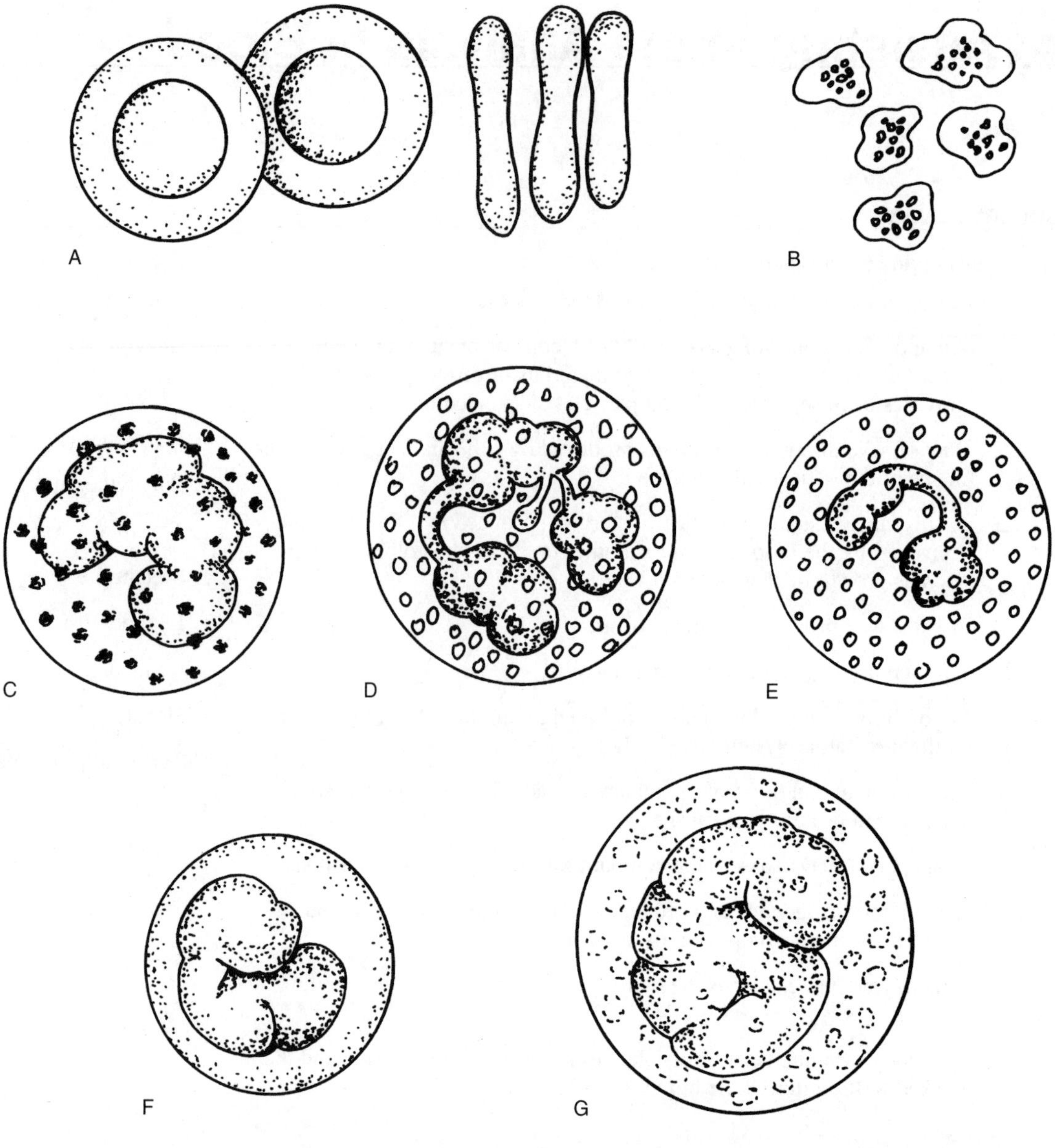

a. ____________________

b. ____________________

c. ____________________

d. ____________________

e. ____________________

f. ____________________

g. ____________________

Copyright © 2011, 2007, 2003 by Saunders, an imprint of Elsevier Inc. All rights reserved.

Fill in the blanks.

4. Whole blood is composed of formed elements suspended in a clear, yellow liquid portion called ________________. It makes up approximately 55% of the blood by volume. The remaining 45% consists of the formed cellular elements, which are the ________________ (red blood cells), ________________ (white blood cells), and ________________ (platelets).
5. ________________ on the RBC carries oxygen throughout the body.
6. The life span of an erythrocyte is about ________________ days, and once matured an erythrocyte has a(n) ________________ shape.
7. The granular leukocytes are called *polymorphonuclear leukocytes* and include the ________________, ________________, and ________________.
8. The agranular leukocytes are the ________________ and ________________, both of which have clear cytoplasm and a solid nucleus.
9. The purpose of the ________________ cell count is to analyze and quantitate the types of WBCs found in a sample of blood.
10. Explain the function of the following WBCs.

    neutrophils ____

    bands ____

    eosinophils ____

    basophils ____

    lymphocytes ____

    monocytes ____

11. Explain the characteristics of a good wedge smear and how it should be dried.

    ____

    ____

    ____

12. What are the normal ranges for an adult differential?

    ____

    ____

13. Explain the characteristics of red blood cell morphology:

    ____

    ____

    ____

14. What factors might affect an ESR result?

    ____

    ____

    ____

Copyright © 2011, 2007, 2003 by Saunders, an imprint of Elsevier Inc. All rights reserved.

15. ________________ are the smallest formed elements of the blood.

16. The platelets produce a substance that combines with ________________ ions in the blood to form, which in turn converts the protein into thrombin in a complex series of reactions. Thrombin, an enzyme, converts fibrinogen, a protein substance, into ________________, an insoluble protein that forms an intricate network of minute threadlike structures called *fibrils* and causes the blood plasma to gel.

17. The ________________ test is used to monitor the condition of patients taking warfarin (Coumadin).

18. Explain the relationship between the PT test and INR levels when following a patient on anticoagulant therapy. What is considered a therapeutic INR level?

____

____

____

19. Vacutainer tubes containing ________________ are used for hematology testing. Why?

____

____

Match the following T cells with their function.

a. Cytotoxic or killer T cells
b. Helper T cells
c. Suppressor T cells
d. Memory T cells
e. Natural killer cells

20. ______ Respond quickly to the presentation of the same antigen at a later date; have a long life span

21. ______ Most numerous type of T cell; stimulate the activity of other T cells

22. ______ Kill foreign, virus-infected, and tumor cells; produce proteins called *perforins* that induce cell death by punching holes in the cell membrane

23. ______ Inhibit the activity of other T cells

24. ______ Cells infected with viruses and tumor cells without prior sensitization

Fill in the blanks.

25. B cells are formed in the ________________.

26. When stimulated, B cells differentiate into ________________, which produce specific antibodies against an antigen.

27. Antibodies are protein molecules that attach to ________________.

28. Destroying pathogens requires three specific steps: ________________, ________________, and ________________.

29. List and describe five commonly used blood chemistry tests.

a. ____

____

b. ____

____

c. ____

____

d. ____

____

e. ____

____

 Copyright © 2011, 2007, 2003 by Saunders, an imprint of Elsevier Inc. All rights reserved.

30. Explain how HbA_{1c} tests are used to manage diabetes mellitus.

____

____

____

31. Complete the following table with the correct reference ranges for a CBC.

Test	Neonates	Infants (6 mo)	Children	Men	Women
RBCs	4.8–7.1 million/mm³	3.8–5.5 million/mm³	4.5–4.8 million/mm³		
Hematocrit (Hct)		30%–40%	35%–41%		
Hemoglobin (Hgb)	17–23 g/dL		11–16 g/dL		
WBCs	9,000–30,000/mm³				
WBC Differential					
Neutrophils	≥45% by 1 wk of age	32%			
Bands	—	—	—		
Eosinophils	—	—	0–3%		
Basophils	—	—	1–3%		
Monocytes	—	—	4–9%		
Lymphocytes	≥41% by age 1 wk	61%	59% for children 2 yr or older		
Platelets		200,000–473,000/mm³	150,000–450,000/mm³		

32. What are the corresponding blood glucose levels for the HbA_{1c} levels in the following table?

Glycosylated Hemoglobin (percent)	Blood Glucose (mg/dL)
14	
13	
12	
11	
10	
9	
8	
7	
6	

Copyright © 2011, 2007, 2003 by Saunders, an imprint of Elsevier Inc. All rights reserved.

CASE STUDIES

1. Dana, the medical assistant, is to perform a microhematocrit procedure on a patient. Explain to the patient the purpose of the microhematocrit and how the procedure will be done. What are the normal values for both men and women? What might a low hematocrit level indicate? What might a high hematocrit level indicate?

2. Dana is drawing blood for an ESR determination on a patient. Define the ESR. What type of conditions can the test indicate? As Dana performs the ESR test, what factor should she be aware of as a source of error?

3. One of the patients in the office has just discovered she is pregnant. Because she is Rh negative, she is very concerned about the welfare of her baby. How will she be managed to prevent any risk to the fetus?

4. Gus Langton, age 54, is scheduled for cholesterol screening. Mr. Langton has a family history of hypercholesterolemia and is very confused about the importance of HDL and LDL levels. Explain their significance to Mr. Langton.

WORKPLACE APPLICATIONS

1. The hemacytometer in the office recently was replaced by an automated blood cell counting machine. Explain the principle behind automated blood cell counting.

2. Blood grouping is extremely specific to prevent agglutination. Dana must be prepared to explain the different blood types to her patients. Answer the following questions about blood grouping and the Rh factor.

   a. The universal donor is ____.

   b. The universal recipient is ____.

   c. A patient who is type AB+ may receive ________________________________ blood type.

   d. A patient who is type B– may receive ________________________________ blood type.

   e. A patient who is O+ may receive ________________________________ blood type.

INTERNET ACTIVITY

1. Blood donation is extremely important. Search the Internet for locations in your area to donate blood. Are there opportunities to volunteer your services? If so, what types of duties can volunteers provide?

2. Research online the most recent developments in HbA_{1c}. What equipment is available to perform this important test, and how is it used?

MEDICAL RECORDS ACTIVITIES

1. You are reporting test results to a patient. The patient's hemoglobin level is 15 g/dL. Explain to the patient the role of hemoglobin in the body and what the level indicates. What factors can cause the level to vary? Document the patient teaching intervention.

2. The physician has ordered a CBC and differential for a patient. Explain to the patient the different tests included in the CBC. Why might the physician have ordered the differential? Document the patient interaction.

Copyright © 2011, 2007, 2003 by Saunders, an imprint of Elsevier Inc. All rights reserved.

55 Assisting in Microbiology and Immunology

VOCABULARY REVIEW

Fill in the blanks with the correct terms.

1. ________________ Pertaining to or originating in the hospital; said of an infection not present or incubating before admission to the hospital
2. ________________ An agent that causes disease, especially a living microorganism such as a bacterium or fungus
3. ________________ A bacterial or fungal culture that contains a single organism
4. ________________ A differentiated structure within a cell, such as a mitochondrion, vacuole, or chloroplast, which performs a specific function
5. ________________ One billionth ($1/10^{-9}$) of a meter
6. ________________ An organism of microscopic or submicroscopic size
7. ________________ A single-celled or multicellular organism in which each cell contains a distinct, membrane-bound nucleus
8. ________________ Requiring specialized media or growth factors to grow
9. ________________ A small, capsulelike sac that encloses certain organisms in their dormant or larval stage
10. ________________ A sample, as of tissue, blood, or urine, used for analysis and diagnosis
11. ________________ A unicellular organism that lacks a membrane-bound nucleus
12. ________________ A drug used to treat a broad range of infections
13. ________________ Refers to conditions outside a living body
14. ________________ The process of removing pathogenic microorganisms or protecting against infection by such organisms
15. ________________ The molecules needed for metabolism: carbohydrates, lipids, proteins, and nucleic acids
16. ________________ The technique or process of keeping tissue alive and growing in a culture medium
17. ________________ A drug used to treat infection
18. ________________ A group of like or different atoms held together by chemical forces
19. ________________ A medium used to keep an organism alive during transport to the laboratory
20. ________________ Capable of living, developing, or germinating under favorable conditions
21. ________________ A slide preparation in which a drop of liquid specimen or the like is covered with a coverslip and examined with a microscope
22. ________________ A chemical released from cells that causes smooth muscle contraction and pain
23. ________________ Glycoproteins produced by cells infected with a virus or another intracellular parasite that can be used medically as antiviral or anticancer therapeutics
24. ________________ A protein produced by certain white blood cells that regulates immune responses by activating lymphocytes and initiating fever
25. ________________ Cloudiness of a liquid, caused by the presence of suspended particles, which increases with the concentration of particles

Copyright © 2011, 2007, 2003 by Saunders, an imprint of Elsevier Inc. All rights reserved.

26. ________________ A category of microorganisms below genus in rank; a genetically distinct group

27. ________________ Microbes that live on or in the body that perform vital functions and protect the body against infection

28. ________________ A breakdown of a family of microorganisms

SKILLS AND CONCEPTS

1. Identify the four shapes of bacteria shown in the figure.

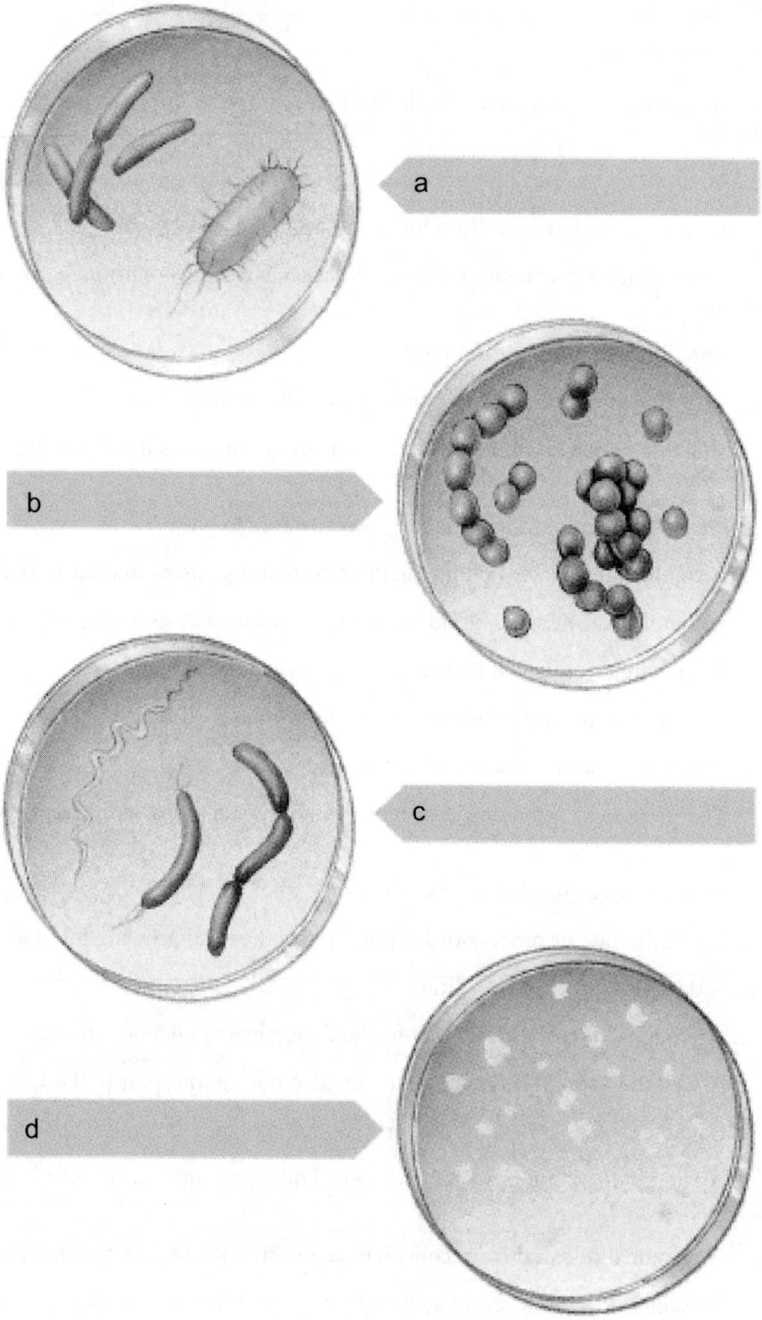

a. ____

b. ____

c. ____

d. ____

Copyright © 2011, 2007, 2003 by Saunders, an imprint of Elsevier Inc. All rights reserved.

2. Identify the four types of disease-causing protozoa shown in the figure.

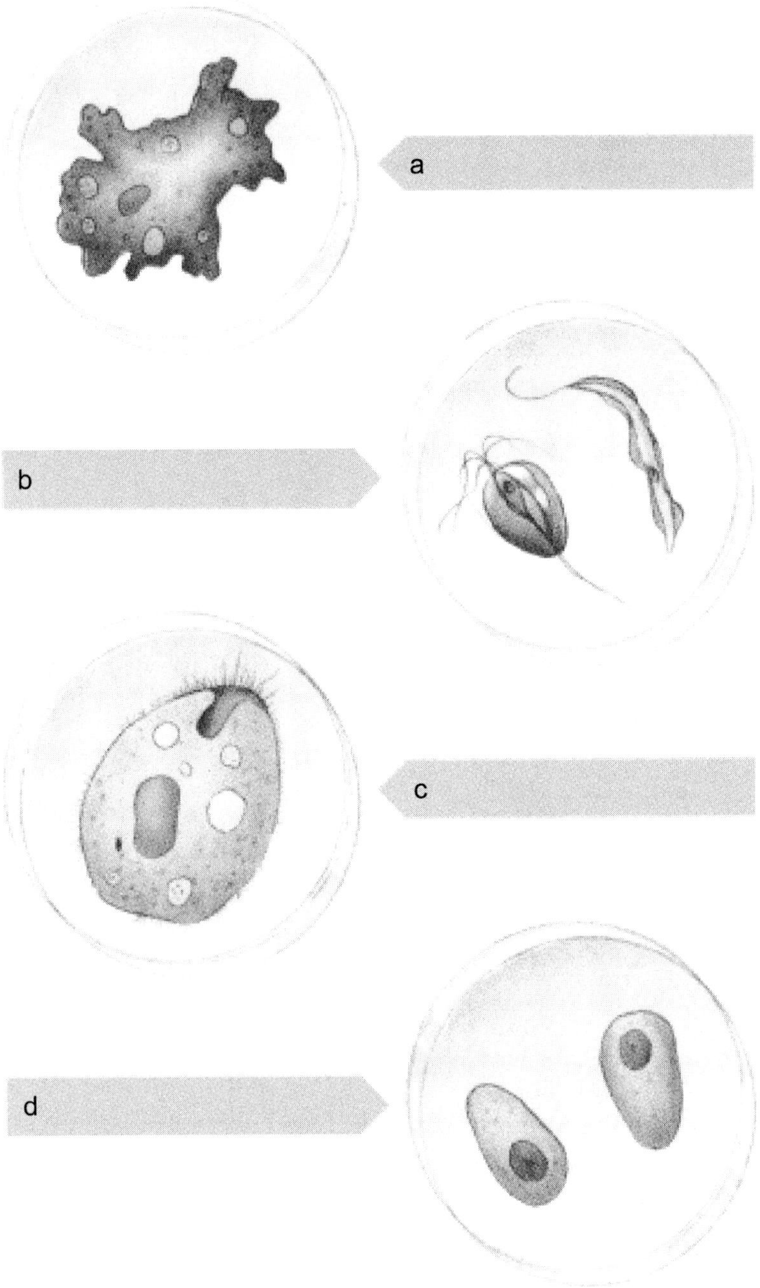

a. ______________________________

b. ______________________________

c. ______________________________

d. ______________________________

Copyright © 2011, 2007, 2003 by Saunders, an imprint of Elsevier Inc. All rights reserved.

3. Identify the three pathogenic animals shown in the figure.

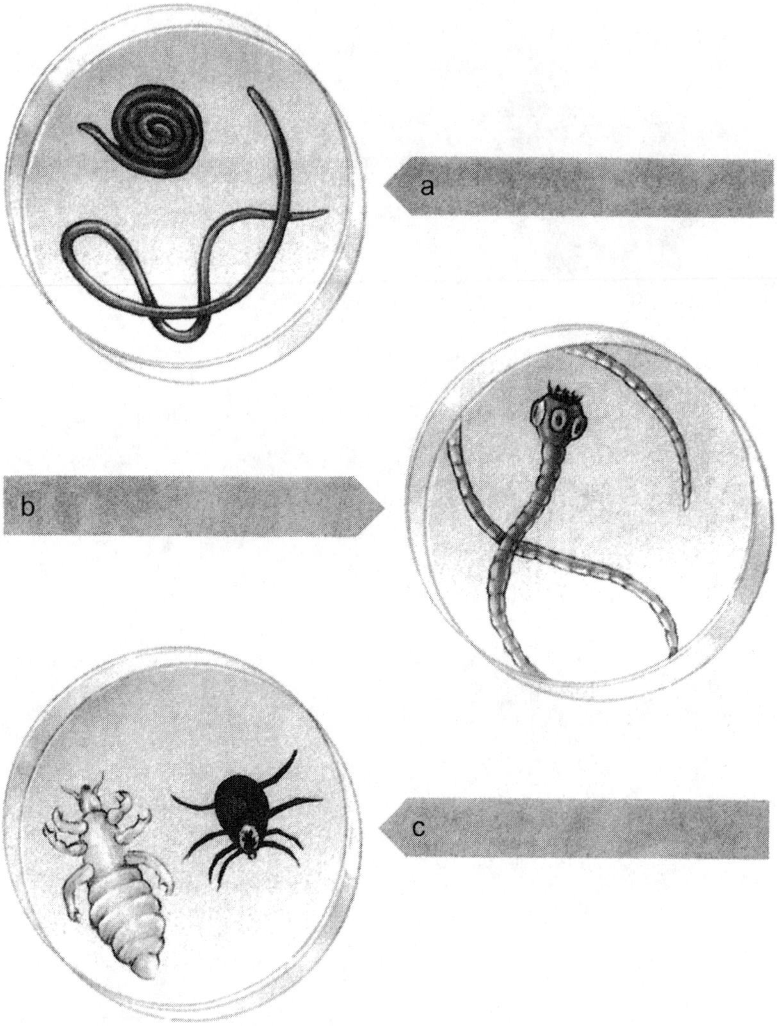

a. ______________________________

b. ______________________________

c. ______________________________

Copyright © 2011, 2007, 2003 by Saunders, an imprint of Elsevier Inc. All rights reserved.

4. Identify the two fungi shown in the figure.

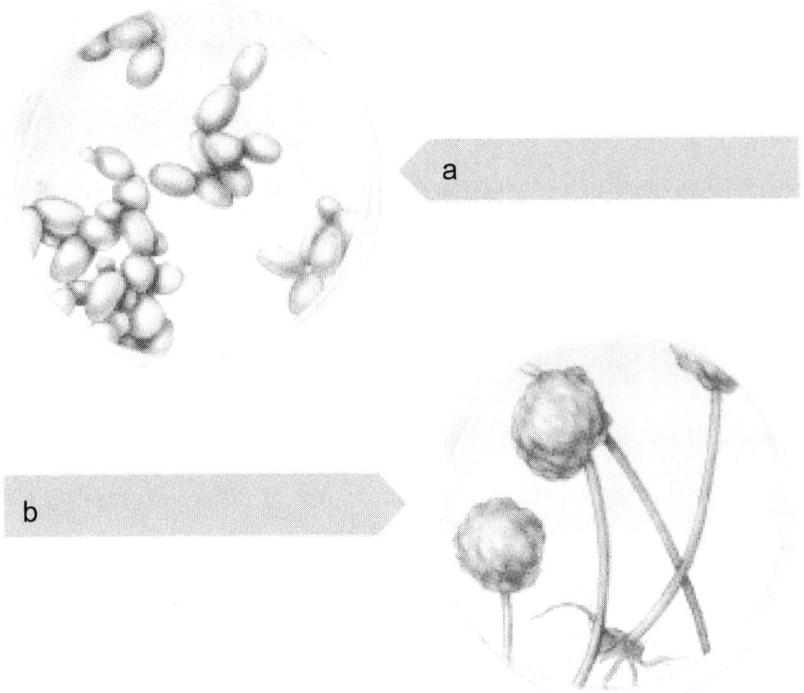

a. ______________________________

b. ______________________________

5. Describe the four different classifications of media.

a. All-purpose or nutritive ______________________________

b. Selective ______________________________

c. Differential ______________________________

d. Enriched ______________________________

6. Draw the pattern you should make when you prepare a *Streptococcus pyogenes* culture on an agar plate.

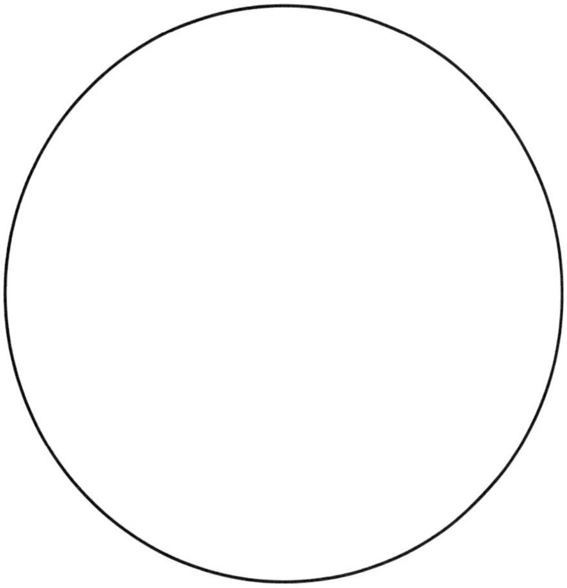

Copyright © 2011, 2007, 2003 by Saunders, an imprint of Elsevier Inc. All rights reserved.

7. Compare and contrast the throat culture for *Streptococcus pyogenes* with the rapid strep test.

____

____

____

8. Each colony that grows on a urine culture plate represents ______________________.

9. The acid-fast stain is used in the identification protocol for ______________________.

10. Explain the methods for performing HIV screening.

____

____

____

____

11. The medical assistant is responsible for collecting specimens from patients and preparing them properly for transport. Complete the following table with the missing information.

Specimen	Container	Patient Preparation	Storage Before Processing
Blood		Disinfect venipuncture site with alcohol swab and Betadine	
Stool	Clean, leakproof container		
Sputum	Sterile, screw-cap container		
Throat	Transport swab		
Ova and parasite (O&P)	O&P transport device (with formalin and PVA)		
Urine	Sterile, screw-cap container		
Superficial wound			Transport and plate within 24 hours; room temperature storage
Deep wound or abscess		Wipe area with sterile saline or alcohol prep pad before collection	

12. Provide the missing information in the following tables.

Common Diseases Caused by Viruses

Disease	Virus	Transmission	Symptoms	Prevention
Infectious mononucleosis				Avoid direct contact with affected individuals
Influenza	Myxovirus (influenza A and B)		Fever, body aches, cough	
Rabies	Rhabdovirus			Vaccine available; have pets vaccinated
Common cold			Headache, fever, runny nose, congestion	Good hygiene (hand washing)

Copyright © 2011, 2007, 2003 by Saunders, an imprint of Elsevier Inc. All rights reserved.

Common Diseases Caused by Bacilli

Disease	Organism	Transmission	Symptoms	Tests and Specimens
Tuberculosis		Inhalation		
Urinary tract infections	*Escherichia coli, Proteus sp. Klebsiella sp., Pseudomonas aeruginosa*		*Cystitis:* Frequency, burning bloody urine *Pyelonephritis:* Flank pain, fever	
Legionnaires' disease	*Legionella pneumophila*			Sputum; blood
Tetanus (lockjaw)			Toxin affects motor nerves; muscle spasms, convulsions, rigidity	
Botulism	*Clostridium botulinum*		Neurotoxin affects speech, swallowing, vision; paralysis of respiratory muscles, death	
Whooping cough	*Bordetella pertussis*			Swabs for culture
Plague	*Yersinia pestis*		Fever, chills, delirium; enlarged, painful lymph nodes	

Common Diseases Caused by Cocci

Disease	Organism	Transmission	Symptoms	Tests and Specimens
Pneumonia	*Streptococcus pneumoniae*		Productive cough, fever, chest pain	
Strep throat		Direct contact, droplets, fomites		
Wound infection, abscesses, boils		Direct contact, fomites, carriers; poor hand washing		
Staphylococcal food poisoning		Poor hygiene and improper refrigeration of food	Vomiting, abdominal cramps, diarrhea	
Meningococcal meningitis		Respiratory tract secretions		

Common Diseases Caused by Spirilla

Disease	Organism	Transmission	Symptoms	Tests and Specimens
Syphilis		Sexually; congenitally	*Primary:* Painless sore (chancre) *Secondary:* Generalized rash involving palms and soles of feet *Congenital:* Birth defects	
Lyme disease		Tick bite	Fever, joint pain, red bull's-eye rash	
Pyloric ulcers			Burning pain in stomach, especially between meals	

Copyright © 2011, 2007, 2003 by Saunders, an imprint of Elsevier Inc. All rights reserved.

Diseases Caused by Rickettsiae, Chlamydiae, and Mycoplasmas

Disease	Organism	Transmission	Symptoms	Tests and Specimens
Rocky Mountain spotted fever	*Rickettsia rickettsii*		Headache, chills, fever, characteristic rash on extremities and trunk	
Typhus	*Rickettsia prowazekii*		Fever, rash, confusion	
Nongonococcal urethritis and vaginitis	*Chlamydia trachomatis*		May be asymptomatic	

Common Diseases Caused by Fungi

Disease	Organism	Predisposing Conditions and Transmission	Symptoms	Tests and Specimens
Thrush (oral yeast), vulvovaginal candidiasis, or monilia (vaginal yeast)		*Oral:* During birth *Other:* After antibiotic therapy; with oral birth control, severe diabetes		
Athlete's foot, jock itch, ringworm (tinea)	*Trichophyton sp., Microsporum sp.,* and others (skin fungi)		Hair loss; thickening of skin and nails; itching; red, scaly patches	
Histoplasmosis	*Histoplasma capsulatum*		Mild, flulike or systemic	
Pneumocystis pneumonia			Pneumonia-like	

Copyright © 2011, 2007, 2003 by Saunders, an imprint of Elsevier Inc. All rights reserved.

Common Protozoal and Parasitic Diseases

Disease	Organism	Transmission	Symptoms	Tests and Specimens
Malaria	*Plasmodium* species (protozoa)		Chills, fever (cyclic)	
Toxoplasmosis	*Toxoplasma gondii* (protozoa)		Febrile illness, rash; *Congenital:* Jaundice, enlarged liver and spleen, brain abnormalities	
Amebic dysentery	*Entamoeba histolytica* (protozoa)		Bloody diarrhea, cramping, fever	
Giardiasis			Asymptomatic to severe diarrhea and abdominal discomfort	
Trichinosis	*Trichinella spiralis* (roundworm)		Nausea, fever, diarrhea, muscle pain and swelling, edema of the face	
Tapeworm	*Taenia* species		Abdominal discomfort, diarrhea, weight loss	
Pinworm	*Enterobius vermicularis* (roundworm)		Severe rectal itching, restlessness, insomnia	
Scabies			Nocturnal itching, skin burrows	
Lice			Intense itching, skin lesions	

CASE STUDIES

1. A patient has been instructed to provide a stool sample. What type of patient education should be included to ensure proper collection?

2. Anna, the medical assistant, works in an office in which some rapid testing is performed. Describe three microbiology tests that use a rapid identification technique.

3. A 5-year-old patient is brought to the office with pinworms. How do people usually become infested with pinworms? Provide the patient education for specimen collection.

4. Anna is educating a patient on the importance of infection control. What factors should Anna be sure to cover?

WORKPLACE APPLICATIONS

1. Anna is preparing to obtain a sample for testing. What should she keep in mind as she is collecting the specimen? The specimen is an anaerobe. What elements are required for growth?

2. Describe some of the different equipment found in the microbiology laboratory.

3. What steps should Anna follow while performing a rapid strep test?

4. List and describe the three CLIA-waived immunology tests that Anna may perform in the POL.

INTERNET ACTIVITY

Go to the American Biological Safety Association Web site at *www.absa.org*. Become familiar with the site. What tools does the site have to help you maintain a safe laboratory environment?

Copyright © 2011, 2007, 2003 by Saunders, an imprint of Elsevier Inc. All rights reserved.

56 Surgical Supplies and Instruments

VOCABULARY REVIEW

Fill in the blanks with the appropriate terms.

1. ________________ The act of scraping a body cavity with a surgical instrument, such as a curette
2. ________________ Opening or widening the circumference of a body orifice with a dilating instrument
3. ________________ A sheet or band of fibrous tissue deep in the skin that covers muscles and body organs
4. ________________ An abnormal, tubelike passage between internal organs or from an internal organ to the body surface
5. ________________ Open space, such as within a blood vessel, the intestine, a needle, or an examining instrument
6. ________________ A rigid tube that surrounds a blunt trocar or a sharp, pointed trocar inserted into the body; when withdrawn, fluid may escape from the body through it, depending on where it is inserted
7. ________________ A metal rod with a smooth, rounded tip that is placed into hollow instruments to minimize the damage to body tissues during insertion
8. ________________ A localized collection of pus, under the skin or deep within the body, that causes tissue destruction
9. ________________ Open condition of a body cavity or canal
10. ________________ Tumors with stems, frequently found on mucous membranes
11. ________________ A metal probe that is inserted into or passed through a catheter, needle, or tube to clear it or to facilitate passage into a body orifice
12. ________________ To cut or separate tissue with a cutting instrument or scissors

SKILLS AND CONCEPTS

1. List two medications that help control bleeding.

   a. ________________________________

   b. ________________________________

2. What is the purpose of combining epinephrine in a local anesthetic?

   ____

   ____

3. List four groups of surgical instruments and give an example of each.

   a. ________________________________

   b. ________________________________

   c. ________________________________

   d. ________________________________

Copyright © 2011, 2007, 2003 by Saunders, an imprint of Elsevier Inc. All rights reserved.

Name the instruments pictured in the following figures.

4.

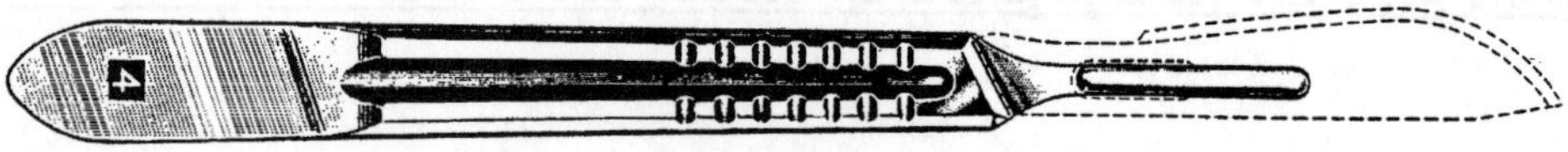

5.

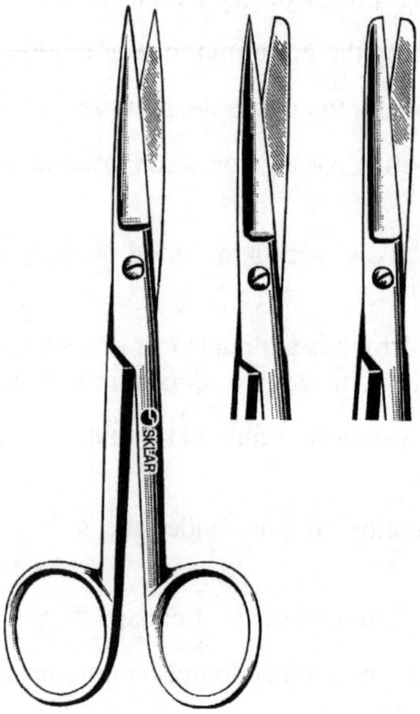

6.

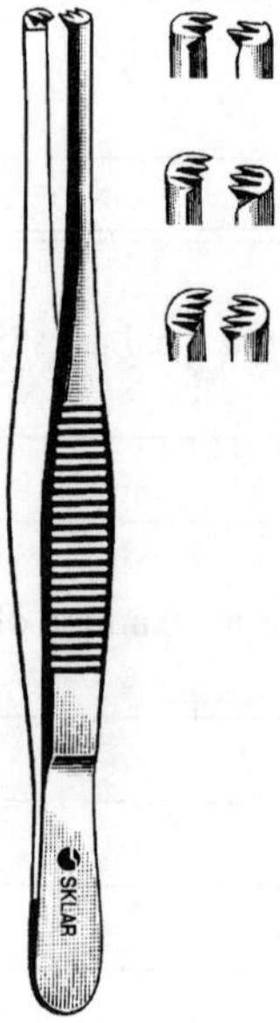

Copyright © 2011, 2007, 2003 by Saunders, an imprint of Elsevier Inc. All rights reserved.

7.

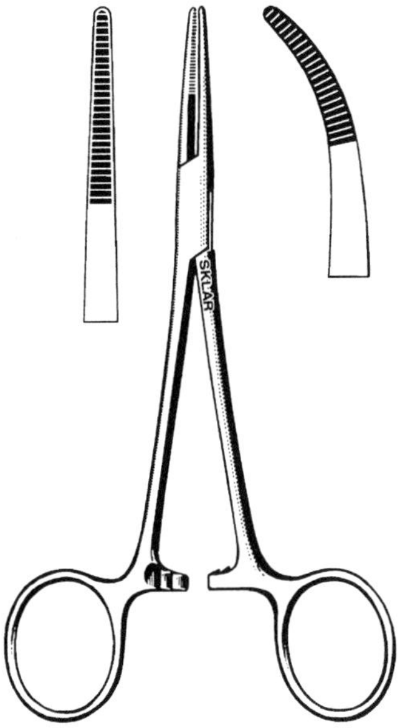

8.

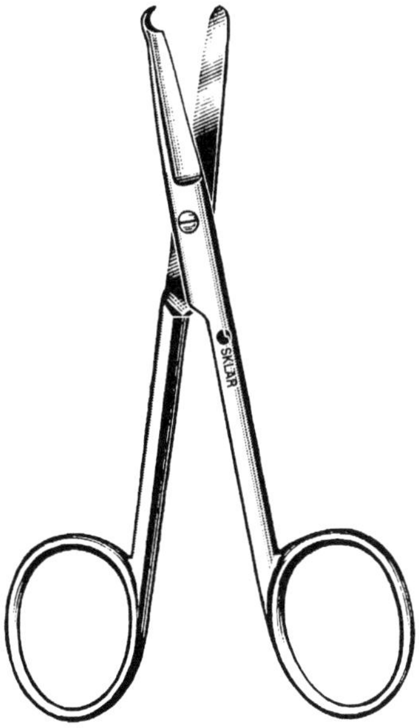

Copyright © 2011, 2007, 2003 by Saunders, an imprint of Elsevier Inc. All rights reserved.

9.

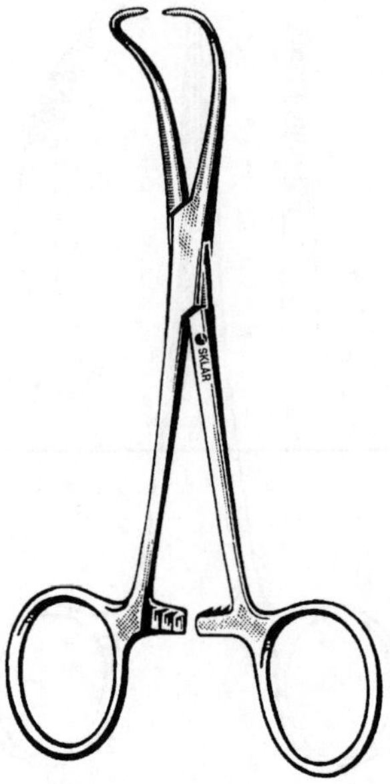

10.

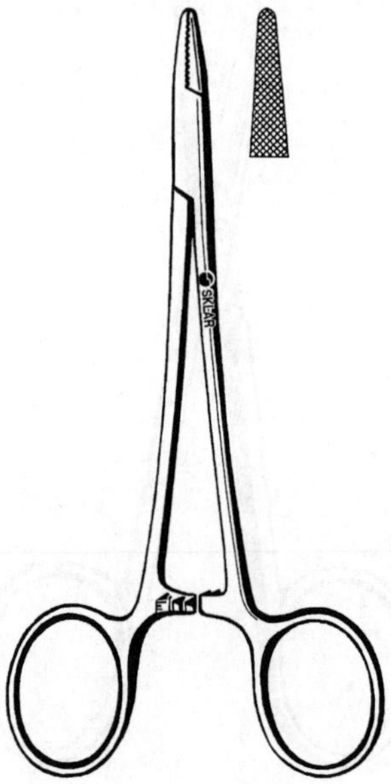

 Copyright © 2011, 2007, 2003 by Saunders, an imprint of Elsevier Inc. All rights reserved.

11.

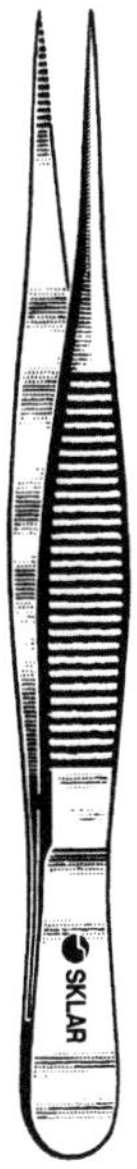

12.

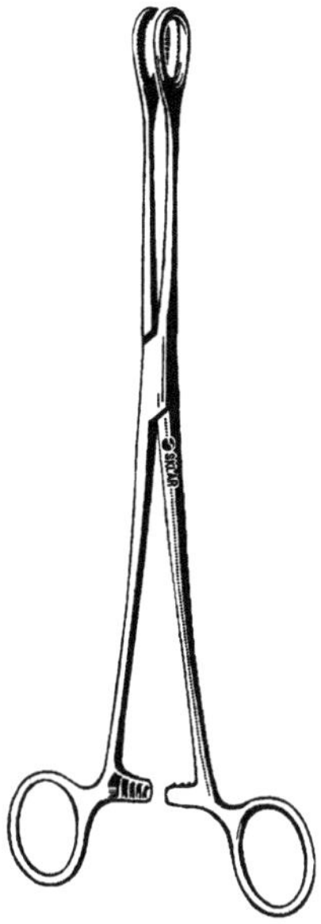

Copyright © 2011, 2007, 2003 by Saunders, an imprint of Elsevier Inc. All rights reserved.

13.

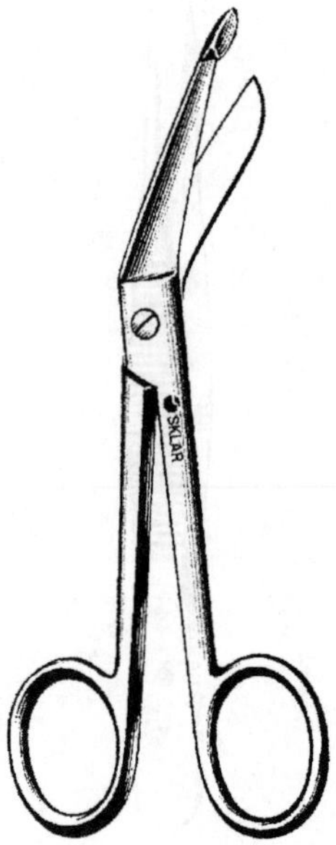

____

Indicate which statements are true (T) and which are false (F).

14. ______________ An instrument should always be unlocked before immersion in the chemical decontaminate to permit cleansing of the entire surface area.

15. ______________ Instruments are always named after the person who designed them.

16. ______________ Scissors have ratchets.

17. ______________ "Mosquito" and "Kelly" are names of hemostats.

18. ______________ All tissues removed from the patient are sent to the pathology laboratory for analysis.

19. ______________ Topical silver nitrate solution is used to control epistaxis.

20. ______________ Ratchets are located just below the ring handles and are used to lock an instrument into position.

Match the following descriptions and instruments.

21. ________ Have a beak or hook to slide under sutures
22. ________ Jaws are shorter and look stronger than hemostat jaws
23. ________ Design and construction vary; have a fine tip for foreign object retrieval
24. ________ Have very sharp hooks
25. ________ Valves can be spread to facilitate viewing
26. ________ Probe tip is blunt
27. ________ Smooth tipped, manufactured in different lengths, and used to insert packing into or remove objects from the nose and ear

a. Bayonet forceps
b. Towel forceps (towel clamp)
c. Littauer stitch or suture scissors
d. Needle holders
e. Splinter forceps
f. Nasal specula
g. Bandage scissors

Copyright © 2011, 2007, 2003 by Saunders, an imprint of Elsevier Inc. All rights reserved.

28. Describe some characteristics of ideal suture material.

a. ______

b. ______

c. ______

d. ______

29. Explain the difference between absorbable and nonabsorbable sutures. When would each type of suture be used?

______

30. Explain the purpose of four different types of additional surgical supplies that may be used in minor surgical procedures in the physician's office.

______

31. Describe the method of identifying the gauge of suture material.

______

______

32. Explain how surgical instruments are handled after a surgical procedure is complete.

______

______

______

CASE STUDIES

1. You are assisting Dr. Samanski during a procedure. The physician has asked you to ensure three local anesthetics are available in the room. List them.

2. Tom is preparing an instrument and supply pack for a cervical biopsy. What instruments should be included for autoclaving?

WORKPLACE APPLICATIONS

1. Tom is in charge of establishing a room in the office for minor surgery. What features should be included in this room?

2. Tom is stocking the supplies in the surgery room. List four types of surgical solutions commonly used.

3. Tom is showing a new employee the various instruments in the office. What should Tom tell the new employee about the care and inspection of the instruments?

INTERNET ACTIVITY

Search the Internet for surgical instruments. How expensive are they? Print out the descriptions of the instruments and bring them to class. Compare your findings with a classmate.

Copyright © 2011, 2007, 2003 by Saunders, an imprint of Elsevier Inc. All rights reserved.

57 Surgical Asepsis and Assisting with Surgical Procedures

VOCABULARY REVIEW

Match the following terms with their definitions.

1. _______ Invasion of body tissues by microorganisms, which proliferate and damage tissues
2. _______ Living organisms that can be seen only with a light microscope
3. _______ Disease-causing microorganisms
4. _______ Allowing a substance to pass or soak through
5. _______ Reducing the number of microorganisms to a relatively safe level
6. _______ A thick-walled, dormant form of bacteria very resistant to disinfection measures
7. _______ Complete destruction of all forms of microbial life
8. _______ A substance that kills microorganisms
9. _______ Becoming nonsterile by contact with any nonsterile material
10. _______ A pathologic process having a descriptive set of signs and symptoms
11. _______ Destruction of pathogens by physical or chemical means
12. _______ Swelling between layers of tissue

a. Permeable
b. Contamination
c. Disease
d. Infection
e. Antiseptic
f. Edema
g. Spores
h. Pathogens
i. Sterilization
j. Disinfection
k. Microorganisms
l. Sanitization

SKILLS AND CONCEPTS

1. Describe the differences among sanitization, disinfection, and sterilization and how each is performed.

____

____

____

____

____

2. Describe the following types of sterilization indicators. Which is considered the best method for checking whether instrument packs are being sterilized when autoclaved?

   a. Chemical

   ____

   ____

   b. Biologic

   ____

   ____

Copyright © 2011, 2007, 2003 by Saunders, an imprint of Elsevier Inc. All rights reserved.

3. The medical assistant is responsible for making sure no problems occur with autoclave procedures. Complete the following table, which outlines methods for improving autoclave techniques.

Problem	Causes	Corrective Measures
Damp linens		
Stained linens		
Corroded instruments		
Spotted or stained instruments		
Instruments that have soft hinges or joints		
Ebullition, or caps that blow off solutions		
Steam leakage		
Chamber door does not open		

4. Describe the following common surgical procedures done in the physician's office.

   a. Cryosurgery

   ____

   ____

   b. Microsurgery?

   ____

   ____

   c. Endoscopic procedures?

   ____

   ____

   d. Electrosurgery?

   ____

   ____

   e. Laser?

   ____

   ____

 Copyright © 2011, 2007, 2003 by Saunders, an imprint of Elsevier Inc. All rights reserved.

5. Explain the importance of skin preparation and describe how it is done.

____

____

____

Indicate which statements are true (T) and which are false (F).

6. ________ Air currents carry bacteria, so body motions over a sterile field and talking should be kept to a minimum.
7. ________ Infection can cause death in some circumstances.
8. ________ A sterile field can get wet but remain microorganism free.
9. ________ Sterile team members should always face each other.
10. ________ You should always keep the sterile field in your view.
11. ________ You should never turn your back on a sterile field or wander away from it.
12. ________ When autoclaving, you should place a gauze sponge around the tips of sharp instruments to prevent them from piercing the wrapping material.
13. ________ Nonsterile individuals should never reach over a sterile field.
14. ________ All hinged instruments are wrapped in the closed position to allow full steam penetration of the joint.
15. ________ When using sterilizing bags, you should insert the grasping end of the instruments first.

16. Describe the three phases of wound healing.

    a. ____

    b. ____

    c. ____

17. Describe first and second intention healing and give an example of each.

____

____

____

____

18. What are the reasons for applying a sterile dressing?

    a. ____

    b. ____

    c. ____

    d. ____

19. What is the purpose of a bandage? Does it have to be sterile?

____

____

____

Copyright © 2011, 2007, 2003 by Saunders, an imprint of Elsevier Inc. All rights reserved.

20. Explain the difference between surgical and medical asepsis. When is each performed?

____

____

____

____

21. What is the shelf life of sterilized packs?

____

____

CASE STUDIES

1. Melissa, the medical assistant, is preparing instruments for the autoclave. What rules must she follow when wrapping instruments for the autoclave?

2. Minor surgical procedures, such as the removal of moles, are commonly done in Melissa's office. What is Melissa's role in these procedures?

3. Melissa is preparing a patient for a procedure, and the patient seems very anxious and worried. What can Melissa do to support the patient?

WORKPLACE APPLICATIONS

1. One of Melissa's duties is maintaining the autoclave. What types of PPE should she wear when loading, operating, and unloading the autoclave? Why?

2. What guidelines should be followed when the autoclave is unloaded?

3. A patient is scheduled for a surgical procedure in the office. What details should Melissa attend to before the appointment?

4. The physician has ordered an open wound healing. What does this mean? How does healing occur? What are some of the advantages of this type of healing process?

INTERNET ACTIVITY

One of your duties is to purchase supplies for minor office procedures. Search the Internet for equipment and supplies typically needed to perform such procedures. Print a list of materials and prices. Share the information with your classmates. Did you find anything surprising?

MEDICAL RECORDS ACTIVITIES

1. After a surgical procedure, the medical assistant should provide the patient with postoperative instructions. Give five reasons a patient should call the office after a procedure. Document the patient instructions.

2. A patient comes to the office for suture removal. The area, the left forearm, is covered with bandages. How should the patient be prepared for the procedure? What setup is required for this procedure? Document the case, including the patient's vital signs.

3. Ms. Maria Idione was seen today for removal of a cyst from her left forearm. The physician asks you to reinforce patient education about the healing process. Document your interaction with Ms. Idione, including the factors that may affect healing and indicators of wound infection.

Copyright © 2011, 2007, 2003 by Saunders, an imprint of Elsevier Inc. All rights reserved.

58 Career Development and Life Skills

VOCABULARY REVIEW

Fill in the blanks with the correct vocabulary terms from this chapter.

1. Jerri wrote a(n) ________________ of the facts that she knew related to the theft of petty cash.
2. June found Daniel's attitude to be ________________ and finally made a complaint to the office manager.
3. Because Allen was continuing his studies at night and was taking 12 credit hours, he was able to place his student loan in ________________.
4. Medical assisting is one of the most versatile ________________ a person can enter.
5. The physician asked Merri to ________________ the documents for grammar and spelling.
6. Andrea found that ________________ provided her with many more job leads than simply looking in the newspaper.
7. Ms. Moore, the office manager, attempted to get the employees to bring up only the ________________ facts related to the conflict.
8. Joel tried to ________________ his error by placing an amendment in the medical record.
9. Dr. McDonald gave the information to Selinda to rewrite, because she could take the regulations and convert them into a(n) ________________, clear document.
10. Mack called his lender to report that he had returned to school full-time so that he would not ________________ on his loan.

SKILLS AND CONCEPTS

Part I: Short Answers

1. List three ways job search training helps the newly graduated medical assistant.

   a. ____

   b. ____

   c. ____

2. What are employers' three basic desires when looking for a new employee?

   a. ____

   b. ____

   c. ____

3. Define *job skills* and give two examples.

____

____

Copyright © 2011, 2007, 2003 by Saunders, an imprint of Elsevier Inc. All rights reserved.

4. Define *self-management skills* and give two examples.

____

____

5. Define *transferable skills* and give two examples.

____

____

6. What is meant when it is said that a medical assistant knows his or her personal needs?

____

____

7. List and define the two best job search methods.

   a. ____

   b. ____

8. Explain at least three ways the Internet can be helpful in a job search.

   a. ____

   b. ____

   c. ____

9. List five items that should be included on a résumé.

   a. ____

   b. ____

   c. ____

   d. ____

   e. ____

10. List two things that should never be included on a résumé.

   a. ____

   b. ____

Copyright © 2011, 2007, 2003 by Saunders, an imprint of Elsevier Inc. All rights reserved.

Part II: Cover Letters

Write a professional cover letter, following the suggestions in the textbook. Turn in the cover letter to the instructor, along with the assignment in Part III.

Part III: Job Applications

1. Complete the job application found on the following pages. Make sure it is legible, accurate, and complete.

DIAMONTE HOSPITAL

APPLICATION FOR EMPLOYMENT

This application is not a contract. It is intended to provide information for evaluating your suitability for employment. Please read each question carefully and give an honest and complete answer. Qualified applicants receive consideration for employment without unlawful discrimination because of sex, religion, race, color, national origin, age, disability, or other classification protected by law. Applications will remain active for three months.

PLEASE TYPE OR PRINT ALL INFORMATION

Date: ______________________

Position(s) applying for: ____

How did you learn about us? ☐ Walk-in ☐ Friend ☐ Relative ☐ Job hotline ☐ Employee ☐ Other
☐ Advertisement (Please state name of publication) ______________________ Referred by: ____________

Name: ____
Last *First* *Middle initial*

Mailing address: ____
City *State* *Zip code*

Phone: (____) ______________ (____) ______________ Social Security #: ______________
Home *Message*

If related to anyone in our employ, state name and department: ______________________

If you have been employed under another name, please list here: ______________________

Are you under 18 years of age? ☐ Yes ☐ No

Are you currently employed? ☐ Yes ☐ No

May we contact your present employer? ☐ Yes ☐ No

Do you have legal rights to work in this country?
(Proof of legal rights to work in this country will be required upon employment) ☐ Yes ☐ No

Have you ever been employed with us before? ☐ Yes ☐ No *If "yes," give date(s):* ____________

Are you available to work: ☐ Full-time ☐ Part-time ☐ Shift work ☐ Temporary

Are you available to work overtime if required? ☐ Yes ☐ No

How flexible are you in accepting varying scheduled hours? ☐ Very flexible ☐ Somewhat flexible
☐ Need set schedule

Minimum salary desired: ______________________

Have you ever been discharged from a job or forced to resign? ☐ Yes ☐ No
Explain: ____

Have you ever been convicted of a felony?
If "yes," please explain: ☐ Yes ☐ No
Criminal convictions are not an absolute bar to employment but will be considered with respect to the specific requirements of the job for which you are applying. ______________________

Copyright © 2011, 2007, 2003 by Saunders, an imprint of Elsevier Inc. All rights reserved.

EDUCATION

High school: ____________________ High school graduate/GED: ☐ Yes ☐ No
____________________ Date: __________

College: ____________________ Graduated: ☐ Yes ☐ No
Major/field(s) of study: ____________________ Degree: __________
Date: __________

College: ____________________ Graduated: ☐ Yes ☐ No
Major/field(s) of study: ____________________ Degree: __________
Date: __________

Technical, business, or correspondence school: ____________________ Graduated: ☐ Yes ☐ No
Major/field(s) of study: ____________________ Degree: __________
Date: __________

Describe any specialized training, apprenticeship, and skills such as computer, office equipment, etc. ____________________

LICENSES AND CERTIFICATIONS

Type of license(s)/certification(s): ____________________ Expiration date: __________
Type of license(s)/certification(s): ____________________ Expiration date: __________
Type of license(s)/certification(s): ____________________ Expiration date: __________
Verified by: __________
Date: __________

REFERENCES

(Give name, address, and telephone number of three references that you have known for at least one year who are not related to you.)

Name: ____________________ Phone: __________ Years acquainted: ______
Address: ____________________ Business: __________

Name: ____________________ Phone: __________ Years acquainted: ______
Address: ____________________ Business: __________

Name: ____________________ Phone: __________ Years acquainted: ______
Address: ____________________ Business: __________

Copyright © 2011, 2007, 2003 by Saunders, an imprint of Elsevier Inc. All rights reserved.

EMPLOYMENT EXPERIENCE

(Please list all employment experience, with most recent employment first. If more space is needed, please use the Additional Employment form.)

Employer: ______________________ Duties and skills performed: ______________________
Address: ______________________
Phone number(s) ______________________
Job title: ______________________
Supervisor's name/title: ______________________
Reason for leaving: ______________________
Salary received: ______________ *hourly / weekly / monthly*
Employed from: ______________ to ______________
month / year *month / year*

Employer: ______________________ Duties and skills performed: ______________________
Address: ______________________
Phone number(s) ______________________
Job title: ______________________
Supervisor's name/title: ______________________
Reason for leaving: ______________________
Salary received: ______________ *hourly / weekly / monthly*
Employed from: ______________ to ______________
month / year *month / year*

Employer: ______________________ Duties and skills performed: ______________________
Address: ______________________
Phone number(s) ______________________
Job title: ______________________
Supervisor's name/title: ______________________
Reason for leaving: ______________________
Salary received: ______________ *hourly / weekly / monthly*
Employed from: ______________ to ______________
month / year *month / year*

Do you expect any of the employers listed above to give you a poor reference? ☐ *Yes* ☐ *No*
If yes, explain: ______________________

Copyright © 2011, 2007, 2003 by Saunders, an imprint of Elsevier Inc. All rights reserved.

APPLICANT'S STATEMENT

I hereby certify that the statements and information provided are true, and I understand that any false statements or omissions are cause for termination. I agree to submit to a drug test and physical following any conditional offer of employment, and I grant permission to Diamonte Hospital to investigate my criminal history, education, prior employment history, and references, and hereby release all persons or agencies from all liability or any damage for issuing this information.

I understand that this application is current for only **three months**. At the end of that time, if I do not hear from Diamonte Hospital and still wish to be considered for employment, it will be necessary to update my application.

______________________________ ______________________________

Signature of Applicant *Date*

____

Print Name

DIAMONTE
HOSPITAL

Copyright © 2011, 2007, 2003 by Saunders, an imprint of Elsevier Inc. All rights reserved.

Part IV: Résumés

1. Write a professional résumé, following the suggestions in the textbook. Turn in the résumé and cover letter to your instructor.

Part V: Interviews

1. Set up an interview with a physician's office. Perhaps the interview can lead to an externship or a position after graduation. Use the *Record of a Job Lead* form and the *Record of an Interview* form to record pertinent information.

Part VI: Follow-up Activities

1. Write a thank you card to the person with whom you interviewed. If a job opportunity exists, continue follow-up activities with the clinic.

Part VII: Goals

1. Set some realistic goals for your career in medical assisting by answering the following questions.

   a. Where am I today?

   ____

   ____

   ____

   b. Where will I be in 5 years?

   ____

   ____

   ____

   c. Where will I be in 10 years?

   ____

   ____

   ____

   d. What additional skills do I need to get to where I want to be?

   ____

   ____

   ____

   ____

Copyright © 2011, 2007, 2003 by Saunders, an imprint of Elsevier Inc. All rights reserved.

Part VIII: Budgeting

1. Plan a budget for yourself using your actual living expenses.

The Guideline Budget

MONTHLY INCOME	AMOUNT
Net Income	
Spouse Net Income	
Child Support	
Other Income	

MONTHLY EXPENSES	AMOUNT
Rent	
Gas	
Electric	
Home/Renters Insurance	
Water/Sewage	
Trash	
Home Telephone	
Cell Telephone	
Pager	
Cable TV/Satellite	
Internet/DSL	
Child Care	
Lawn Care	
Clothing	
Food-Home	
Food-Work or School	
Food-Eating Out	
Laundry/Dry Cleaning	
Medical Expenses	
Dental Expenses	
Life Insurance	
Medical Insurance	
Dental Insurance	
Eyeglasses	
Prescriptions	
Automobile Payment	
Automobile Insurance	
Repairs	
Gas/Oil	
Furniture	
Beauty/Barber Shop	
Pet Expenses	
Student Loan	
Other Loans	
Credit Cards	
Church/Charities	
Birthdays	
Anniversaries	
Christmas	
Vacation Planning	
Entertainment	

Part IX: Mail Address

1. Open an e-mail account that reflects a professional electronic address using a free service (e.g., Yahoo!, MSN, Hotmail). Make sure the mail address you choose is appropriate for professional resumes and job applications.

Copyright © 2011, 2007, 2003 by Saunders, an imprint of Elsevier Inc. All rights reserved.

CASE STUDY

Monica was an exceptional student during school and graduated with a high GPA. After a successful externship and 1 month looking for employment, she has been unable to secure a job. She calls the placement officer at her school, who sends her on several interviews, which are also unsuccessful. The placement officer asks Monica to come to the school dressed for an interview and to bring her résumé. The placement officer is impressed with Monica's appearance and her communications skills during the interview. However, when she looks down at Monica's résumé, she realizes why Monica has not been hired. What problem did the placement officer probably discover? What can Monica do to be more likely to secure employment?

WORKPLACE ACTIVITIES

Make a list of 20 potential employers. Use the Internet to obtain information about the facilities. Make a list of five points about each potential employer that could be discussed in an interview. Also, find five ways you qualify for a position in the facility. If appropriate, visit the facilities and make appointments for interviews. Obtain and complete a job application from each facility. Submit the application and a résumé if you are close to the end of your training.

INTERNET ACTIVITIES

1. Research potential employers in your geographic area. Find out as much information about the employers as possible. Keep a record of the information using the job lead forms provided in the text.

2. Use the Internet to locate potential job opportunities. Have your résumé in electronic form ready to attach so that you can apply for the jobs that interest you.

3. Look for job search sites other than those in the textbook. Share the sites with your classmates.

4. Form a group on a social networking site, such as Facebook, that includes each classmate. Share e-mails and stay in touch with one another after graduation. Share leads that might result in employment.

Copyright © 2011, 2007, 2003 by Saunders, an imprint of Elsevier Inc. All rights reserved.

English-Spanish Terms for the Medical Assistant

abscess A localized collection of pus that causes tissue destruction and may be either under the skin or deep within the body.
absceso Cantidad de pus localizada en un lugar que puede estar bajo la piel o a más profundidad en el interior del cuerpo y causa la destrucción de los tejidos.

academic degree A title conferred by a college, university, or professional school after completion of a program of study.
grado académico Título concedido por una, universidad o escuela profesional, tras completar un programa de estudios.

accommodation Adjustment of the eye for seeing various sizes of objects at different distances.
acomodación Ajuste del ojo para ver distintos tamaños de objetos a distancias diferentes.

account A statement of transactions during a fiscal period and the resulting balance.
cuenta Estado de transacciones durante un periodo fiscal y el saldo resultante.

account balance The amount owed or on hand in an account.
saldo de la cuenta Suma que se debe o que está en una cuenta.

accounts receivable ledger A record of the income and payments due from creditors on an account.
libro mayor de cuentas por cobrar Registro de cargos y pagos asentados en una cuenta.

accreditation The process by which an organization is recognized for adhering to a group of standards that meet or exceed the expectations of the accrediting agency.
acreditación Proceso por el cual se reconoce a una organización por su cumplimiento de ciertos estándares en un grado que cumple o sobrepasa las expectativas de la agencia que la acredita.

act The formal product of a legislative body; a decision or determination by a sovereign, a legislative council, or a court of justice.
ley Producto formal de un cuerpo legislativo; decisión o determinación por un soberano, un consejo legislativo o un tribunal de justicia.

acute Having a rapid onset and severe symptoms.
agudo Que tiene un comienzo rápido y síntomas serios.

adage A saying, often in metaphoric form, that embodies a common observation.
refrán Dicho, con frecuencia metafórico, que refleja una observación común.

adhesions Bands of scar tissue that bind together two anatomic surfaces that normally are separate.
adhesiones Bandas de tejido de una cicatriz que unen dos superficies anatómicas que están normalmente separadas.

adrenocorticotropic hormone (ACTH) A hormone released by the anterior pituitary gland that stimulates the production and secretion of glucocorticoids.
hormona adrenocorticotropina (ACTH) Hormona, liberada por la glándula pituitaria anterior, que estimula la producción y secreción de glucocorticoides.

advent A coming into being or use.
advenimiento Próximo a ser o a usarse.

advocate One who pleads the cause of another; one who defends or maintains a cause or proposal.
abogado Persona que defiende la causa de otro; aqel que defiende o apoya una causa o propuesta.

affable Being pleasant and at ease in talking to others; characterized by ease and friendliness.
afable Que es agradable y tiene un trato fácil con los demás; caracterizado por su trato fácil y amistoso.

agenda A list or outline of things to be considered or done.
agenda Lista o resumen de cosas a considerar o a hacer.

aggression A forceful action or procedure intended to dominate; hostile, injurious, or destructive behavior, especially when caused by frustration.
agresión Acción o procedimiento forzado, con la intención de dominar; comportamiento hostil, injurioso o destructivo, en especial cuando es causado por frustración.

albuminuria Abnormal presence of albumin in the urine.
albuminuria Presencia anómala de albúmina en la orina.

Copyright © 2011, 2007, 2003 by Saunders, an imprint of Elsevier Inc. All rights reserved.

aliquot A portion of a well-mixed sample removed for testing.
alícuota Porción de una muestra bien mezclada, separada para ser analizada.

allegation A statement of what a party to a legal action undertakes to prove.
alegación Declaración por una de las partes implicadas en un proceso legal para apoyar lo que dicha parte intenta probar.

allied health fields Areas of healthcare delivery or related services in which professionals assist physicians with the diagnosis, treatment, and care of patients in many different specialty areas.
campos relacionados con la salud Áreas del cuidado de la salud y servicios relacionados en los cuales profesionales ayudan a los médicos en el diagnóstico, tratamiento y atención de los pacientes en muchas áreas diferentes.

allocating Apportioning for a specific purpose or to particular persons or things.
distribuir Asignar a un fin específico o a personas o cosas en particular.

allopathy A method of treating a disease by introducing a condition that is intended to cause a pathologic reaction that will be antagonistic to the condition being treated.
alopatía Método de tratar una enfermedad provocando una afección con el fin de causar una reacción patológica, la cual será opuestaa la enfermedad que se está tratando.

allowed charge The maximum amount of money that many third-party payors will pay for a specific procedure or service. Often based on the UCR fee.
cargo permitido Cantidad máxima de dinero que muchos pagadores intermediarios pagan por una práctica o servicio especifico; con frecuencia se basa en el cargo UCR.

alopecia Partial or complete lack of hair.
alopecia Pérdida de cabello, parcial o total.

alphabetic filing Any system that arranges names or topics according to the sequence of the letters in the alphabet.
archivo alfabético Cualquier sistema que ordena los nombres o temas siguiendo la secuencia de las letras del alfabeto.

alphanumeric Systems made up of combinations of letters and numbers.
alfanumérico Sistema constituido por combinaciones de letras y números.

ambiguous Capable of being understood in two or more possible senses or ways; unclear.
ambiguo Que puede entenderse de dos o más maneras; que no es claro.

amblyopia Reduction or dimness of vision with no apparent organic cause; often referred to as *lazy eye syndrome*.
ambliopía Reducción o disminución de la visión sin causa orgánica aparente; con frecuencia se conoce como *síndrome del ojo vago*.

ambulatory Able to walk about and not be bedridden.
ambulatorio Capaz de caminar y no tiene que estar postrado en la cama.

amenity Something conducive to comfort, convenience, or enjoyment.
amenidad Algo que proporciona confort, comodidad o placer.

amino acids Organic compounds that form the chief constituents of protein and are used by the body to build and repair tissues.
aminoácidos Compuestos orgánicos que son los constituyentes principales de la proteína y son usados por el cuerpo para formar y reparar tejidos.

amorphous Lacking a defined shape.
amorfo Que carece de forma definida.

analyte The substance or chemical being analyzed or detected in a specimen.
analito La sustancia o producto químico que se analiza o que se detecta en una muestra.

anaphylaxis Exaggerated hypersensitivity reaction that in severe cases leads to vascular collapse, bronchospasm, and shock.
anafilaxia Reacción de hipersensibilidad exagerada, la cual, en casos graves, conduce a colapso vascular, broncospasmo y choque.

anastomosis The surgical joining together of two normally distinct organs.
anastomosis Unión quirúrgica de dos órganos normalmente diferentes.

ancillary Subordinate; auxiliary.
auxiliar Subordinado, complementario.

ancillary diagnostic services Services that support patient diagnoses (e.g., laboratory or x-ray).
servicios de diagnóstico auxiliares Servicios que apoyan el diagnóstico del paciente (como laboratorio o rayos x).

Copyright © 2011, 2007, 2003 by Saunders, an imprint of Elsevier Inc. All rights reserved.

"and" In the context of ICD-9-CM, the word "and" should be interpreted as "and/or."
"y" En el contexto de ICD-9-CM, la palabra "y" debe interpretarse como "y/o."

anemia A condition marked by deficiency of red blood cells.
anemia Enfermedad caracterizada por una deficiencia de glóbulos rojos en la sangre.

angiocardiography Radiography of the heart and great vessels using an iodine contrast medium.
angiocardiografía Radiografía del corazón y los vasos sanguíneos mayores usando un medio de contraste yodado.

angiography Radiography of blood vessels using an iodine contrast medium.
angiografía Radiografía de los vasos sanguíneos usando un medio de contraste yodado.

angioplasty Interventional technique using a catheter to open or widen a blood vessel to improve circulation.
angioplastia Técnica quirúrgica que usa un catéter para abrir o hacer más ancho un vaso sanguíneo a fin de mejorar la circulación.

animate Full of life; to give spirit and support to expressions.
animar Dar vida; dar ánimo y apoyo a las manifestaciones.

annotating To furnish with notes, which are usually critical or explanatory.
anotar Añadir notas, por lo general, críticas o explicatorias.

annotation A note added by way of comment or explanation.
anotación Nota añadida a modo de comentario o explicación.

anomalies Faulty development of the fetus resulting in deformities or deviations from normal.
anomalías Desarrollo defectuoso del feto que tiene como resultado deformidades o desviaciones de lo normal.

anorexia Lack or loss of appetite for food.
anorexia Falta o pérdida del apetito.

anoxia Absence of oxygen in the tissues.
anoxia Ausencia de oxígeno en los tejidos.

anteroposterior (AP) Frontal projection in which the patient is supine or facing the x-ray tube.
anteroposterior (AP) Proyección frontal en la cual el paciente está en posición supina o frente al tubo de rayos x.

antibody Immunoglobulin produced by the immune system in response to bacteria, viruses, or other antigenic substances.
anticuerpo Inmunoglobulina producida por el sistema inmunológico en respuesta a bacterias, virus u otras substancias antigénicas.

anticoagulant A chemical added to the blood after collection to prevent clotting.
anticoagulante Producto químico que se añade a la sangre después de extraerla para que no forme coágulos.

antidiuretic hormone (ADH) A hormone secreted at the posterior pituitary gland that causes water retention in the kidneys and elevates the blood pressure; also known as *vasopressin*.
hormona antidiurética (ADH) Hormona secretada por la glándula pituitaria posterior y que provoca retención de agua en los riñones y aumento de la presión sanguínea. Es conocida también como *vasopresina*.

antigen A foreign substance that causes the production of a specific antibody.
antígeno Substancia extraña que provoca la producción de un anticuerpo específico.

antimicrobial agent A drug that is used to treat infection.
agente antimicrobiano Substancia que se usa para tratar infecciones.

antiseptic Pertaining to substances that inhibit the growth of microorganisms (e.g., alcohol and Betadine).
antiséptico Perteneciente o relativo a las substancias que inhiben el crecimiento de microorganismos como el alcohol y la Betadina.

antiseptic A substance that kills microorganisms.
antiséptico Substancia que mata microorganismos.

antiseptic An agent that inhibits bacterial growth and can be used on human tissue.
antiséptico Agente que inhibe el crecimiento bacteriano y que puede usarse en los tejidos humanos.

aortogram A radiographic image of the aorta made with the use of an iodine contrast medium.
aortograma Radiografía de la aorta usando un medio de contraste yodado.

apnea Absence or cessation of breathing.
apnea Ausencia o cese de la respiración.

appeal A legal proceeding by which a case is brought before a higher court for review of the decision of a lower court.
apelación Procedimiento legal por el cual un caso se lleva ante un tribunal superior para obtener una revisión de la decisión de un tribunal inferior.

Copyright © 2011, 2007, 2003 by Saunders, an imprint of Elsevier Inc. All rights reserved.

appellate Having the power to review the judgment of another tribunal or body of jurisdiction; for example, an appellate court reviews the rulings of a lower court.
de apelación Que tiene el poder de revisar el veredicto de otro tribunal o cuerpo jurídico, como una corte de apelación.

applications Software programs designed to perform specific tasks.
aplicaciones Programas informáticos diseñados para realizar tareas específicas.

appraisal An expert judgment of the value or merit of something; judging as to quality.
evaluación Acción de emitir un juicio experto sobre el valor o mérito de algo; juzgar la calidad de algo; evaluar el rendimiento en el trabajo.

arbitration The hearing and determination of a cause in controversy by a person or persons either chosen by the parties involved or appointed under statutory authority.
arbitraje Vista y resolución de una causa en conflicto por una persona o personas elegida/s por las partes implicadas o designadas por la autoridad establecida por ley.

arbitrator A neutral person chosen to settle differences between two parties in a controversy.
árbitro Persona neutral seleccionada para poner fin a las diferencias entre dos partes involucradas en un conflicto.

archaic Of, relating to, or characteristic of an earlier or more primitive time.
arcaico Perteneciente o relativo a una época anterior o más primitiva; que tiene las características de dicha época.

archive To file or collect records or documents in or as if in an archive.
archivar Guardar o recoger informes o documentos en un archivo o de manera similar.

arrhythmia An abnormality or irregularity in the heart rhythm.
arritmia Anomalía o irregularidad en el ritmo cardiaco.

arteriography Radiography of the arteries in which an iodine contrast medium is used.
arteriografía Radiografía de las arterias usando un medio de contraste yodado.

arthritis Inflammation of a joint.
artritis Inflamación de una articulación.

arthrogram A fluoroscopic image of the soft tissue components of a joint for which a contrast medium is injected directly into the joint capsule.
artrografía Examen fluoroscópico de los componentes de los tejidos blandos de las articulaciones con una inyección directa de un medio de contraste en la cápsula de la articulación.

articular Pertaining to a joint.
articulatorio Perteneciente o relativo a una articulación.

artificial intelligence The aspect of computer science that deals with computers taking on the attributes of humans. An example is an expert system, which is capable of making decisions; this might be software designed to help a physician diagnose an illness when given a set of symptoms. Game-playing programming and programs designed to recognize human language are other examples of artificial intelligence.
inteligencia artificial Parte de la informática que se ocupa de la incorporación de atributos humanos a las computadoras. Un ejemplo de esto es un sistema práctico capaz de tomar decisiones, como los programas informáticos diseñados para ayudar a los médicos a diagnosticar a un paciente dado un conjunto de síntomas. Los programas de juegos y otros programas diseñados para reconocer el lenguaje humano son otros ejemplos.

ASCII (American Standard Code for Information Interchange) A code representing English characters as numbers, with each given a number from 0 to 127.
ASCII (Estándar Americano de Codificación para el-Intercambio de Información) Un código que representa carácteres ingleses como números, en el cual a cada uno se le asigna un número de 0 a-127.

asepsis The process or state of making or keeping something free of infection or infectious materials; the state of being free of pathogens.
asepsia Que está libre del infecciones.

assault An intentional, unlawful attempt to do bodily injury to another by force.
asalto Intento ilícito de causar daño físico a otro usando la fuerza.

assent To agree to something, especially after thoughtful consideration.
asentir Aceptar algo, especialmente cuando se hace tras una detenida reflexión.

asystole Absence of a heartbeat.
asistolia Ausencia de latidos del corazón.

ataxia Failure or irregularity of muscle actions and coordination.

Copyright © 2011, 2007, 2003 by Saunders, an imprint of Elsevier Inc. All rights reserved.

ataxia Fallo o irregularidad del movimiento y coordinación musculare.

atherosclerosis A form of arteriosclerosis distinguished by fatty deposits within the inner layers of larger arterial walls.
aterosclerosis Forma de arteriosclerosis que se distingue por la presencia de depósitos de grasa en las capas internas de las paredes de las arterias mayores.

atria The two upper chambers of the heart.
aurículas Las dos cavidades superiores del corazón.

atrioventricular (AV) node A part of the cardiac conduction system located between the atria and the ventricles.
nódulo aurioventricular (AV) Parte del sistema cardiaco que se encuentra entre las aurículas y los ventrílculos.

atrophy A decrease in the size of a normally developed organ.
atrofia Disminución del tamaño de un órgano desarrollado de forma normal.

atrophy To waste away or decrease in size.
atrofia Desgastado, disminuido en tamaño.

attenuated Weakening or a change in virulence of a pathogenic microorganism.
atenuado Cambio o debilitación en la virulencia de un microorganismo.

audiologist An allied healthcare professional who specializes in the evaluation of hearing function, detection of hearing impairment, and determination of the anatomic site of impairment.
audiólogo Profesional del cuidado de la salud que se especializa en evaluar la función auditiva, detectar las dificultades auditivas y determinar el-lugar físico en el que se produce el problema auditivo.

audit A formal examination of an organization's or individual's accounts or financial situation; a methodic examination and review.
auditoría Análisis formal de las cuentas o estado financiero de una organización o un individuo; examen y revisión sistemáticos.

augment To make greater, more numerous, larger, or more intense.
aumentar Hacer mayor, más numeroso, más grande o más intenso.

aura A peculiar sensation that precedes the appearance of a more definite disturbance.
aura Sensación peculiar que precede a la aparición de un trastorno definido.

authorization A term used by managed care for an approved referral.
autorización Término usado en el cuido administrado para referirse a la aprobación de la referencia de un paciente de un médico a otro profesional del cuidod o de la salud.

autoimmune Referring to the development of an immune response to one's own tissues; action against one's own cells that causes localized and systemic reactions.
autoinmune Desarrollo de una respuesta inmunológica a los propios tejidos; actuar contra sus propias células para originar reacciones sistémicas localizadas.

autoimmune disorder A disturbance in the immune system in which the body reacts against its own tissue. Examples of autoimmune disorders include multiple sclerosis, rheumatoid arthritis, and systemic lupus erythematosus.
trastorno autoinmune Trastorno del sistema inmunológico en el cual el cuerpo reacciona contra sus propios tejidos. Algunos ejemplos de trastornos autoinmunes incluyen la esclerosis múltiple, la artritis reumatoide y el lupus eritematoso sistémico.

axial projection A radiograph taken with a longitudinal angulation of the x-ray beam; sometimes referred to as a *semiaxial projection.*
proyección axial Radiografía que se toma con un ángulo longitudinal del haz de rayos x; a veces se llama *proyección semi-axial.*

azotemia Retention of excessive amounts of nitrogenous wastes in the blood.
azotemia Retención en la sangre de cantidades de desperdicios nitrogenados.

backup Any type of storage of files to prevent their loss in the event of hard disk failure.
copia de seguridad Cualquier tipo de almacenamiento de archivos para evitar que se pierdan en caso de que ocurrra un fallo en el disco duro.

bailiff An officer of some U.S. courts who usually serves as a messenger or usher and keeps order at the request of the judge.
alguacil Funcionario de algunos tribunales estadounidenses que suele servir como mensajero o ujier y que se ocupa de mantener el orden a petición del juez.

bank reconciliation The process of proving that a bank statement and checkbook balance are in agreement.

Copyright © 2011, 2007, 2003 by Saunders, an imprint of Elsevier Inc. All rights reserved.

reconciliación bancaria Proceso por el cual se prueba que un estado bancario y un saldo de una libreta de cheques concuerdan.

banners Also called *banner ads;* advertisements often found on a Web page that can be animated to attract the user's attention in hopes the person will click on the ad, be redirected to the advertiser's home page, and make a purchase from the site or gain information.
viñetas Viñetas o anuncios de viñetas; anuncios, a veces animados, que se hallan, con frecuencia en las páginas web; su fin es atraer la atención del usuario con la esperanza de que éste haga clic en el anuncio, y así sea llevado a la página principal del anunciante para que compre algo en ese sitio o para que obtenga información sobre el mismo.

battery Willful, unlawful use of force or violence on the person of another; offensive touching or use of force on a person without that person's consent.
golpiza Uso de la fuerza o violencia en contra de la persona de otro, de manera intencional e ilegítima. Tocar de manera ofensiva a una persona o usar la fuerza en contra de ella sin su consentimiento.

beneficence The act of doing or producing good, especially performing acts of charity or kindness.
beneficencia Acción de hacer o producir el bien, en especial llevando a cabo obras caritativas o bondadosas.

beneficiary The person who receives the benefits of an insurance policy. The "insured" person on a Medicare claim.
beneficiario Persona que recibe los beneficios de una póliza de seguro. La persona "asegurada" en una reclamación de Medicare.

benefits Services or payments provided under a health plan, employee plan, or some other agreement, including programs such as health insurance, pensions, retirement planning, and many other options, that may be offered to employees of a company or organization.
beneficios Servicio o pago proporcionado bajo un plan de salud, un plan de empleados o algún otro acuerdo, incluyendo programas como seguros de salud, pensiones, planes de retiro y muchas otras opciones que pueden ser ofrecidas a los empleados de una compañía u organización.

benefits The amount payable by the insurance company for a monetary loss to an individual insured by that company, under each coverage.
beneficios Suma que ha de pagar la compañía aseguradora por una pérdida monetaria a un individuo asegurado por dicha compañía, bajo cada cobertura.

benign Not cancerous and not recurring.
benigno No canceroso y no recurrente.

bevel The angled tip of a needle.
bisel Punta de aguja en ángulo.

bifurcate To divide from one into two branches.
bifurcar Dividir una unidad en dos ramas.

bifurcation The point of forking or separation into two branches.
bifurcación Lugar en el que se separan dos ramas.

bilirubin An orange pigment in bile; the accumulation of bilirubin leads to jaundice.
bilirrubina Pigmento de color naranja que se encuentra en la bilis; cuando se acumula produce ictericia.

bilirubinuria The presence of bilirubin in the urine.
bilirrubinuria Presencia de bilirrubina en la orina.

biophysical Pertaining to the science that deals with the application of physical methods and theories to biologic problems.
biofísico Perteneciente o relativo a la ciencia que trata de la aplicación de métodos y teorías físicas a los problemas biológicos.

birthday rule An insurance rule that states that when an individual is covered under two insurance policies, the insurance plan of the policyholder whose birthday comes first in the calendar year (month and day—not year) becomes primary.
regla del cumpleaños Cuando un individuo está cubierto bajo dos pólizas de seguro, el plan de seguro del titular de la póliza cuya fecha de cumpleaños esté antes en el año civil (mes y día, no año) se convierte en el plan primario.

blatant Completely obvious, conspicuous, or obtrusive, especially in a crass or offensive manner; brazen.
flagrante Completamente obvio, notorio o inoportuno, en especial de una manera torpe u-ofensiva; desvergonzado.

bond A durable, formal paper used for documents.
obligación Papel duradero y formal usado para documentos.

bounding pulse A pulse that feels full because of increased power of cardiac contractions or increased blood volume.
pulso saltón Pulso que se siente lleno debido a un aumento de potencia en las contracciones cardiacas o debido a un aumento del volumen de la sangre.

bradycardia A slow heartbeat; a pulse below 60 beats per minute.

Copyright © 2011, 2007, 2003 by Saunders, an imprint of Elsevier Inc. All rights reserved.

bradicardia Latido lento; pulso por debajo de 60 pulsaciones por minuto.

bradypnea Respirations that are regular in rhythm but slower than normal in rate.
bradipnea Respiración que tiene un ritmo regular pero es más lenta de lo normal.

broad-spectrum antimicrobial agent A drug used to treat a broad range of infections.
agente antimicrobiano de amplio espectro Sustancia que se usa para tratar una amplia gama de infecciones.

bronchiectasis Dilation of the bronchi and bronchioles associated with a secondary infection or ciliary dysfunction.
broncoectasia Dilatación de los bronquios y bronquiolos asociada con una infección secundaria o disfunción ciliar.

bronchoconstriction Narrowing of the bronchiole tubes.
broncoconstricción Estrechamiento de los bronquiolos.

bruit An abnormal sound or a murmur heard on auscultation of an organ, vessel, or gland.
ruido Sonido o murmullo anómalo que se oye al auscultar un órgano, vaso sanguíneo o glándula.

bucky A moving grid device that prevents scatter radiation from fogging the radiographic film.
bucky Dispositivo de rejilla móvil que evita que la difusión de la radiación empañe la película.

bundle of His Fibers that conduct electrical impulses from the AV node to the ventricular myocardium.
haz de His Fibras que conducen impulsos eléctricos del nódulo aurioventricular al miocardio ventricular.

burnout Exhaustion of physical or emotional strength or motivation, usually as a result of prolonged stress or frustration.
agotamiento Llegar al fin de la fortaleza o motivación física o emocional, por lo general como resultado un prolongado estado de estrés o frustración.

bursa A fluid-filled, saclike membrane that provides for cushioning and frictionless motion between two tissues.
bursa Membrana con forma de saco llena de fluido que proporciona amortiguación y movimiento sin fricción entre dos tejidos.

byte A unit of data that contains 8 binary digits.
byte Unidad de información que contiene ocho dígitos binarios.

C&S (culture and sensitivity) A procedure performed in the microbiology laboratory in which a specimen is cultured on artifical media to detect bacterial or fungal growth, followed by appropriate screening for antibiotic sensitivity.
C&S (cultivo y sensibilidad) Procedimiento llevado a cabo en el laboratorio de microbiología en el cual se cultiva un espécimen en un medio artificial para detectar el crecimiento de bacterias u hongos y después investigar su sensibilidad los antibióticos.

cache A special high-speed storage area that can be part of the computer's main memory or a separate storage device. One function of the cache is to store in the computer's memory the Web sites visited; this allows faster recall the next time the Web site is requested.
caché Almacenamiento especial de alta velocidad que puede formar parte de la memoria principal de la computadora o puede ser un dispositivo de almacenamiento separado. Una función del caché es almacenar las páginas Web visitadas en la memoria de la computadora para llegar a ellas con mayor rapidez la próxima vez que desee ver la página.

candidiasis An infection, caused by a yeastlike fungus, that typically affects the vaginal mucosa and skin.
candidiasis Infección causada por una levadura (una especie de hongo) que típicamente afecta la mucosa y la piel vaginal.

cannula A rigid tube that surrounds a blunt or a sharp, pointed trocar that is inserted into the body; when the trocar is withdrawn, fluid may escape from the body through the cannula, depending on the insertion site.
cánula Tubo rígido que envuelve un trocar romo o un trocar de punta afilada que se inserta en el cuerpo; cuando se saca, puede salir fluido corporal a través de la cánula, según en donde haya sido insertada.

caption A heading, title, or subtitle under which records are filed.
leyenda Encabezamiento, título o subtítulo bajo el cual se archivan los informes.

carbohydrates Chemical substances that contain only carbon, oxygen, and hydrogen; they include sugars, glycogen, starches, dextrins, and celluloses.
carbohidratos Sustancias químicas, en las que se incluyen azúcares, glucógenos, almidones, dextrinas y celulosas, y están formadas sólo por carbono, oxígeno e hidrógeno.

carcinogenic A substance that is known to cause cancer.
cancerígeno Sustancia que se sabe que produce cáncer.

Copyright © 2011, 2007, 2003 by Saunders, an imprint of Elsevier Inc. All rights reserved.

carcinogens Substances or agents that cause the development or increase the incidence of cancer.
carcinógeno Sustancia o agente que origina el desarrollo de cáncer o aumenta su incidencia.

cardiac arrest Complete cessation of cardiac contractions.
paro cardiaco Detención completa de las contracciones cardiacas.

cardiac arrhythmia An irregular heartbeat caused by a malfunction in the heart's electrical system.
arritmias cardiacas Pulso irregular que es resultado de un mal funcionamiento del sistema eléctrico del corazón.

cardioversion The use of electroshock to convert an abnormal cardiac rhythm to a normal one.
cardioversión Utilización de un electrochoque para normalizar un ritmo cardiaco anómalo.

cartilage The rubbery, smooth, somewhat elastic connective tissue that covers the ends of bones.
cartílago Tejido de unión similar a la goma, suave y un tanto elástico, que cubre los extremos de los huesos.

case management The process of assessing and planning patient care, including referral and follow up, to ensure continuity of care and quality management.
administración de casos Proceso de evaluación y planificación de la atención al paciente, incluyendo envío de pacientes a especialistas y seguimiento del caso para asegurar la continuidad del tratamiento y la calidad de la administración.

cash on delivery (COD) The method of payment used when an article or item is delivered; payment is expected before the item is released.
contra reembolso (COD) Método de pago usado cuando se entrega un artículo u objeto y el destinatario ha de pagar antes de recibirlo.

casts A fibrous or proteinaceous material, molded to the shape of the part in which it accumulated, that is thrown off into the urine in kidney disease.
cálculos Materiales fibrosos o proteínicos que han tomado la forma de la parte del cuerpo en la que han sido acumulados y que se expulsan a través de la orina en los casos de enfermedades renales.

categorically Placed in a specific division of a system of classification.
categorizado Colocado en un lugar específico dentro de una división de un sistema de clasificación.
caustic (1) A sarcastic remark or phrase. (2) A substance that burns or destroys tissue by chemical action.
cáustico (1) Comentario o frase dicha con sarcasmo. (2) Substancia que quema o destruye tejidos por acción química.

CD burner A CD writer that can write data onto a blank CD or copy data from a CD to a blank CD.
grabador de CD Dispositivo que puede escribir datos en un CD en blanco o copiar datos de un CD a otro CD en blanco.

centrifuge An apparatus consisting essentially of a compartment that spins around a central axis to separate contained materials of different specific gravities or to separate colloidal particles suspended in a liquid.
centrifugadora Aparato que consiste básicamente de un compartimiento que gira alrededor de un eje central para separar materiales con diferentes pesos específicos, o para separar partículas coloidales suspendidas en un líquido.

cerebrospinal fluid The fluid within the subarachnoid space, the central canal of the spinal cord, and the four ventricles of the brain.
fluido cerebroespinal Fluido del interior del espacio subaracnoideo, el canal central de la médula espinal y los cuatro ventrículos del cerebro.

certification Attested as being true as represented or as meeting a standard; to have been tested, usually by a third party, and awarded a certificate based on proven knowledge.
certificación Atestiguar que algo es verdadero en cuanto a lo que representa, o al cumplimiento de un estándar; que ha sido examinado, por lo general por una tercera parte, y que se le ha concedido un certificado basándose en el conocimiento del que ha dado prueba.

cerumen A waxy secretion in the ear canal, commonly called *ear wax*.
cerumen Secreción cerosa del canal del oído, comúnmente se conoce como *cera de los oídos*.

cervical Referring to the region of the neck that contains the seven cervical vertebrae.
cervical Región del cuello en la que hay siete vértebras cervicales.

chain of command A series of executive positions in order of authority.
cadena de mando Serie de puestos ejecutivos en orden de autoridad.

channels A means of communication or expression; a way, course, or direction of thought.
canales Medios de comunicación o de expresión; vía, curso o dirección del pensamiento.

characteristic A distinguishing trait, quality, or property.
característica Rasgo, cualidad o propiedad distintiva.

Copyright © 2011, 2007, 2003 by Saunders, an imprint of Elsevier Inc. All rights reserved.

chief complaint The reason for seeking medical care.
problema principal Razón por la cual un paciente solicita atención médica.

chiropractic A medical discipline; the chiropractic physician focuses on the nervous system and manually and painlessly adjusts the vertebral column to affect the nervous system, resulting in healthier patients.
quiropráctica Disciplina médica en la que los médicos quiroprácticos se centran en el sistema nervioso y ajustan la columna vertebral manualmente y sin dolor, para lograr un efecto sobre el sistema nervioso, dando como resultado pacientes más sanos.

cholesterol A substance produced by the liver and also found in plant and animal fats that can cause fatty deposits or atherosclerotic plaques in the blood vessels.
colesterol Ustancia que produce el hígado y que se halla en las grasas animales y vegetales, y que puede producir depósitos grasos o placas ateroscleróticas en los vasos sanguíneos.

chronic Persisting for a prolonged period.
crónico Que persiste por largo tiempo.

chronic bronchitis Recurrent inflammation of the membranes lining the bronchial tubes.
bronquitis crónica Inflamación recurrente de-las membranas que recubren los tubos bronquiales.

chronologic order Of, relating to, or arranged in or according to the order of time.
orden cronológico Perteneciente o relativo al orden en el tiempo; organizado según el orden en el tiempo.

circumvent To manage to avoid something, especially by ingenuity or stratagem.
circunvenir Lograr evitar algo usando ingeniosidad o estratagemas.

cite To quote by way of example, authority, or proof, or to mention formally in commendation or praise.
cita Que se nombra para servir de ejemplo, autoridad o prueba o para hacer una mención formal como recomendación o alabanza.

claims clearinghouse A centralized facility (sometimes called a *third-party administrator,* or TPA) to which insurance claims are transmitted; the clearinghouse checks and redistributes claims electronically to various insurance carriers.
centro de reclamaciones Establecimiento centralizado (algunas veces conocido como *administrador mediador* o TPA) al cual se transmiten las reclamaciones de seguros y que se encarga de verificar y redistribuir las reclamaciones electrónicamente a varias compañías de seguros.

clarity The quality or state of being clear.
claridad Calidad o estado de claro.

clause A group of words containing a subject and a predicate that functions as part of a complex or compound sentence.
cláusulas Conjunto de palabras que incluye un sujeto y un predicado y que funciona como miembro de una oración compuesta.

clean claim An insurance claim form that has been completed correctly (with no errors or omissions) and can be processed and paid promptly.
reclamación limpia Formulario de reclamación de seguro que ha sido llenado correctamente (sin errores ni omisiones) y que puede procesarse y pagarse prontamente.

clearinghouses Networks of banks that exchange checks with one another.
sistema de compensación Redes bancarias que intercambian cheques entres sí.

clinical trials Research studies that test how well new medical treatments or other interventions work in the subjects, usually human beings.
ensayos clínicos Estudio de investigación que prueba cómo actúan los nuevos tratamientos médicos u otras intervenciones en los sujetos, normalmente en los seres humanos.

clitoris The small, elongated, erectile body situated above the urinary meatus at the superior point of the labia minora.
clítoris Órgano eréctil pequeño y alargado situado sobre el meato urinario a la altura de los labios menores.

clubbing Abnormal enlargement of the distal phalanges (fingers and toes) that is associated with cyanotic heart disease or advanced chronic pulmonary disease.
hipocratismo digital (dedos en palillo de tambor) Engrosamiento anómalo de las falanges distales (en los dedos de las manos y de los pies), relacionado con una enfermedad cardiaca cianótica o una enfermedad pulmonar crónica avanzada.

coagulate To form into clots.
coagular Formar coágulos.

"code also" In ICD-9-CM coding, when more than one code is necessary to identify a given condition fully, "code also" or "use additional code" is used.
"código adicional" Cuando se necesita más de un código para identificar por completo una afección (enfermedad) determinado, se usa "código adicional" o "usar código adicional."

Code of Federal Regulations (CFR) The Code of Federal Regulations (CFR) is a coded delineation of the rules and regulations published in the *Federal Register* by the various departments and agencies of the federal

Copyright © 2011, 2007, 2003 by Saunders, an imprint of Elsevier Inc. All rights reserved.

government. The CFR is divided into 50 titles, which represent broad subject areas, and further into chapters, which provide specific detail.
Código de Regulaciones Federales (CFR) El Código de Regulaciones Federales (CFR) es un resumen codificado de las normas y regulaciones publicadas en el Registro Federal por los diferentes departamentos y agencias del gobierno federal. El CFR se divide en 50 Títulos que representan amplias áreas temáticas, los cuales, a su vez, se subdividen en capítulos que proporcionan detalles específicos.

cognitive Pertaining to the operation of the mind; the process by which a person becomes aware of perceiving, thinking, and remembering.
cognitivo Perteneciente o relativo a la operación del proceso mental por el cual nos damos cuenta de cómo, percibimos, pensamos y recordamos.

cohesive Sticking together tightly; exhibiting or producing cohesion.
cohesivo El estado de estar estrechamente unidos; mostrar o producir cohesión.

coitus Sexual union between male and female; also known as *intercourse*.
coito Unión sexual entre un macho y una hembra.

collagen The protein that forms the inelastic fibers of tendons, ligaments, and fascia.
colágeno Proteína que forma las fibras no elásticas de los tendones, los ligamentos y la fascia.

collodion A preparation of cellulose nitrate that dries to a strong, thin, protective, transparent film when applied to the skin.
colodión Preparación de nitrato de celulosa que, cuando se aplica a la piel, se seca formando una película fina resistente, protectora y transparente.

colloidal Pertaining to a gluelike substance.
coloidal Perteneciente o relativo a una substancia parecida a la cola.

colostrum The thin, yellow, milky fluid secreted by the mammary glands a few days before and after delivery.
calostro Fluido lácteo poco espeso y amarillo que segregan las glándulas mamarias unos días antes y después del parto.

coma An unconscious state from which the patient cannot be aroused.
coma Estado inconsciente del cual el paciente no puede ser despertado.

comfort zone A mental state in which an individual feels safe and confident.
zona de bienestar Un lugar en la mente en el que un individuo se siente seguro y confiado.

commensurate Corresponding in size, amount, extent, or degree; equal in measure.
equiparable Que es equivalente en tamaño, cantidad o grado; de igual medida.

commercial insurance Plans (sometimes called *private insurance*) that reimburse the insured (or his or her dependents) for monetary losses resulting from illness or injury according to a specific schedule as outlined in the insurance policy and on a fee-for-service basis. Individuals insured under these plans normally are not limited to any one physician and usually can see the healthcare provider of their choice.
seguro comercial Planes (a veces llamados *seguros privados*) que reembolsan al asegurado (o a sus dependendientes) por pérdidas monetarias debidas a enfermedad o lesión siguiendo una escala específica que se explica en la póliza de seguro y cobrando un cargo por cada servicio. Los individuos asegurados bajo estos planes, por lo general, no están limitados a un solo médico y suelen poder acudir al proveedor del cuidado de la salud que elijan.

co-morbidities Pre-existing conditions that, because of their presence with a specific principal diagnosis, increase the length of stay in a healthcare facility by at least 1 day in approximately 75% of cases.
patologías coexistentes Enfermedades preexistentes que, debido a su presencia junto al diagnóstico principal, causan un aumento en la duración de la estadía de al menos un día en aproximadamente 75% de los casos.

competence The quality or state of being competent; having adequate or requisite capabilities.
competencia Capacidad o aptitud de quien es competente en algo; tener las capacidades necesarias o cumplir con los requisitos necesarios para hacer algo.

competent Having adequate abilities or qualities; having the capacity to function or perform in a certain way.
competente Que tiene ciertas capacidades o cualidades; que tiene la capacidad de funcionar o actuar de un modo determinado.

complications Conditions that arise during the hospital stay that prolong the length of stay by at least 1 day in approximately 75% of the cases.
complicaciones Condiciones que surgen durante la permanencia en el hospital que prolongan el tiempo de la estadía en al menos un día en aproximadamente 75% de los casos.

compression The state of being pressed together.
compresión Condición de estar apretado.

Copyright © 2011, 2007, 2003 by Saunders, an imprint of Elsevier Inc. All rights reserved.

computed tomography (CT) A computerized x-ray imaging modality that provides axial and three-dimensional scans.
tomografía asistida por computadora (TAC) Modalidad de formación computarizada de imágenes de rayos x que proporciona imágenes de escáner axiales y tridimensionales.

computer A machine designed to accept, store, process, and give out information.
computadora (u ordenador) Máquina diseñada para aceptar, almacenar, procesar y emitir información.

concise Expressing much in brief form.
conciso Que expresa mucho en forma breve.

concurrently Occurring at the same time.
concurrente Que ocurre al mismo tiempo.

cones Structures in the retina that make the perception of color possible.
conos Estructuras que se encuentran en la retina y que hacen posible la percepción del color.

congruence Consistency between the verbal expression of the message and the sender's nonverbal body language.
congruencia Expresión verbal del mensaje que corresponde al lenguaje corporal no verbal del emisor.

congruent Being in agreement, harmony, or correspondence; conforming to the circumstances or requirements of a situation.
congruente Que está en acuerdo, armonía o correspondencia; conforme a las circunstancias o requisitos de una situación.

connotation An implication; something suggested by a word or thing.
connotación Implicación; lo que sugiere una palabra o una cosa.

contaminate To make impure or unclean; to make unfit for use by the introduction of unwholesome or undesirable elements.
contaminación Volver impuro o sucio; hacer que algo sea inadecuado para el uso por la introducción de elementos insalubres o indeseables.

contaminated Soiled with pathogens or infectious material; nonsterile.
contaminado Manchado con materiales patógenos o infecciosos; no estéril.

contamination Becoming nonsterile through contact with any nonsterile material.
contaminación Pasar al estado de no estéril por contacto con cualquier material no estéril.

continuation pages The second and following pages of a letter.
paginas de continuación En una carta, la segunda página y las siguientes.

continuing education credits (CEUs) Credits for courses, classes, or seminars related to an individual's profession that are designed to promote education and to keep the professional up-to-date on current procedures and trends in the field; CEUs often are required to maintain licensure.
créditos de educación continua (CEU) Créditos por cursos, clases o seminarios relacionados con la profesión de un individuo y que tienen la finalidad de promocionar la educación y mantener al profesional al corriente de los procedimientos y tendencias actuales en su campo; con frecuencia son obligatorios para obtener una licencia.

continuity of care Care that continues smoothly from one provider to another so that care is not interrupted and the patient receives the most benefit.
continuidad de la atención Atención que continúa sin interrupciones de un proveedor a otro, de manera que el paciente recibe los máximos beneficios sin que haya una interrupción de la atención sanitaria.

contralateral Pertaining to the opposite side of the body.
colateral Perteneciente o relativo a la parte opuesta del cuerpo.

contrast media Substances used to enhance visualization of soft tissues in imaging studies.
medios de contraste Substancias usadas para mejorar la visualización de los tejidos blandos en estudios de formación de imágenes.

contributory negligence Statutes in some states that may prevent a party from recovering damages if the person contributed in any way to the injury or condition.
negligencia concurrente Estatutos existentes en algunos estados que impiden que una parte sea recompensada por daños si esta parte ha contribuido en algún modo a provocar la lesión o enfermedad.

cookies Messages sent to the hard drive from the Web server that identify users and allow preparation of custom Web pages for them, possibly displaying their name on return to the site.
cookies Mensaje que se envía al navegador de la red desde el servidor, el cual identifica a los usuarios y puede preparar páginas web especiales para ellos, posiblemente, mostrando su nombre la próxima vez que visiten el sitio.

coordination of benefits The mechanism used in group health insurance to designate the order in which multiple carriers are to pay benefits to prevent duplicate payments.

Copyright © 2011, 2007, 2003 by Saunders, an imprint of Elsevier Inc. All rights reserved.

coordinación de beneficios Mecanismo usado en seguros de enfermedad de grupo para designar el orden en el que varias compañías de seguros tienen que pagar los beneficios para evitar pagos dobles.

co-payment Also called *co-insurance;* a policy provision frequently found in medical insurance whereby the policyholder and the insurance company share the cost of covered losses in a specified ratio (e.g., 80/20: 80% by the insurer and 20% by the insured).
co-pago Un co-pago (o *co-seguro*) es una provisión frecuente de la póliza en los seguros médicos, por la que el titular de la póliza y la compañía aseguradora comparten el costo de las pérdidas cubiertas en una proporción determinada (ej.: 80/20: 80% por parte del asegurador y 20% por parte del asegurado).

COPD (chronic obstructive pulmonary disease) A progressive, irreversible lung condition that results in diminished lung capacity.
COPD (enfermedad pulmonar obstructiva crónica) Enfermedad pulmonar progresiva e irreversible que conlleva una reducción de la capacidad pulmonar.

copulation Sexual intercourse.
copulación Cópula sexual.

coronal plane The plane that divides the body into anterior and posterior parts.
plano coronal Plano que divide el cuerpo en una anterior y una posterior.

corticosteroids Natural or synthetic antiinflammatory hormones.
corticosteroides Hormonas antiinflamatorias, naturales o sintéticas.

costal Pertaining to the ribs.
costal Perteneciente o relativo a las costillas.

coulombs per kilogram (C/kg) The international unit of radiation exposure.
culombios por kilogramo (C/kg) Unidad internacional de exposición a la radiación.

counteroffer A return offer made by one who has rejected an offer or a job.
contraoferta Oferta-respuesta hecha por quien ha rechazado una oferta o trabajo.

creatinine Nitrogenous waste from muscle metabolism that is excreted in the urine.
creatinina Residuo nitrogenado del metabolismo muscular que se excreta en la orina.

credentialing The act of extending professional or medical privileges to an individual; the process of verifying and evaluating that person's credentials.
concesión de credenciales Acción de conceder privilegios profesionales o médicos a un individuo; proceso de verificar y evaluar los credenciales de esa persona.

credibility The quality or power of inspiring belief.
credibilidad Calidad de creíble; facilidad para ser creído.

credit An entry on an account constituting an addition to a revenue, net worth, or liability account; the balance in a person's favor in an account.
crédito Dato que se entra en una cuenta y que constituye una adición a los ingresos, ganancia neta o cuenta de pasivo; saldo a favor de una persona en una cuenta.

crenate Forming notches or leaflike, scalloped edges on an object.
crenar Formar muescas o bordes en forma de concha o de hoja en un objeto.

crepitation A dry, crackling sound or sensation.
crepitación Sonido o sensación seca y crujiente.

critical thinking The constant practice of considering all aspects of a situation when deciding what to believe or what to do.
razonamiento crítico Práctica constante de considerar todos los aspectos de una situación al decidir qué creer o qué hacer.

cross-training Training in more than one area so that a multitude of duties may be performed by one person or so that substitutions of personnel may be made when necessary or in emergencies.
entrenamiento cruzado Entrenamiento en más de un área, de modo que una persona pueda desempeñar varias labores o que se puedan realizar sustituciones de personal cuando sea necesario o en caso de emergencia.

cryosurgery The technique of exposing tissue to extreme cold to produce a well-defined area of cell destruction.
criocirugía Técnica que consiste en exponer los tejidos a un frío extremo para producir una destrucción de células en un área bien definida.

cryptogenic Hidden origin.
criptogénico De origen oculto.

cultivate To foster the growth of; to improve by labor, care, or study.
cultivar Promover el desarrollo; mejorar algo por medio de trabajo, cuidado o estudio.

curettage The act of scraping a body cavity with a surgical instrument, such as a curette.

Copyright © 2011, 2007, 2003 by Saunders, an imprint of Elsevier Inc. All rights reserved.

curetaje Acción de raspar una cavidad corporal con un instrumento quirúrgico, como una cureta o cucharilla cortante.

cursor A symbol that appears on the computer monitor to show where the next character to be typed will appear.
cursor Símbolo que aparece en el monitor y que muestra el lugar donde aparecerá el próximo carácter que se escriba.

curt Marked by rude or peremptory shortness.
cortante Caracterizado por una interrupción ruda o perentoria.

cyanosis A blue discoloration of the mucous membranes and body extremities caused by lack of oxygen.
cianosis Color azul de las membranas mucosas y las extremidades provocado por una falta de oxígeno.

cyberspace The nonphysical space of the online world of computer networks.
ciberespacio Palabra que se usa para describir el espacio no-físico del mundo en linea de las redes informáticas.

cyst A small, capsulelike sac that encloses certain organisms in their dormant or larval stage.
quiste Pequeño saco en forma de cápsula que encierra ciertos organismos en estado letárgico o larval.

damages Loss or harm resulting from injury to person, property, or reputation; monetary compensation imposed by law for losses or injuries.
daños Pérdidas o perjuicios que resultan de injuriar a una persona, atentar contra una propiedad o una reputación; compensación monetaria impuesta por ley en casos de pérdidas o injurias.

database A collection of related files that serves as a foundation for retrieving information.
base de datos Conjunto de archivos relacionados que sirven de base para la recuperación de información.

debit An entry on an account constituting an addition to an expense or asset balance or a deduction from a revenue, net worth, or liability balance.
débito Dato que se entra en una cuenta y que constituye una adición a los gastos o a una cuenta de activo o una deducción de un ingreso, ganancia neta o cuenta de pasivo.

debit card A card similar to a credit card with which money may be withdrawn or the cost of purchases paid directly from the holder's bank account without the payment of interest.
tarjeta de débito Tarjeta similar a la de crédito pero con la cual se puede retirar dinero o pagar compras directamente de la cuenta bancaria del titular sin tener que pagar intereses.

debridement The removal of foreign material and dead, damaged tissue from a wound.
desbridamiento Eliminación de materiales extraños y tejidos muertos y deteriorados de una herida.

decedent A legal term used to represent a deceased person.
difunto Término legal usado para referirse a una persona muerta.

decode To convert, as in a message, into intelligible form; to recognize and interpret.
decodificar Convertir la información, como en un mensaje, de modo que sea inteligible; reconocer e interpretar.

decubitus ulcer A sore or ulcer over a bony prominence caused by ischemia from prolonged pressure; a bed sore.
úlcera por decúbito Llaga o úlcera sobre una prominencia ósea debida a una isquemia por presión prolongada; escara.

deductible A specific amount of money a patient must pay out of pocket, up front, before the insurance carrier begins paying. Often this amount ranges from $100 to $1,000. The deductible amount must be met on a yearly or per incident basis.
deducible Cantidad de dinero específica que un paciente debe pagar de su bolsillo antes de que la compañía de seguros comience a pagar. Con frecuencia esta suma está entre 100 y 1000 dólares. Esta cantidad deducible ha de satisfacerse—anualmente o por caso.

default To fail to pay financial debts, especially a student loan.
incumplimiento Dejar de pagar deudas financieras, especialmente en un préstamo de estudiante.

defense mechanisms Psychological methods of dealing with stressful situations that are encountered in day-to-day living.
mecanismos de defensa Métodos psicológicos de hacer frente a situaciones tensas que surgen en la vida diaria.

deferment A postponement, especially of payment of a student loan.
aplazamiento Postergación de un pago, especialmente en un préstamo de estudiante.

defibrillator A machine used to deliver an electrical shock to the heart through electrodes placed on the chest wall.

Copyright © 2011, 2007, 2003 by Saunders, an imprint of Elsevier Inc. All rights reserved.

desfibrilador Máquina usada para dar un electrochoque al corazón por medio de electrodos colocados en la pared torácica.

deficiencies Conditions caused by a below-normal intake of a particular substance.
deficiencias Estados causados por un consumo menor del normal de una sustancia específica.

demeanor Behavior toward others; outward manner.
conducta Comportamiento hacia los demás; comportamiento que se exterioriza.

demographic The statistical characteristics of human populations (as in age or income), used especially to identify markets.
dato demográfico Característica estadística de la población humana (como edad o ingresos), que se usa sobre todo para identificar mercados.

detrimental Harmful or damaging.
perjudicial Que es obvio que causa daño o perjuicio.

device driver A computer program or set of commands that enables a device connected to the computer to function. For instance, a printer may come equipped with software that must be loaded onto the computer first so that the printer will work.
controlador de dispositivo Programa que controla un dispositivo conectado a una computadora y que hace que dicho dispositivo pueda funcionar. Por ejemplo, una impresora puede estar equipada con un programa que primero ha de cargarse en la computadora para que ésta funcione.

diabetes mellitus type 2 A condition in which the body is unable to use glucose for energy because of a lack of insulin production in the pancreas or because of resistance to insulin on the cellular level.
diabetes mellitus tipo 2 Incapacidad de utilizar la glucosa para producir energía, debido a una falta de producción de insulina en el páncreas o a una resistencia a la insulina en el nivel celular.

diagnose To determine the nature of a disease, injury, or congenital defect.
diagnóstico Determinación del origen de una enfermedad, lesión o defecto congénito.

diagnosis The concise technical description of the cause, nature, or manifestations of a condition or problem. *Initial diagnosis:* The physician's temporary impression, sometimes called a *working diagnosis. Differential diagnosis:* A comparison of two or more diseases with similar signs and symptoms. *Final diagnosis:* The conclusion reached by the physician after evaluating all findings, including laboratory and other test results.
diagnóstico Descripción técnica y concisa de la causa, naturaleza o manifestaciones de una enfermedad o problema. *Inicial:* Impresión momentánea del médico, a veces se llama diagnóstico de trabajo.
Diagnóstico diferenciado: comparación de dos o más enfermedades con signos y síntomas similares. *Final:* Conclusión médica a la que se llega tras evaluar todos los datos, incluyendo los resultados de análisis de laboratorio y otras pruebas.

diaphoresis The profuse excretion of sweat.
diaforesis Excreción profusa de sudor.

diaphysis The middle portion of a long bone, which contains the medullary cavity.
diafisis Parte intermedia de un hueso largo en la que está la cavidad medular.

dictation The act or manner of uttering words to be transcribed.
dictado Acción de pronunciar palabras para que sean transcritas.

diction The choice of words, especially with regard to clearness, correctness, and effectiveness.
dicción Acción de elegir las palabras, especialmente para lograr claridad, corrección y eficacia en el discurso.

digestion The process of converting food into chemical substances that can be used by the body.
digestión Proceso de transformar alimentos en sustancias químicas que pueden ser usadas por el cuerpo.

Digital Subscriber Lines (DSL) High-speed, sophisticated modulation schemes that operate over existing copper telephone wiring systems; often referred to as "last mile technologies" because DSL is used for connections from a telephone switching station to a home or office and not between switching stations.
Línea de Abonado Digital (DSL) Sofisticado sistema de modulación de alta velocidad que opera en sistemas de cableado telefónicos de cobre ya existentes; con frecuencia se habla del DSL como "tecnología de las últimas millas" porque se utiliza para conexiones entre un centro de conmutación telefónica y un hogar u oficina, y no entre centros de conmutación.

Digital Versatile Disk (DVD) An optical disk that holds approximately 28 times more information than a CD and is most commonly used to hold full-length movies. A CD holds approximately 600 megabytes, whereas a DVD can hold approximately 4.7 gigabytes.
Disco Digital Versátil (DVD) El DVD es un disco óptico con capacidad para almacenar unas 28 veces más información que un CD; su uso más común es para guardar películas de larga duración. Mientras que un CD puede almacenar unos 600 megabytes, un DVD tiene una capacidad aproximada de almacenamiento de 4.7 gigabytes.

Copyright © 2011, 2007, 2003 by Saunders, an imprint of Elsevier Inc. All rights reserved.

dilation (1) Opening or widening the circumference of a body orifice with a dilating instrument. (2) The opening of the cervix through the process of labor, measured as 0 to 10 centimeters dilated.
dilatación (1) Proceso de abrir o ensanchar un orificio corporal con un instrumento dilatador. (2) Ensanchamiento del cuello del útero durante el proceso del parto, se mide en centímetros, de 0 a 10.

dilation and curettage (D&C) The procedure in which the cervix is widened and the endometrial wall of the uterus is scraped.
dilatación y curetaje (D&C) Proceso de hacer más ancho el cuello del útero y raspar su pared endometrial.

diluent A liquid used to dilute a specimen or reagent.
diluyente Líquido usado para diluir un espécimen o un reactivo.

dingy claim A claim that is put on hold because it lacks certain adjunction that allows it to be processed, often because of system changes.
reclamación oscura Reclamación en espera de ser procesada debido a que se necesita alguna información o elemento adicional, con frecuencia, debido a cambios en el sistema.

diplopia Double vision.
diplopía Visión doble.

direct filing system A filing system in which materials can be located without consulting an intermediary source of reference.
sistema directo de archivo Sistema de archivo en el cual los materiales pueden ser localizados sin consultar una fuente de referencia intermedia.

dirty claim Claims that contain errors or omissions and that cannot be processed or must be processed by hand because of OCR scanner rejection.
reclamación sucia Reclamación con errores u omisiones que no puede procesarse o que debe procesarse manualmente debido a que el escáner OCR la rechaza.

disbursements Funds paid out.
desembolsos Dinero o fondos que se pagan.

discretion The quality of being discrete; having or showing good judgment or conduct, especially in speech.
discreción Calidad de discreto; tener sensatez o tacto al obrar, especialmente al hablar.

disease A pathologic process having a descriptive set of signs and symptoms.
enfermedad Proceso patológico que tiene una serie descriptiva de signos y síntomas.

disinfection The destruction of pathogens by physical or chemical means.
desinfección Destrucción de agentes patógenos con medios físicos o químicos.

disk A magnetic surface capable of storing computer programs.
disco Superficie magnética capaz de almacenar programas de computadora.

disk drives Devices that load a program or data stored on a disk into the computer.
unidades de discos Dispositivos que cargan en la computadora un programa o datos almacenados en un disco.

disorder Disruption of normal system functions.
trastorno Interrupción de las funciones normales de un sistema.

disparaging Speaking slightingly about something or someone, with a negative or degrading tone.
menospreciar Hablar con desdén de algo o alguien, con un tono negativo o degradante.

disposition The tendency of something or someone to act in a certain manner under given circumstances.
disposición Tendencia de algo o alguien a actuar de un modo específico en determinadas circunstancias.

disruption A breaking down, or throwing into disorder.
disrupción Interrupción o creación de un estado de trastorno.

dissect To cut or separate tissue with a cutting instrument or scissors.
diseccionar Cortar o separar tejidos con tijeras u otro instrumento cortante.

dissection The cutting or separating of a specimen into pieces and exposing the parts for scientific examination.
disección Separar en piezas y dejar las partes a la vista para realizar un estudio científico.

disseminate To disperse throughout.
diseminar Dispersar, esparcir.

disseminate To disburse; to spread around.
diseminado Suelto, esparcido.

diurnal rhythm Patterns of activity or behavior that follow day-night cycles.
ritmo diurno Patrones de actividad o comportamiento que siguen a los ciclos nocturnos.

Copyright © 2011, 2007, 2003 by Saunders, an imprint of Elsevier Inc. All rights reserved.

docket A formal record of judicial proceedings; a list of legal causes to be tried.
orden del día Registro formal de procesos judiciales; lista de causas legales a juzgar.

domestic mail Mail sent within the boundaries of the United States and its territories.
correo nacional Correo que se envía dentro de los límites de Estados Unidos y sus territorios.

dosimeter A badge for monitoring the exposure of personnel to radiation.
dosímetro Placa para controlar la exposición a la radiación del personal.

drawee The bank or facility on which a check is drawn or written.
librado Banco o entidad contra la que se gira o emite un cheque.

due process A fundamental, constitutional guarantee that all legal proceedings will be fair and that one will be given notice of the proceedings and an opportunity to be heard before the government acts to take away life, liberty, or property; a constitutional guarantee that a law will not be unreasonable or arbitrary.
proceso debido Garantía fundamental constitucional de que todos los procesos legales serán justos, que las partes implicadas serán notificadas de los procedimientos y que se les dará la oportunidad de ser escuchados rantes que el gobierno les quite su vida, libertad o propiedad; garantía constitucional de que la ley no irá en contra de la razón ni será arbitraria.

duty Obligatory tasks, conduct, service, or functions that arise from one's position, as in life or in a group.
deber Tareas, conducta, servicio o funciones de carácter obligatorio que conlleva el ocupar un puesto, en la vida o como miembro de un grupo.

dyspnea Difficult or painful breathing.
disnea Respiración difícil o dolorosa.

e-banking Electronic banking via computer modem or over the Internet.
banca electrónica Operaciones bancarias a través del módem de una computadora o en Internet.

ecchymosis A hemorrhagic skin discoloration, commonly called *bruising*.
equimosis Descoloramient o hemorrágico de la piel comúnmente conocido como *magulladura*.

e-commerce A term used to describe the sale and purchase of goods and services over the Internet; doing business over the Internet; an abbreviation for *electronic commerce*.
comercio electrónico Expresión que se usa para describir la compra y venta de bienes y servicios a través de Internet; hacer negocios a través de Internet. Se conoce también con la abreviatura de *comercio-e*.

edema An abnormal accumulation of fluid in the interstitial spaces of tissue; swelling between layers of tissue.

edema Acumulación anómala de fluido en los espacios intersticiales de los tejidos; inflamación entre capas de tejidos.

effacement The thinning of the cervix during labor, measured in percentages from 0% to 100% effaced.
borramiento Adelgazamiento del cuello del útero durante el parto. Se mide en porcentaje, borrado de 0 a 100 por ciento.

elastic pulse A pulse with regular alterations of weak and strong beats, without changes in cycle.
pulso elástico Pulso con alteraciones regulares de latidos fuertes y débiles sin cambios en el ciclo.

elastin An essential part of elastic connective tissue that is flexible and elastic when moist.
elastina Parte esencial del tejido conectivo elástico que cuando está húmedo es flexible y elástico.

electrodesiccation Destructive drying of cells and tissue by means of short, high-frequency electrical sparks.
electrodesecación Secado destructivo de células y tejidos por medio de cortas descargas eléctricas de alta frecuencia.

electrolytes Small molecules that conduct an electrical charge. Electrolytes are necessary for proper functioning of muscle and nerve cells.
electrolitos Pequeñas moléculas que conducen una carga eléctrica. Los electrolitos son necesarios para un funcionamiento correcto de los músculos y las células nerviosas.

electronic claims Claims submitted to insurance processing facilities using a computerized medium, such as direct data entry, direct wire, dial-in telephone digital fax, or personal computer download and upload.
reclamación electrónica Reclamaciones enviadas al lugar de procesamiento de la compañía aseguradora usando un sistema computarizado, tales como entrada de datos directa, cable directo, fax digital con marcado telefónico, o a través de una computadora personal.

e-mail Communications transmitted via computer using a modem.

Copyright © 2011, 2007, 2003 by Saunders, an imprint of Elsevier Inc. All rights reserved.

correo electrónico Comunicaciones transmitidas a través de una computadora usando un módem.

emancipated minor A person under legal age who is self-supporting and living apart from parents or a guardian.
menor emancipado Persona que no ha alcanzado la mayoría de edad legal y que se mantiene a sí misma y vive sin la custodia de padres o tutores.

embezzlement Stealing from an employer; appropriation without permission of goods, services, or funds for personal use.
desfalco Robo a un empleador; apropiación sin permiso de bienes, servicios o fondos para uso personal.

embolization An interventional technique in which a catheter is used to block off a blood vessel, thereby preventing hemorrhage.
embolización Técnica de intervención usando un catéter para bloquear un vaso sanguíneo y evitar una hemorragia.

embolus Foreign material that blocks a blood vessel, frequently a blood clot that has broken away from some other part of the body.
émbolo Material extraño que bloquea un vaso sanguíneo, con frecuencia un coágulo de sangre procedente de otra parte del cuerpo.

emetic A substance that causes vomiting.
emético Sustancia que causa vómito.

emisor The person who writes a check.
emisor Persona que emite un cheque.

empathy Sensitivity to the individual needs and reactions of patients.
empatía Sensibilidad ante las necesidades y reacciones individuales de los pacientes.

emphysema The pathologic accumulation of air in the tissues or organs; in the lungs, the bronchioles become plugged with mucus and lose elasticity.
enfisema Acumulación patológica de aire en los tejidos u órganos; en los pulmones, los bronquiolos se obstruyen con mucosidade y pierden elasticidad.

emulsification Dispersion of ingested fats into small globules by bile.
emulsionamiento Dispersión (llevada a cabo por la bilis) en pequeños glóbulos de las grasas ingeridas.

encode To convert from one system of communication to another; to convert a message into code.
codificar Convertir de un sistema de comunicación a otro; convertir un mensaje en un código.

encounter Any contact between a healthcare provider and a patient that results in treatment or evaluation of the patient's condition; not limited to in-person contact.
encuentro Cualquier contacto entre un proveedor de atención sanitaria y un paciente que resulta en un tratamiento o evaluación del estado del paciente; no se limita a un contacto personal.

encroachment To advance beyond the usual or proper limits.
intrusiones Ir más allá de los límites habituales o apropiados.

endemic A disease or microorganism that is specific to a particular geographic area.
endémico Enfermedad o microorganismo que-es específico de una zona geográfica en particular.

endocervical curettage The scraping of cells from the wall of the uterus.
curetaje endocervical Raspado de células de la pared uterina.

endorser The person who signs his or her name on the back of a check for the purpose of transferring title to another person.
endosante Persona que firma en la parte posterior de un cheque a fin de transferir la propiedad del mismo a otra persona.

enteric coated A term referring to a special compound used to coat some oral medications; the coating resists the effects of stomach juices and does not dissolve, releasing the medication, until the tablet is exposed to the fluids of the small intestine.
cubierta entérica Capa exterior que se añade a un medicamento que se toma por vía oral, la cual es resistente a los efectos de los jugos gástricos; recubrimiento diseñado para que la medicina sea absorbida en el intestino delgado; formulación usada en medicinas en la cual las tabletas se recubren con un componente especial que no se disuelve hasta que la tableta es expuesta a los fluidos del intestino delgado.

enunciate To utter articulate sounds; to be very distinct in speech.
articular Pronunciar los sonidos de manera cuidada; hablar de una forma muy clara.

enunciation The utterance of articulate, clear sounds; the act of being very distinct in speech.
articulación Pronunciación cuidada, con sonidos claros.

Copyright © 2011, 2007, 2003 by Saunders, an imprint of Elsevier Inc. All rights reserved.

enzymatic reaction A chemical reaction controlled by an enzyme.
reacción enzimática Reacción química controlada por una enzima.

enzyme Any of several complex proteins that are produced by cells and that act as catalysts in specific biochemical reactions.
enzima Cualquiera de las varias proteínas complejas que producen las células y que actúan como catalíticos en reacciones bioquímicas específicas.

epiphysis The end of a long bone.
epífisis Extremo de un hueso largo.

erythropoietin A substance released from the kidney and the liver that promotes red blood cell formation.
eritropoyetina Sustancia liberada por los riñones y el hígado y que promueve la formación de glóbulos rojos.

essential hypertension Elevated blood pressure of unknown cause that develops for no apparent reason; sometimes called *primary hypertension*.
hipertensión esencial Presión sanguínea alta de causa desconocida que surge sin razón aparente; a veces se llama *hipertensión primaria*.

established patients Patients who are returning to the office and who have previously seen the physician.
pacientes establecidos Pacientes que regresan al consultorio médico que ya han sido atendidos por el médico con anterioridad.

etiology The cause of a disorder, as determined for the purpose of classifying a claim.
etiología Clasificación de una reclamación según la causa del trastorno.

eukaryote A single-cell or multicellular organism in which the cell or cells have a distinct, membrane-bound nucleus.
eucariote Organismo unicelular o multicelular cuyas células tienen un núcleo diferenciado rodeado por una membrana.

euthanasia The act or practice of killing or permitting the death of hopelessly sick or injured individuals in a relatively painless way for reasons of mercy.
eutanasia Acción o práctica de matar o permitir la muerte de enfermos o heridos en estado terminal, de una forma relativamente sin dolor, por razones de piedad.

exacerbation An increase in the seriousness of a disease marked by greater intensity of the signs and symptoms; worsening of disease symptoms.
exacerbación Aumento en la gravedad de una enfermedad, caracterizado por una mayor intensidad de los signos y síntomas. Empeoramiento de los síntomas de una enfermedad.

"excludes" In insurance claims, exclusion terms are always written in italics, and the word "Excludes" is enclosed in a box to draw particular attention to these instructions. Exclusion terms may apply to a chapter, a section, a category, or a subcategory. The applicable code number usually follows the exclusion term.
"excluye" Las expresiones de exclusión siempre se escriben en cursiva y la palabra "Excluye" se encierra en una casilla para llamar la atención acerca de estas instrucciones. Los términos de exclusión pueden ser aplicables a un capítulo, una sección, una categoría o una subcategoría. El número de código correspondiente por lo general sigue al término de exclusión.

expediency Haste or caution; a means of achieving a particular end.
prontitud Situación que requiere actuar con prisa o precaución; un medio de alcanzar un fin específico.

expert witness A person who provides testimony to a court as an expert in a certain field or subject to verify facts presented by one or both sides in a lawsuit. An expert witness often is compensated and is used to refute or disprove the claims of one party.
testigo perito Persona que da testimonio ante un tribunal como perito o experto en cierto campo o tema para verificar los hechos presentados por una o ambas partes en litigio, a menudo, cobrando una retribución económica, y cu yo testimonio suele usarse para refutar o impugnar las demandas de una de las partes.

external noise Noise outside the brain that interferes with the communication process.
ruido externo Ruido producido fuera del cerebro y que interfiere con el proceso de comunicación.

externalization Attribution of an event or occurrence to causes outside oneself.
exteriorización Acción de atribuir a un suceso o acontecimiento causas externas al mismo.

externship/internship A training program that is part of the course of study of an educational institution and that is taken in the actual business setting in that field of study; the two terms often are used interchangeably with regard to medical assisting.
prácticas internas/externas Programa de entrenamiento que es parte de un curso de estudio de una institución educativa y se sigue en un lugar real de trabajo en el campo de estudio; estos términos se intercambian cuando se refieren a los asistentes médicos.

exudates Fluids with a high concentration of protein and cellular debris that has escaped from the blood vessels and has been deposited in tissues or on tissue surfaces.
exudados Fluidos con una alta concentración de proteínas y restos celulares extravasados de los vasos

Copyright © 2011, 2007, 2003 by Saunders, an imprint of Elsevier Inc. All rights reserved.

sanguíneos y depositados en los tejidos o en sus superficies.

familial Occurring in or affecting members of a family more than would be expected to occur by chance.
familiar Que sucede o afecta a miembros de una familia más de lo que podría esperarse por azar.

fascia A sheet or band of fibrous tissue located deep in the skin that covers muscles and body organs.
fascia Lámina o banda de tejido fibroso localizada bajo la piel y que cubre los músculos y los órganos.

fastidious With regard to laboratory cultures, an organism that requires specialized media or growth factors to grow.
exigente Que requiere un medio o factores especiales para crecer.

fat A substance stored as adipose tissue in the body that serves as a concentrated energy reserve.
grasa Sustancia que se almacena como tejido adiposo en el cuerpo y sirve como reserva de energía concentrada.

fax The abbreviation for the term *facsimile;* a document sent using a fax machine.
fax Abreviatura de facsímile; documento que se envía usando una máquina de fax.

febrile Pertaining to an elevated body temperature.
febril Perteneciente o relativo a una temperatura corporal elevada.

fecalith A hard, impacted mass of feces in the colon.
fecaloma Masa de heces endurecidas e impactadas en el colon.

fee profile A compilation or average of physicians' fees over a given period.
perfil de cargos Recopilación o porcentaje de cargos médicos en un periodo de tiempo dado.

fee schedule A compilation of pre-established fee allowances for given services or procedures.
escala de cargos Recopilación de asignaciones de cargos preestablecidos para servicios o procedimientos dados.

feedback The transmission of evaluative or corrective information about an action, event, or process to the original or controlling source.
reacciones y comentarios Envío de información de evaluación o corrección a la fuente original o a la que ejerce el control sobre una acción, suceso o proceso.

felony A major crime, such as murder, rape, or burglary, that is punishable by a more stringent sentence than that given for a misdemeanor, or lesser crime.
crimen Delito mayor, como asesinato, violación o robo; se penaliza con una sentencia más severa que un delito menor o falta.

fermentation An enzymatically controlled transformation of an organic compound.
fermentación Transformación de un compuesto orgánico controlada por enzimas.

fervent Exhibiting or marked by great intensity of feeling.
ferviente Que posee sentimientos de gran intensidad o que da muestra de ellos.

fibrillation Rapid, random, ineffective contractions of the heart.
fibrilación Contracciones cardiacas rápidas, aleatorias e inefectivas.

fidelity Faithfulness to something to which one is bound by pledge or duty.
fidelidad Fe en algo a lo que se está unido por juramento o deber.

filtrate The fluid that remains after a liquid is passed through a membranous filter.
filtrado Fluido que queda después de pasar un líquido a través de un filtro membranoso.

fine A sum imposed as punishment for an offense; a forfeiture or penalty paid to an injured party or the government in a civil or criminal action.
multa Suma impuesta como penalización por un delito menor; suma que se paga a una parte a la que se ha perjudicado o dañado, o al gobierno, en un proceso civil o penal.

fiscal agent An organization or private plan under contract to the government to act as a financial representative in handling insurance claims from providers of health care; also referred to as a *fiscal intermediary*.
agente fiscal Organización o plan privado bajo contrato con el gobierno para actuar como representantes financieros en la administración de reclamaciones de seguros por parte de proveedores de atención sanitaria; también se conoce como *intermediario fiscal*.

fiscal intermediary An organization that contracts with the government and other insuring entities to handle and mediate insurance claims from medical facilities.
intermediario fiscal Organización que establece un contrato con el gobierno y otras entidades aseguradoras para administrar reclamaciones de seguro provenientes de centros médicos y para mediar en ellas.

fissures Narrow slits or clefts in the abdominal wall.

Copyright © 2011, 2007, 2003 by Saunders, an imprint of Elsevier Inc. All rights reserved.

fisuras Grietas o hendiduras estrechas en la pared abdominal.

fistulas Abnormal, tubelike passages within the body tissue, usually between two internal organs or from an internal organ to the body surface.
fístulas Pasajes anómalos en forma de tubos entre los tejidos corporales, por lo general entre dos órganos internos, o de un órgano interno a la superficie del cuerpo.

flagged Marked in some way to serve as a reminder that specific action needs to be taken.
señalado Marcado de alguna forma para recordar que se necesita que se tomen medidas al respeto.

Flash Animation technology often used on the opening page of a Web site to draw the attention of, excite, and impress the user.
Flash Tecnología de imágenes animadas que se usa con frecuencia en la página inicial de un sitio web para llamar la atención del usuario, entusiasmarlo e impresionarlo.

flatus Gas expelled through the anus.
flato Gas expulsado a través del ano.

fluoroscopy Direct observation of an x-ray image in motion.
fluoroscopía Observación directa de una imagen de rayos x en movimiento.

flush Directly abutting or immediately adjacent to, such as set even with the edge of a page or column; having no indention.
alineado Directamente contiguo o inmediatamente adyacente, ordenado de forma regular en relación con un borde de una página o columna; sin sangría o espacios en blanco.

follicle-stimulating hormone (FSH) A hormone secreted by the anterior pituitary that stimulates oogenesis and spermatogenesis.
hormona foliculoestimulante (FSH) Hormona que segrega la pituitaria anterior y que estimula los procesos de formación y desarrollo de óvulos y de espermatozoides.

font A design, as in typesetting, for a set of characters.
fuente tipográfica Diseño similar al de la composición para un conjunto de caracteres.

format To magnetically create tracks on a disk in which information will be stored; formatting usually is done by the manufacturer of the disk.
formatear Crear pistas magnéticas en un disco destinado a almacenar información; por lo general, el fabricante del disco es quien se encarga de hacerlo.

fovea centralis A small pit in the center of the retina that is considered the center of clearest vision.
fóvea central Pequeña concavidad en el centro de la retina que se cree que es el centro de visión más claro.

frontal projection The radiographic view in which the coronal plane of the body or body part is parallel to the film plane; AP or PA.
proyección frontal Vista radiográfica en la cual el plano coronal del cuerpo o de la parte del cuerpo está paralelo al plano de la película; AP o PA.

gait The manner or style of walking.
andares Forma o estilo de caminar.

gamete A mature male or female germ cell, which usually has a haploid chromosome set and can initiate the formation of a new diploid individual.
gameto Célula germinal madura, tanto masculina como femenina, que por lo general tiene un conjunto cromosómico haploide y es capaz de iniciar la formación de un nuevo individuo diploide.

gangrene The death of body tissue, as a result of the loss of nutritive supply, and subsequent bacterial invasion and putrefaction.
gangrena Muerte de tejido corporal debido a la pérdida de suministro de nutrientes por invasión bacteriana y putrefacción.

gantry The doughnut-shaped portion of a scanner than surrounds the patient and functions at least in part to gather imaging data.
gantry Parte de un escáner con forma de rosquilla que rodea al paciente y funciona, al menos en parte, reuniendo datos de formación de imágenes.

generic Not protected by trademark.
genéricas Medicinas que no están protegidas por una marca registrada.

genome The genetic material of an organism.
genoma El material genético de un organismo.

genuineness Expressing sincerity and honest feeling.
autenticidad Expresión de sentimientos sincera y honrada.

germicides Agents that destroy pathogenic organisms.
germicidas Agentes químicos que destruyen o matan organismos patógenos.

gigabyte Approximately 1 billion bytes.
gigabyte Aproximadamente, mil millones de bytes.

girth A measure around a body or item.
contorno Medida alrededor de un cuerpo o artículo.

glean To gather information or material bit by bit; to pick over in search of relevant material.

Copyright © 2011, 2007, 2003 by Saunders, an imprint of Elsevier Inc. All rights reserved.

recopilar Reunir información o material pedazo a pedazo; examinar en busca de material pertinente.

glucagon A hormone produced by the alpha cells of the pancreatic islets that stimulates the liver to convert glycogen into glucose.
glucagón Hormona producida por las células alfa de los islotes pancreáticos; estimula al hígado para que convierta el glucógeno en glucosa.

glucosuria The abnormal presence of glucose in the urine.
glucosuria Presencia anómala de glucosa en la orina.

glycogen The sugar (starch) that is formed from glucose and stored mainly in the liver.
glucógeno Azúcar (almidón) formado a partir de la glucosa y almacenado principalmente en el hígado.

glycohemoglobin (hemoglobin A_{1c}) A type of hemoglobin that is made slowly during the 120-day life span of the red blood cell (RBC). Glycohemoglobin makes up 3% to 6% of hemoglobin in a normal RBC; in individuals with diabetes mellitus, it makes up to 12%.
glucohemoglobina (hemoglobina A_{1c}) Tipo de hemoglobina que se produce lentamente durante el periodo de los 120 días de vida de los glóbulos rojos (RBC). La glucohemoglobina constituye de un 3% a un 6% de la hemoglobina en un RBC normal; en los casos de diabetes mellitus constituye hasta un 12%.

glycosuria The presence of glucose in the urine.
glucosuria Presencia de glucosa en la orina.

goniometer An instrument used to measure the degrees of motion in a joint.
goniómetro Instrumento para medir los grados de movimiento de una articulación.

government plan An insurance or healthcare plan sponsored and/or subsidized by the state or federal government, such as Medicaid and Medicare.
plan del gobierno Seguro o plan de atención sanitaria patrocinado y subvencionado por el gobierno estatal o federal, como Medicaid y Medicare.

grammar The study of the classes of words, their inflections, and their functions and relations in a sentence; the study of what is preferred and what should be avoided in inflection and syntax.
gramática Estudio de las clases de palabras, sus desinencias y sus funciones y relaciones en la oración; estudio del uso que se prefiere y de lo que hay que evitar en cuanto a desinencias y sintaxis.

gray (Gy) The international unit of radiation dose.
gray (Gy) Unidad internacional de dosis de radiación.

grief An unfortunate outcome; deep distress caused by bereavement.
pesar Resultado desafortunado; profunda aflicción causada por la pérdida de un ser querido.

group policy Insurance written under a policy that covers a number of people under a single master contract, which is issued to their employer or to an association with which they are affiliated.
póliza de grupo Seguro contratado bajo una póliza que cubre a varias personas bajo un único contrato maestro establecido con su empleador o con una asociación a la que estén afiliados.

growth hormone (GH) The hormone that stimulates tissue growth and restricts tissue glucose dependence when nutrients are not available; also called *somatotropic hormone*.
hormona del crecimiento (GH) También llamada *hormona somatotrópica,* estimula el crecimiento de los tejidos y restringe la dependencia de la glucosa de los tejidos cuando no hay nutrientes disponibles.

guarantor A person who makes or gives a guarantee of payment for a bill.
garante Persona que paga una factura o que garantiza su pago.

guardian ad litem The legal representative of a minor.
tutor ad litem Representante legal de un menor.

hard copy The readable paper copy or printout of information.
copia impresa Copia impresa en papel o impresión de la información.

harmonious Marked by accord in sentiment or action; having the parts agreeably related.
armonioso Caracterizado por una armonía en los sentimientos o acciones; partes de un todo relacionadas de forma agradable.

health insurance Protection, in return for periodic premiums, that provides reimbursement of monetary losses resulting from illness or injury. Included under this heading are various types of insurance, such as accident insurance, disability income insurance, medical expense insurance, and accidental death and dismemberment insurance. Also known as *accident and health insurance* or *disability income insurance*.
seguro de enfermedad Cobertura a cambio del pago de primas periódicas, la cual proporciona el reembolso de las pérdidas monetarias debidas a enfermedad o lesión. Bajo este nombre se incluyen varios tipos de seguros como seguro de accidente, seguro de incapacidad, seguro de gastos médicos y seguro en caso de muerte y pérdida de extremidades. También se conoce como *seguro de accidente y enfermedad* o *seguro de incapacidad.*

hematemesis Vomiting of bright red blood, which indicates rapid upper gastrointestinal bleeding and is associated with esophageal varices or a peptic ulcer.

Copyright © 2011, 2007, 2003 by Saunders, an imprint of Elsevier Inc. All rights reserved.

hematemesis Vómito de sangre roja brillante que indica hemorragia rápida del sistema gastrointestinal superior, relacionado con varices esofágicas o úlcera péptica.

hematocrit The percentage by volume of packed red blood cells in a given sample of blood after centrifugation; the volume percentage of erythrocytes in whole blood.
hematocrito Porcentaje por volumen de glóbulos rojos en una muestra de sangre dada después de ser centrifugada. Porcentaje del volumen de eritrocitos en la sangre completa.

hematoma A sac filled with blood that may be the result of trauma.
hematoma Saco lleno de sangre que puede ser el resultado de una lesión.

hematuria Blood in the urine.
hematuria Sangre en la orina.

hemoconcentration A condition in which the concentration of blood cells is increased in proportion to the plasma.
hemoconcentración Situación en la cual la concentración de glóbulos rojos ha aumentado en proporción al plasma.

hemoglobin A protein in erythrocytes that transports molecular oxygen in the blood.
hemoglobina Proteína que se encuentra en los eritrocitos que transportan el oxígeno en la sangre.

hemolysis The destruction or dissolution of red blood cells, with subsequent release of hemoglobin.
hemolisis Destrucción o disolución de los glóbulos rojos, con la subsiguiente liberación de hemoglobina.

hemolyzed A term used to describe a blood sample in which the red blood cells have ruptured.
hemolizado Término usado para describir una muestra de sangre en la cual los glóbulos rojos se han roto.

hepatomegaly Abnormal enlargement of the liver.
hepatomegalia Agrandamiento anómalo del hígado.

hereditary Pertaining to a characteristic, condition, or disease transmitted from parent to offspring on the DNA chain.
hereditario Perteneciente o relativo a una característica, estado o enfermedad transmitida de padres a hijos en la cadena de ADN.

hermetically sealed Sealed such that no air may enter or escape.
herméticamente sellado Sellado de forma que el aire no pueda entrar o escapar.

HMO An organization that provides a wide range of comprehensive healthcare services for a specified group at a fixed periodic payment. HMOs may be sponsored by the government, medical schools, hospitals, employers, labor unions, consumer groups, insurance companies, and hospital medical plans.
HMO Organización que proporciona una amplia gama de servicios completos de atención sanitaria para un grupo específico por un pago periódico fijado. Las HMO puedes estar patrocinadas por el gobierno, facultades de medicina, hospitales, patronos, sindicatos laborales, grupos de consumidores, compañías aseguradoras y planes médico-hospitalarios.

holder The person who presents a check for payment.
portador Persona que presenta un cheque para cobrarlo.

holistic Related to or concerned with all of the body's systems as a whole, rather than as separate parts.
holístico Relacionado con todos los sistemas corporales y no dividido en partes.

homeostasis The maintenance of constant internal ambient conditions compatible with life.
homeostasis Mantenimiento de unas condiciones ambientales internas constantes compatibles con la vida.

homeostatic Maintaining a constant internal environment.
homeostático Que mantiene un ambiente interno constante.

hormone A substance, usually a peptide or steroid, produced by one tissue and conveyed by the bloodstream to another to effect physiologic activity, such as growth or metabolism; a chemical transmitter produced by the body and transported to a target tissue or organs by the bloodstream.
hormona Sustancia química transmisora, por lo general un péptido o un esteroide, que es producida por un tejido y transportada por la corriente sanguínea hasta el tejido u órgano—objetivo para provocar un efecto en la actividad fisiológica, como el crecimiento o el metabolismo.

HTML Abbreviation for *hypertext markup language,* the language used to create documents for the Internet.
HTML Abreviatura de *lenguaje de marcas de hipertexto,* que es el lenguaje que se emplea para crear documentos destinados a usarse en Internet.

HTTP Abbreviation for *hypertext transfer protocol,* which designates how messages are defined and transmitted over the Internet; when a URL is entered into the computer, an HTTP command tells the Web server to retrieve the requested Web page.
HTTP Abreviatura de *protocolo de transporte de hipertexto,* que define cómo se interpretan y transmiten los mensajes en Internet; cuando un URL entra en la computadora, una orden de HTTP manda la señal al servidor web para que busque la página web que se solicita.

Copyright © 2011, 2007, 2003 by Saunders, an imprint of Elsevier Inc. All rights reserved.

hub A common connection point for devices in a network containing multiple ports; it often is used to connect segments of an LAN.
nodo Punto de conexión común para dispositivos en una red de conexiones de varios puertos; suele usar se para conectar segmentos de una LAN (red de área local).

hydrocephaly Enlargement of the cranium caused by the abnormal accumulation of cerebrospinal fluid in the cerebral system.
hidrocefalia Agrandamiento del cráneo causado por una acumulación anómala de fluido cerebroespinal en el interior del sistema cerebral.

hydrogenated Combined with, treated with, or exposed to hydrogen.
hidrogenado Combinado con hidrógeno, tratado con él o expuesto a él.

hyperlipidemia An excess of fats or lipids in the blood plasma.
hiperlipemia Exceso de grasas o lípidos en el plasma sanguíneo.

hyperplasia An increase in the number of cells.
hiperplasia Aumento del número de células.

hyperpnea An increase in the depth of breathing.
hiperpnea Aumento en la profundidad de la respiración.

hypertension High blood pressure (i.e., a systolic pressure consistently above 140 mm Hg and a diastolic pressure above 90 mm Hg).
hipertensión Presión sanguínea alta (presión sistólica continuamente por encima de 140 mm Hg y presión diastólica por encima de 90 mm Hg).

hyperventilation Abnormally prolonged and deep breathing, usually associated with acute anxiety or emotional tension.
hiperventilación Respiración profunda anómalamente prolongada, que suele estar asociada con una ansiedad aguda o con tensión emocional.

hypotension Blood pressure that is below normal (i.e., a systolic pressure below 90 mm Hg and a diastolic pressure below 50 mm Hg).
hipotensión Presión sanguínea que está por debajo de lo normal (presión sistólica por debajo de 90 mm Hg y presión diastólica por debajo de 50 mm Hg).

icon A picture, often on the desktop of a computer, that represents a program or an object. By clicking on the icon, the user is directed to the program.
icono Dibujo, con frecuencia colocado en el escritorio de la computadora, que representa un programa o un objeto. Al hacer clic sobre el icono, el usuario es llevado a dicho programa.

idealism The practice of forming ideas or living under the influence of ideas.
idealismo Práctica de formarse ideas o vivir bajo la influencia de ideas.

idiopathic Of unknown cause.
idiopático Causa desconocida.

ileocecal valve The valve at the opening between the ileum and the cecum; also called the *ileocolic valve.*
válvula ileocecal Válvula que controla la abertura entre el íleo y el intestino ciego; también se llama *válvula ileocólica.*

ileostomy The surgical formation of an opening of the ileum onto the surface of the abdomen, through which fecal material is emptied.
ileostomía Formación quirúrgica de una abertura del íleo en la superficie del abdomen, a través de la cual se vacían los materiales fecales.

immigrant A person who comes to a country to take up permanent residence.
inmigrante Persona que va a un país para vivir allí de forma permanente.

immunotherapy The administration of repeated injections of diluted extracts of a substance that causes an allergic reaction; also called *desensitization.*
inmunoterapia Administración de repetidas inyecciones de extractos diluidos de la substancia que provoca una alergia; también se conoce como *desensibilización.*

impenetrable Incapable of being penetrated or pierced; not capable of being damaged or harmed.
impenetrable Que no puede ser penetrado o traspasado; que no puede ser dañado o perjudicado.

implied consent Presumed consent, such as when a patient offers an arm for a phlebotomy procedure.
consentimiento tácito Consentimiento que se supone que ha sido dado, como cuando un paciente presenta el brazo para que se le extraiga sangre.

in vitro Refers to conditions outside of a living body.
in-vitro Expresión que se refiere a condiciones exteriores de un ser vivo.

incentive Something that incites or spurs to action; a reward or reason for performing a task.
incentivo Algo que incita o impulsa a actuar; recompensa o razón para llevar a cabo una tarea.

"includes" In insurance claims, when this term appears under a subdivision such as a category (three digit) code or a two-digit procedure code, this indicates that the code and title include these terms. Other terms also classified to that particular code and title are listed in the Alphabetic Index.

Copyright © 2011, 2007, 2003 by Saunders, an imprint of Elsevier Inc. All rights reserved.

"incluye" La presencia de esta expresión, cuando aparece bajo una subdivisión, como una categoría (código de tres dígitos) o como un código de procedimiento de dos dígitos, indica que el código y el título incluyen estos términos. En los Índices alfabéticos se enumeran otros términos también clasificados para este código específico.

incontinence The inability to control excretory functions.
incontinencia Incapacidad de controlar las funciones excretoras.

indemnity plan The traditional health insurance plan that pays for all or a share of the cost of covered services, regardless of which doctor, hospital, or other licensed healthcare provider is used. Policyholders of indemnity plans and their dependents choose when and where to get healthcare services.
plan de indemnización Plan de seguro de enfermedad tradicional que paga todo o parte del costo de los servicios que cubre, sin importar a qué médico, hospital u otro proveedor de atención sanitaria licenciado se acuda. Los titulares de pólizas de planes de indemnización y las personas que dependen de estos titulares escogen cuándo y dónde recibir atención médica.

indicators An important point or group of statistical values that, when evaluated, indicates the quality of care provided in a healthcare institution.
indicadores Importante punto o grupo de valores estadísticos que al ser evaluados indican la calidad del servicio que se proporciona en una institución de atención sanitaria.

indict To charge with a crime by the finding or presentment of a jury according to due process of law.
acusado Que se le imputa con un cargo criminal por conclusión o acusación de un jurado con el proceso legal debido.

indigent Totally lacking in something necessary.
indigente Que carece totalmente de algo necesario.

indirect filing system A filing system in which an intermediary reference, such as a card file, must be consulted to locate specific files.
sistema indirecto de archivo Sistema de archivo en el cual debe consultarse una fuente de referencia intermedia, como un fichero, para localizar documentos específicos.

individual policy An insurance policy designed specifically for the use of one person (and his or her dependents); a policy that is not associated with the amenities of a group policy, such as lower premiums. Often referred to as "personal insurance."
póliza individual Póliza de seguros destinada específicamente a ser usada por una persona (y quienes dependan de ella) y que no conlleva los beneficios de una póliza de grupo y tiene primas más altas. Con frecuencia se le llama "seguro—personal."

induration An abnormally hard, inflamed area.
induración Área anómalamente dura, inflamada.

infarction Area of tissue that has died because of lack of blood supply.
infarto Área de tejido que ha muerto debido a una falta de suministro de sangre.

infection Invasion of body tissues by microorganisms, which then proliferate and damage tissues.
infección Invasión de los tejidos corporales por microorganismos, los cuales entonces proliferan y dañan los tejidos.

infertile Not fertile or productive; not capable of reproducing.
estéril Que no es fértil o productivo; que no tiene la capacidad de reproducirse.

inflammation A tissue reaction to trauma or disease that includes redness, heat, swelling, and pain.
inflamación Reacción de los tejidos ante una lesión o enfermedad que incluye enrojecimiento, calentamiento, hinchazón y dolor.

inflection A change in the pitch or loudness of the voice.
inflexión Cambio en el tono o volumen de la voz.

informed consent Consent given because the patient understands the proposed treatment and the risks involved, the reasons it should be done, and alternative treatments available (including no treatment) and their attendant risks.
consentimiento informado Consentimiento que implica la comprensión del tratamiento al que se va a ser sometido y de los riesgos que conlleva, del porqué de dicho tratamiento, así como la comprensión de los tratamientos alternativos disponibles (incluyendo la ausencia de tratamiento) y los riesgos que conllevan.

infraction A minor offense against rules or regulations.
infracción Incumplimiento de la ley; delito menor contra las normas establecidas.

initiate To introduce; to cause or start something.
iniciativa El causar o facilitar el comienzo de algo; el hacer que algo comience a ocurrir.

Copyright © 2011, 2007, 2003 by Saunders, an imprint of Elsevier Inc. All rights reserved.

innate Existing in, belonging to, or determined by factors present in an individual since birth.
innato Que existe en un individuo, que le pertenece o que está determinado por factores existentes en ese individuo desde el momento de su nacimiento.

input Information entered into a computer and used to produce output.
entrada Información introducida en una computadora y que la computadora utiliza.

instigate To goad or urge forward; to provoke.
instigar Incitar, exhortar, provocar.

insubordination Disobedience to authority.
insubordinación Desobediencia a la autoridad.

insulin A hormone secreted by the beta cells of the pancreatic islets in response to increased levels of glucose in the blood.
insulina Hormona que segregan las células beta de los islotes pancreáticos en respuesta a la presencia de altos niveles de glucosa en la sangre.

insured A person or organization covered by an insurance policy, along with any other parties for whom protection is provided under the policy terms.
asegurado Persona u organización que está cubierta por una póliza de seguro junto con cualquier otro a quien se proporcione cobertura bajo los términos de la póliza.

intangible Incapable of being perceived, especially by touch; incapable of being precisely identified or realized by the mind.
intangible Que no se puede percibir, especialmente que no se puede tocar; que no puede ser identificado con precisión ni ser comprendido por la mente.

integral Essential; an indispensable part of a whole.
integral Esencial; parte indispensable de un todo.

interaction A two-way communication; mutual or reciprocal action or influence.
interacción Comunicación bidireccional; acción o influencia recíproca o mutua.

intercom A two-way communication system with a microphone and loudspeaker at each station for localized use.
intercomunicador Sistema de comunicación bidireccional con un micrófono y un altavoz en cada estación para uso local.

intermittent Coming and going at intervals; not continuous.
intermitente Que va y viene a intervalos; de forma no continua.

intermittent claudication Recurring cramping in the calves caused by poor circulation of blood to the muscles of the lower leg.
cojera intermitente Calambres recurrentes en las pantorrillas causados por una mala circulación de la sangre de los músculos de la parte inferior de la pierna.

intermittent pulse A pulse in which beats occasionally are skipped.
pulso intermitente Pulso en el cual de vez en cuando se salta algún latido.

internal noise Noise inside the brain that interferes with the communication process.
ruido interno Ruido en el interior del cerebro que interfiere con el proceso de comunicación.

International Classification of Diseases, Ninth Revision, Clinical Modification (ICD-9-CM) A system for classifying diseases to facilitate the collection of uniform, comparable health information for statistical purposes and for indexing medical records for data storage and retrieval.
Clasificación Internacional de Enfermedades, Novena Revisión, Modificación clínica (ICD-9-CM) Sistema de clasificación de enfermedades para facilitar la recopilación de información médica uniforme, tanto para fines estadísticos como para indexar informes médicos a fin de almacenar y recuperar datos.

International Classification of Diseases, Tenth Revision (ICD-10) A system marked by the greatest number of changes in the ICD's history. To allow more specific reporting of diseases and newly recognized conditions, the ICD-10 has approximately 5,500 more codes than the ICD-9.
Clasificación Internacional de Enfermedades, Décima Revisión (ICD-10) Sistema que contiene el mayor número de cambios en la historia de la ICD. Para permitir elaborar informes más precisos de las enfermedades y de los estados patológicos que se conocen sólo recientemente, la ICD-10 incluye aproximadamente 5,500 códigos más que la ICD-9.

international mail Mail sent outside the boundaries of the United States and its territories.
correo internacional Correo que se envía fuera de los límites de Estados Unidos y sus territorios.

interval The length of time between events.
intervalo Espacio de tiempo entre dos sucesos.

intolerable Not tolerable or bearable.
intolerable Que no se puede tolerar o soportar.

Copyright © 2011, 2007, 2003 by Saunders, an imprint of Elsevier Inc. All rights reserved.

intravenous urogram (IVU) A radiographic examination of the urinary tract that uses intravenous injection of an iodine contrast medium.
urograma intravenoso (IVU) Examen radiográfico del tracto urinario usando una inyección intravenosa de un medio de contraste yodado.

intrinsic Belonging to the essential nature or constitution of a thing; indwelling, inward.
intrínseco Que pertenece a la naturaleza o constitución básica de una cosa; inherente, interno.

introspection An inward, reflective examination of one's own thoughts and feelings.
introspección Examen de nuestros propios pensamientos y sentimientos.

invariably Consistently; without changing or being capable of change.
invariablemente De forma constante; que no cambia ni puede cambiar.

invasive A term that refers to entry into the living body, as by incision or insertion of an instrument.
invasivo Que entra en un organismo vivo, como por incisión o inserción de un instrumento.

ipsilateral Pertaining to the same side of the body.
isolateral Perteneciente a la misma parte del cuerpo.

irregular pulse A pulse that varies in force and frequency.
pulso irregular Pulso que varía en fuerza y frecuencia.

ischemia Decreased blood flow to a body part or organ, caused by constriction or plugging of the supplying artery; a temporary interruption in blood supply to a tissue or organ.
isquemia Disminución del flujo sanguíneo a una parte del cuerpo u órgano provocada por la constricción o atasco de la arteria suministradora; interrupción temporal del suministro de sangre a un tejido u órgano.

islets (of Langerhans) Cells of the pancreas that produce insulin (beta cells) and glucagon (alpha cells); also called *pancreatic islets*.
islotes (de Langerhans) Células del páncreas que producen insulina (células beta) y glucagón (células alfa); también llamados *islotes pancreáticos*.

jargon The technical terminology or characteristic idiom of a particular group or special activity.
jerga Terminología técnica o lenguaje característico de un grupo específico o una actividad especial.

jaundice Yellowness of the skin and mucous membranes caused by deposition of bile pigment. Jaundice is not itself a disease, but rather a sign of a number of diseases, especially liver disorders.
ictericia Coloración amarilla en la piel y las membranas mucosas causada por deposición del pigmento biliar. No es una enfermedad pero es un síntoma de muchas enfermedades, sobre todo de trastornos hepáticos.

Java An object-oriented, high-level programming language commonly used and well suited for the Internet.
Java Lenguaje de programación de alto nivel y orientado a objetos que es usado ampliamente y es muy adecuado para Internet.

judicial Of or relating to a judgment, the function of judging, the administration of justice, or the judiciary.
judicial Perteneciente o relativo al juicio, los procesos jurídicos, la administración de justicia o a la judicatura.

jurisdiction A power constitutionally conferred on a judge or magistrate to decide cases according to law and to carry sentence into execution. Jurisdiction is *original* when it is conferred on the court in the first instance (original jurisdiction); it is *appellate* when an appeal is given from the judgment of another court (appellate jurisdiction).
jurisdicción Poder constitucional otorgado a un juez o magistrado para resolver casos de acuerdo con la ley y hacer que se cumplan las sentencias. Es jurisdicción *original* cuando se otorga en un tribunal de primera instancia; es jurisdicción en *apelación* cuando existe una apelación al juicio de otro tribunal.

jurisprudence The science or philosophy of law; a system or body of law or the course of court decisions.
jurisprudencia Ciencia o filosofía que trata sobre la ley; sistema o cuerpo legal; línea de decisiones de los tribunales.

keratin A very hard, tough protein found in the hair, nails, and epidermal tissue.
queratina Proteína muy dura que se encuentra en el pelo, uñas y tejidos epidérmicos.

keratinocytes Any one of the skin cells that synthesize keratin.
queratinocitos Cualquiera de las células de la piel que sintetizan queratina.

ketosis The abnormal production of ketone bodies in the blood and tissues as a result of fat catabolism in cells. Ketones accumulate in large quantities when fat, instead of sugar, is used as fuel for energy in cells.
quetosis Producción anormal de cuerpos de quetosis en la sangre y tejidos como resultado de un catabolismo graso en las células. Los quetones se acumulan en grandes cantidades cuando se usa grasa, en lugar de azúcar, como combustible para las células.

Copyright © 2011, 2007, 2003 by Saunders, an imprint of Elsevier Inc. All rights reserved.

kyphosis An abnormal convex curvature of the thoracic spine region.
cifosis Curvatura convexa anómala de la región espinal torácica.

lacrimation The secretion or discharge of tears.
lagrimeo Secreción o descarga de lágrimas.

language barrier Any type of interference that inhibits the communication process and is related to the difference in languages spoken by the people attempting to communicate.
barrera del idioma Cualquier tipo de interferencia que inhibe el proceso de comunicación y que está relacionado con la diferencia en los idiomas que hablan las personas que intentan comunicarse.

laryngoscopy Visual examination of the voice box area through an endoscope equipped with a light and mirrors for illumination.
laringoscopia Examen visual de la laringe por medio de un endoscopio equipado con una luz y espejos.

latent image Invisible changes in exposed film that become a visible image when the film is processed.
imagen latente Cambios invisibles en la película que se convertirán en una imagen visible cuando se procese la película.

law A binding custom or practice of a community; a rule of conduct or action prescribed or formally recognized as binding or enforceable by a controlling authority.
ley Costumbre o práctica obligatoria de una comunidad; norma de comportamiento o proceder prescrita o reconocida formalmente como norma obligatoria o que se puede hacer cumplir por una autoridad encargada.

learning style The way a person perceives and processes information to learn new material.
estilo de aprendizaje Forma en la que un individuo percibe y procesa la información para aprender cosas nuevas.

leukoderma White patches on the skin.
leucodermia Manchas blancas en la piel.

liable Obligated according to law or equity; responsible for an act or circumstance.
responsable Que tiene alguna obligación según la ley o el derecho lato; responsable de un acto o circunstancia.

libel A written defamatory statement or representation that conveys an unjustly unfavorable impression.
libelo Escrito difamatorio que produce una impresión desfavorable injusta.

ligament A tough connective tissue band that holds joints together by attaching to the bones on either side of the joint.
ligamento Banda de tejido conectivo resistente que sostiene las articulaciones uniendo los huesos de cada lado de la articulación.

ligation The process of tying off something to close it (e.g., a blood vessel during surgery) with a tie called a *ligature*.
ligado Proceso de atar algo, por ejemplo, un vaso sanguíneo durante una cirugía, con una atadura llamada *ligadura*.

limited radiography A limited-scope radiography practice, usually in an outpatient setting, that does not require the same credentials as those for professional radiologic technology; also called *practical radiography*.
radiografía limitada Práctica radiográfica de alcance limitado que se suele usar con pacientes externos y que no requiere las mismas credenciales que se necesitan para la tecnología radiográfica profesional. También se llama radiografía práctica.

lithotripsy A procedure for eliminating a stone (as in the bladder) by crushing or dissolving it in situ with high-intensity sound waves.
litotripsia Procedimiento para eliminar una piedra rompiéndola o disolviéndola in-situ por medio del uso de ondas sonoras de alta intensidad.

litigious Prone to engage in lawsuits.
litigioso Propenso a iniciar pleitos y litigios.

loading dose A double dose of medication administered as the first dose. Loading doses usually are given in antibiotic therapy to reach therapeutic drug levels in the blood quickly.
dosis de ataque Dosis doble de una medicación ladministrada como primera dosis. Suele hacerse con terapia antibiótica para alcanzar rápidamente los niveles terapéuticos en sangre.

lordosis An abnormal concave curvature of the cervical and lumbar spines.
lordosis Curvatura cóncava anómala de la espina cervical y lumbar.

lower GI series A fluoroscopic examination of the colon that usually involves rectal administration of barium sulfate (also called a *barium enema*) as a contrast medium.
serie GI inferior Examen fluoroscópico del colon, por lo general usando una administración rectal de

Copyright © 2011, 2007, 2003 by Saunders, an imprint of Elsevier Inc. All rights reserved.

sulfato de bario (también llamado *enema de bario*) como medio de contraste.

lumbar The area of the lower back containing the five lumbar vertebrae.
lumbar Región posterior inferior en la que hay cinco vértebras lumbares.

lumen The open space within a hollow tube such as a blood vessel, the intestine, a needle, or an examining instrument.
lumen Espacio abierto, como en el interior de un vaso sanguíneo, el intestino, una aguja, un tubo o un instrumento para examinar.

luteinizing hormone (LH) A hormone produced by the pituitary gland that promotes ovulation.
hormona luteinizante (LH) Hormona que produce la glándula pituitaria y que promueve la ovulación.

luxation Dislocation of a bone from its normal anatomic location.
luxación Dislocación de un hueso de su ubicación anatómica normal.

lymphadenopathy Any disorder of the lymph nodes or lymph vessels.
linfadenopatía Cualquier trastorno de los nódulos o de los vasos linfáticos.

macromolecules The molecules needed for metabolism: carbohydrates, lipids, proteins, and nucleic acids.
macromoléculas Moléculas que se necesitan para el metabolismo: carbohidratos, lípidos, proteínas y ácidos nucleicos.

magnetic resonance imaging (MRI) An imaging modality that uses a magnetic field and radiofrequency pulses to create computer images of both bones and soft tissues in multiple planes.
formación de imágenes por resonancia magnética (MRI) Modalidad de formación de imágenes en la que se usa un campo magnético y pulsos de radiofrecuencia para crear imágenes computarizadas, tanto de huesos como de tejidos blandos, en planos múltiples.

major diagnostic categories (MDCs) Broad clinical categories differentiated from all others on the basis of body system involvement and cause of disease.
categorías de diagnosis principales (MDCs) Amplias categorías clínicas que se diferencian de todas las demás en base a la inclusión del sistema corporal y la etiología de la enfermedad.

maker (of a check) Any individual, corporation, or legal party who signs a check or any type of negotiable instrument.
signatario (de un cheque) Cualquier individuo, corporación o parte legal que firma un cheque o cualquier tipo de instrumento negociable.

malignant Cancerous.
maligno Canceroso.

managed care An umbrella term for all healthcare plans that provide health care in return for preset monthly payments and that offer coordinated care through a defined network of primary care physicians and hospitals.
atención administrada Término que engloba todos los planes de atención sanitaria que proporcionan atención médica a cambio de pagos mensuales preestablecidos y atención coordinada a través de una red definida de médicos de cabecera y hospitales.

mandated Required by an authority or law.
obligatorio Que lo exige una autoridad o la ley.

mandatory Containing or constituting a command.
obligatorio Que contiene una orden o que es una orden en sí mismo.

manifestation Something easily understood or recognized by the mind.
manifestación Algo que puede ser comprendido o reconocido por la mente con facilidad.

manipulation Moving or exercising a body part by an externally applied force.
manipulación Mover o ejercitar una parte del cuerpo por medio de la aplicación de una fuerza externa.

mastectomy Surgical removal of the breast, usually including the excision of lymph nodes in the axillary region.
mastectomía Eliminación quirúrgica del seno que por lo general incluye la escisión de los nódulos linfáticos de la región axilar.

matrix Something in which a thing originates, develops, takes shape, or is contained; a base on which to build.
matriz Algo donde las cosas se originan, desarrollan, toman forma o están contenidas; base sobre la cual construir.

m-banking Banking through the use of wireless devices, such as cellular phones and wireless Internet services.
banca-m Operaciones bancarias a través de dispositivos inalámbricos, como teléfonos celulares y servicios de comunicaciones inalámbricas.

media The term applied to agencies of mass communication, such as newspapers, magazines, and telecommunications.

Copyright © 2011, 2007, 2003 by Saunders, an imprint of Elsevier Inc. All rights reserved.

medios de comunicación Término que se aplica a las agencias de noticias o de comunicación de masas, como periódicos, revistas y telecomunicaciones.

mediastinum The space in the center of the chest, under the sternum.
mediastino Espacio en el centro del pecho, bajo el esternón.

medical savings account A tax-deferred bank or savings account combined with a low-premium, high-deductible insurance policy, designed for individuals or families who choose to fund their own healthcare expenses and medical insurance.
cuenta de ahorros para gastos médicos Cuenta bancaria o de ahorros de impuestos diferidos combinada con una póliza de seguro con primas bajas y deducibles altos destinada a individuos o familias que eligen financiar ellos mismos sus gastos de atención sanitaria y su seguro médico.

medically indigent An individual who can afford to pay for his or her normal daily living expenses but cannot afford adequate healthcare.
médicamente indigente Individuo que puede pagar sus gastos normales de la vida cotidiana pero que no puede abordar el pago de un servicio de atención sanitaria adecuado.

medically necessary Criteria used by third-party payers to decide whether a patient's symptoms and diagnosis justify specific medical services or procedures; also known as *medical necessity*.
médicamente necesario Criterio usado por pagadores intermediarios para decidir si los síntomas y el diagnóstico de un paciente justifican el uso de procedimientos o servicios médicos específicos; también se conoce como *necesidad médica*.

Medigap A term sometimes applied to private insurance products that supplement Medicare insurance benefits.
Medigap Término que se aplica algunas veces a seguros privados que complementan los beneficios del seguro Medicare.

medullary cavity The inner portion of the diaphysis that contains the bone marrow.
cavidad medular Porción interna de la diafisis que contiene la médula ósea.

megabyte Approximately 1 million bytes.
megabyte Aproximadamente, un millón de bytes.

megahertz (MHz) A measuring unit for microprocessors. A megahertz is 1 million cycles of electromagnetic current alternation per second; it is used as a unit of measure for the clock speed of computer microprocessors. The hertz is a unit of measure named after Heinrich Hertz, a German physicist.
megahercio (MHz) Unidad de medida para microprocesadores, abreviada MHz. Un megahercio es un millón de ciclos de alternancia de corriente electromagnética por segundo y se usa como unidad de medida para la velocidad de los—microprocesadores de computadoras. El hercio recibe su nombre de Heinrich Hertz, un físico alemán.

melena A black, tarry stool containing digested blood; it usually is the result of bleeding in the upper GI tract.
melena Deposición negra y alquitranada que contiene sangre digerida y por lo general es le resultado de una hemorragia en el tracto gastrointestinal superior.

mentor A trusted counselor or guide.
mentor Consejero o guía de confianza.

metabolite A substance produced by metabolism.
metabolito Sustancia producida por el metabolismo.

meticulous Marked by extreme or excessive care in the consideration or treatment of details.
meticuloso Caracterizado por una atención exagerada o excesiva a los detalles.

microcephaly Abnormally small head size in relation to the rest of the body.
microcefalia Tamaño pequeño de la cabeza en relación con el resto del cuerpo.

microfilm A film bearing a photographic record of printed or other graphic matter on a reduced scale.
microfilm Película que contiene una fotografía de un documento impreso u otro elemento gráfico a escala reducida.

microorganism An organism of microscopic or submicroscopic size.
microorganismo Organismo de tamaño microscópico o sub-microscópico.

MIDI The abbreviation for *musical instrument digital interface*. A MIDI interface allows computers to record and manipulate sound.
MIDI Abreviatura para *interfaz digital para instrumentos musicales*. Una interfaz MIDI permite a las computadoras grabar y manipular sonido.

miotic Any substance or medication that causes contraction of the pupil.
miótico Cualquier sustancia o medicamento que produce una contracción de la pupila.

misdemeanor A minor crime punishable by fine or imprisonment in a city or county jail rather than in a penitentiary.

Copyright © 2011, 2007, 2003 by Saunders, an imprint of Elsevier Inc. All rights reserved.

falta Delito menor, por oposición a delito mayor, se penaliza con multa o prisión en una cárcel de una ciudad o condado más bien que con prisión en una penitenciaría.

mock To imitate or practice.
simular Imitar o practicar.

modem The acronym for *modulator demodulator;* a device that allows information to be transmitted over phone lines at speeds measured in bits per second (bps).
módem Abreviatura para modulador desmodulador, un dispositivo que permite transmitir información a través de las líneas telefónicas a velocidades que se miden en bits por segundos (bps).

molecule A group of like or different atoms held together by chemical forces.
molécula Grupo de átomos iguales o diferentes que se mantiene unido por fuerzas químicas.

monochromatic Having or consisting of one color or hue.
monocromático Que tiene un solo color o tonalidad.

mononuclear white blood cell A leukocyte with an unsegmented nucleus, particularly monocytes and lymphocytes.
glóbulo blanco mononuclear Leucocito que tiene un núcleo sin segmentar; en particular los monocitos y linfocitos.

mons pubis The fat pad that covers the symphysis pubis.
monte del pubis Almohadilla de grasa que cubre la sínfisis púbica.

morale The mental and emotional condition (e.g., enthusiasm, confidence, or loyalty) of an individual or group with regard to the function or tasks at hand.
moral Estado mental y emocional (como entusiasmo, lealtad o confianza) de un individuo o grupo en cuanto al puesto que desempeña o el trabajo que realiza.

motivation The process of inciting a person to some action or behavior.
motivación Proceso de incitar a una persona a hacer algo o a comportarse de una forma determinada.

multimedia The presentation of graphics, animation, video, sound, and text on a computer in an integrated way or all at once. CD-ROMs are the most effective multimedia devices.
multimedia Presentación de gráficos, imágenes animadas, video, sonido y texto en una computadora de forma integrada o simultánea. Los CD ROM son los dispositivos de multimedia más eficaces.

multiparous Pertaining to women who have had two or more pregnancies.
multípara Perteneciente o relativo a la mujer que ha tenido dos o más embarazos.

multitasking Performing multiple tasks at one time.
multitarea Realización de varias tareas diferentes al mismo tiempo.

municipal court A court that sits in some cities and larger towns and that usually has civil and criminal jurisdiction over cases arising within the municipality.
Municipal corte Se aplica al juzgado con sede en algunas ciudades y pueblos grandes y que suele tener jurisdicción civil y penal sobre casos que surgen dentro de la municipalidad.

murmur An abnormal sound heard on auscultation of the heart; it may or may not be pathologic.
murmullo Sonido anómalo que se escucha al auscultar el corazón y que puede ser patológico o no.

myelography A fluoroscopic examination of the spinal canal involving spinal injection of an iodine contrast medium.
mielografía Examen fluoroscópico del canal espinal con una inyección espinal de un medio de contraste yodado.

myelomeningocele A herniation of part of the spinal cord and its meninges that protrudes through a congenital opening in the vertebral column.
mielomeningocele Hernia de una parte de la médula espinal y sus meninges que sale hacia fuera a través de una abertura congénita en la columna vertebral.

myocardial Pertaining to the heart muscle.
miocárdico Perteneciente o relativo al músculo cardiaco.

myocardium The heart muscle.
miocardio Músculo cardiaco.

myoglobinuria The abnormal presence of a hemoglobin-like chemical of muscle tissue in the urine; it occurs as a result of muscle deterioration.
mioglobinuria Presencia anómala en la orina de una susbtancia química del tejido muscular parecida a la hemoglobina; es el resultado de una deterioración muscular.

mysticism The experience of seeming to have direct communication with God or the ultimate reality.
misticismo Experiencia de parecer tener comunicación directa con Dios o una realidad superior.

nanometer One billionth ($1/10^{-9}$) of a meter.
nanómetro Una mil millonésima parte (10^{-9}) de metro.

Copyright © 2011, 2007, 2003 by Saunders, an imprint of Elsevier Inc. All rights reserved.

naturopathy An alternative to conventional medicine in which holistic methods are used, as well as herbs and natural supplements, in the belief that the body will heal itself. Currently, naturopathic physicians can be licensed in 12 states.
naturopatía Alternativa a la medicina convencional en la que se usan métodos holísticos, así como hierbas y suplementos naturales, con la creencia de que el cuerpo sanará por sí mismo. En la actualidad, los médicos naturópatas pueden obtener la licencia en doce estados.

necrosis Pertaining to the death of cells or tissue.
necrosis Perteneciente o relativo a la muerte de células o tejidos.

negative feedback mechanism A homeostatic mechanism that responds as a regulator to counteract a change.
mecanismo de respuesta negativa Mecanismo homeostático que responde como regulador para contrarrestar un cambio.

negligence Failure to exercise the care that a prudent person usually exercises; implied inattention to one's duty or business; implied want of due or necessary diligence or care.
negligencia Falta de cuidado en algo que se hace; falta implicita de atención en el deber o trabajo; deseo implicito de una diligencia o cuidado necesario o merecido.

negotiable Legally transferable to another party.
negociable Que se puede transferir legalmente a otra parte.

networking The exchange of information or services among individuals, groups, or institutions; meeting and getting to know individuals in the same or similar career fields and sharing information about available opportunities.
interconexión Intercambio de información o servicios entre individuos, grupos o instituciones; conocer a individuos del mismo campo profesional o de campos similares y compartir información acerca de oportunidades de empleo.

neural tube defect Any of a group of congenital anomalies involving the brain and spinal column that are caused by failure of the neural tube to close during embryonic development.
defecto del tubo neural Cualquiera de las anomalías congénitas que afectan al cerebro y a la médula espinal y que tienen su origen en que el tubo neural no logró cerrarse durante el desarrollo embrionario.

nodule A small lump, lesion, or swelling that is felt when the skin is palpated.
nódulo Pequeña protuberancia, herida o hinchazón que se siente al tocar la piel.

nomogram A graph on which variables are plotted so that a particular value can be read on the appropriate line.
nomograma Gráfica en la que las variables están presentadas de tal manera que se puede leer un valor específico en la línea adecuada.

nonmaleficence Refraining from the act of causing harm or doing evil.
ausencia de maleficencia No hacer el mal.

no-show A person who fails to keep an appointment without giving advance notice.
no-acudió Persona que no acude a una cita médica sin dar previo aviso.

nosocomial infection An infection acquired during hospitalization or in a healthcare setting. These infections often are caused by *Escherichia coli,* hepatitis viruses, *Pseudomonas* organisms, and staphylococci.
infección nosocomial Infección adquirida en un establecimiento de atención sanitaria o durante una hospitalización. Con frecuencia se debe a *E. coli,* virus de hepatitis, pseudomonas y estafilococos.

nosocomial Pertaining to or originating in the hospital; a term for an infection that either was not present or was incubating before the patient was admitted to the hospital.
nosocomial Perteneciente o relativo al hospital, incubado en el hospital, dícese de la infección que no estaba presente ni en estado de incubación antes de ser ingresado al hospital.

"note" In coding manuals, notes are found in both the Alphabetic Index and the Tabular Index as instructions or guides for classification assignments; they define the category content or the use of subdivision codes.
"nota" Las notas se encuentran tanto en los Índices alfabéticos como en las instrucciones o guías en las Asignaciones de clasificación, para definir el contenido de la categoría o el uso de los códigos de subdivisión.

NSAIDs Nonsteroidal antiinflammatory drugs.
NSAIDs Medicamentos antiinflamatorios no esterioides.

nuclear medicine An imaging modality that uses radioactive materials injected or ingested into the body to provide information about the function of organs and tissues.
medicina nuclear Modalidad de la formación de imágenes que usa materiales radioactivos inyectados en el cuerpo o ingeridos para obtener información acerca del funcionamiento de órganos y tejidos.

obesity An excessive accumulation of body fat (usually defined as a weight more than 20% above the recommended body weight).

Copyright © 2011, 2007, 2003 by Saunders, an imprint of Elsevier Inc. All rights reserved.

obesidad Acumulación excesiva de grasa en el cuerpo (se suele definir como más del 20% del peso recomendado).

objective information Information gathered by watching or observing a patient.
información objetiva Información que se recoge vigilando u observando a un paciente.

oblique projection The radiographic view in which the body or part is rotated so that the projection is neither frontal nor lateral.
proyección oblicua Vista radiográfica en la cual que cuerpo o parte del cuerpo se gira de forma que la proyección no es frontal ni lateral.

obliteration Making something indecipherable or imperceptible by obscuring or wearing away.
obliterar Hacer algo indescifrable o imperceptible oscureciéndolo o desgastándolo.

obturator A disk or plate that closes an opening.
obturador Disco o placa que cierra una abertura.

obturator A metal rod with a smooth, rounded tip that is placed inside hollow instruments to reduce damage to body tissues during insertion of the instrument.
obturador Varilla de metal con un extremo redondeado que se coloca en el interior de instrumentos huecos para disminuir la destrucción de los tejidos corporales durante su inserción.

occlusion The complete blocking off of an opening.
oclusión Cierre completo de una abertura.

"omit code" In insurance claims, a term used primarily in volume 3 of the ICD-9-CM when a procedure is the method of approach for an operation.
"omitir código" Esta expresión se usa sobre todo en el tomo 3 cuando el procedimiento es el método de acercamiento a una operación.

opaque Not translucent or transparent.
opaco Que no es translúcido ni transparente.

OPIM (other potentially infectious material) Substances or material other than blood (e.g., body fluids, such as urine and semen) that have the potential to carry infectious pathogens.
OPIM (otras materias potencialmente peligrosas) Sustancias o materias además de la sangre (como, por ejemplo, los fluidos corporales, la orina, el semen).

opinion A formal expression of judgment or advice by an expert; the formal expression of the legal reasons and principles on which a legal decision is based.
opinión Expresión formal de un juicio o consejo dado por un experto; expresión formal de las razones y principios legales sobre los que se basa una decisión legal.

opportunistic infection An infection caused by a normally nonpathogenic organism in a host whose resistance has been decreased.
infección oportunista Infección en una persona con una resistencia a las enfermedades más baja de lo normal, provocada por un organismo que en condiciones normales no resulta patógeno.

optic disc The region at the back of the eye where the optic nerve meets the retina. It is considered the blind spot of the eye, because it contains only nerve fibers and no rods or cones and therefore is insensitive to light.
papila óptica Región en la parte posterior del ojo donde el nervio óptico se une con la retina. Se considera el punto ciego del ojo, ya que allí sólo hay fibras nerviosas y no bastoncillos ni conos, y por tanto es insensible a la luz.

optic nerve The second cranial nerve, which carries impulses for the sense of sight.
nervio óptico Segundo nervio del cráneo que transporta impulsos para el sentido de la vista.

optical character recognition (OCR) Electronic scanning of printed items as images, followed by the use of special software to recognize these images (or characters) as ASCII text.
reconocimiento óptico de caracteres (OCR) Proceso de escanear electrónicamente documentos impresos como si fueran imágenes y después, usando un programa de computadora especial, reconocer esas imágenes (o caracteres) como texto ASCII.

ordinance An authoritative decree or direction; a law set forth by a governmental authority, specifically a municipal regulation.
ordenanza Decreto u orden de la autoridad; ley definida por una autoridad gubernamental, específicamente, una regulación municipal.

organelle A differentiated structure within a cell (e.g., a mitochondrion, vacuole, or chloroplast) that performs a specific function.
organelo Estructura diferenciada dentro de una célula, como un mitocondrio, vacuola o cloroplasto que realiza una función específica.

orthopnea Difficulty breathing in the supine position. The individual must sit or stand to breathe comfortably.
ortopnea Dificultad para respirar estando en posición supina. El individuo debe estar sentado o de pie para respirar con comodidad.

Copyright © 2011, 2007, 2003 by Saunders, an imprint of Elsevier Inc. All rights reserved.

orthostatic (postural) hypotension A temporary fall in blood pressure when a person rapidly changes from a recumbent position to a standing position.
hipotensión ortostática (relacionada con la postura) Baja temporal de la presión sanguínea cuando una persona cambia con rapidez de una posición recostada a una posición en pie.

osteopathy A medical discipline based primarily on the manual diagnosis and holistic treatment of impaired function resulting from loss of movement in all kinds of tissues.
osteopatía Disciplina médica que se basa primordialmente en el diagnóstico manual y el tratamiento holístico de funciones deterioradas como resultado de la pérdida de movilidad en todo tipo de tejidos.

osteoporosis A condition of loss of bone density; lack of calcium intake is a major factor in its development.
osteoporosis Disminución de la densidad de los huesos. La falta de consumo de calcio es uno de los factores principales de su desarrollo.

otitis externa Inflammation or infection of the external auditory canal.
otitis externa Inflamación o infección del canal auditivo externo.

otosclerosis The formation of spongy bone in the labyrinth of the ear, often causing the auditory ossicles to become fixed and unable to vibrate when sound enters the ears.
otosclerosis Formación de huesos parecidos a esponjas en el laberinto del oído, a menudo causando que los huesecillos auditivos queden fijos y que no puedan vibrar cuando el sonido entra en los oídos.

ototoxic Pertaining to a substance or medication that damages the eighth cranial nerve or the organs of hearing and balance.
ototóxico Perteneciente o relativo a una sustancia o medicamento que daña el octavo nervio craneal o los órganos auditivos y del equilibrio.

OUTfolder A folder used to provide space for the temporary filing of materials.
Carpeta OUT Carpeta que se usa para proporcionar espacio para archivar materiales de forma temporal.

OUTguide A heavy guide used to replace a folder that has been temporarily moved from the filing space.
Guía OUT Guía grande que se usa para reemplazar una carpeta que ha sido retirada temporalmente del archivo.

output Information processed by the computer and transmitted to a monitor, printer, or other device.
salida Información procesada por la computadora y enviada a un monitor, impresora u otro dispositivo.

over-the-counter drugs Medications legally sold without a prescription.
medicinas de venta libre Medicinas que se venden sin receta legalmente.

oxytocin A hormone secreted by the posterior pituitary gland that stimulates smooth muscle contractions of the uterus or mammary glands.
oxitocina Hormona que segrega la glándula pituitaria posterior y que estimula las contracciones del útero o de las glándulas mamarias.

palliative An agent that relieves or alleviates symptoms without curing the disease; something that alleviates or eases a painful situation without curing it.
paliativo Agente que calma o alivia los síntomas sin curar la enfermedad; algo que alivia o hace más soportable una situación dolorosa sin curarla.

pandemic Affecting most of the people in a country or a number of countries.
pandémico Que afecta a la mayoría de la población de un país o de varios países.

paper claims Hard copies of insurance claims that have been completed and sent by surface mail.
reclamaciones de papel Copias impresas de reclamaciones de seguros que han sido completadas y enviadas por correo ordinario.

papilledema Bulging of the optic disc and dilated retinal veins, which are seen through ophthalmoscopic examination of the retina. Papilledema is a sign of increased intracranial pressure.
edema papilar Abultamiento de la papila óptica y de las venas retinianas dilatadas que se ven en un examen oftalmoscópico de la retina. La emeda papilar es una señal de un aumento en la presión intracraneal.

paraphrased Pertaining to a text, passage, or work that has been restated to give the meaning in another form.
parafraseado Perteneciente o relativo a un texto, selección u obra que ha sido expresado nuevamente para dar su significado de otra forma.

paraphrasing Expressing an idea in different wording in an effort to enhance communication and clarify meaning.
parafrasear Expresar una idea con palabras diferentes para mejorar la comunicación y hacer más claro su significado.

parenteral Referring to injection or introduction of substances into the body through any route other than the digestive tract (e.g., subcutaneous, intravenous, or intramuscular administration).

Copyright © 2011, 2007, 2003 by Saunders, an imprint of Elsevier Inc. All rights reserved.

parenteral Inyección o introducción de sustancias en el cuerpo a través de cualquier otra vía que no sea el tracto digestivo, como administración subcutánea, intravenosa o intramuscular.

paresthesia An abnormal sensation of burning, prickling, or stinging.
parestesia Sensación anómala de ardor, escozor o aguijoneo.

paroxysmal Pertaining to a sudden, recurrent spasm of symptoms.
paroxístico Perteneciente o relativo a espasmos repentinos recurrentes o a sus síntomas.

participating provider A physician or other healthcare provider who enters into a contract with a specific insurance company or program and by doing so agrees to abide by certain rules and regulations set forth by that particular third-party payer.
proveedor participante Médico u otro proveedor de atención sanitaria que establece un contrato con una compañía o programa de seguro específico, y al hacerlo acepta respetar ciertas normas y regulaciones establecidas por ese pagador intermediario.

parturition The act or process of giving birth to a child.
parto Acción o proceso de dar a luz un niño.

patency The condition of a body cavity or canal that is open or unobstructed.
abertura Estado abierto de un cuerpo, cavidad o canal.

pathogen An agent that causes disease, especially a living microorganism such as a bacterium or fungus; a disease-causing microorganism.
patógeno Agente que causa enfermedades, especialmente microorganismos vivos como bacterias u hongos; microorganismos causantes de enfermedades.

pathogenic Pertaining to disease-causing microorganisms.
patogénico Perteneciente o relativo a los microorganismos causantes de enfermedades.

pathophysiology The study of biologic and physical manifestations of disease as they are related to system abnormalities and physiologic disturbances.
patofisiología Estudio de las manifestaciones biológicas y físicas de las enfermedades y cómo se relacionan con las anomalías del sistema y las alteraciones fisiológicas.

payables The balance due to a creditor on an account.
pendiente de pago Saldo que se le debe al acreedor en una cuenta.

payee The person named on a draft or check as the recipient of the amount shown.
beneficiario Persona que se nombra en una letra de cambio o en un cheque como receptor de la cantidad indicada.

payer The person who writes a check to be cashed by the payee.
pagador Persona que emite el cheque a ser cambiado por el beneficiario.

peer review organization A group of medical reviewers who contract with the Health Care Financing Administration (HCFA) to ensure quality control and the medical necessity of services provided by a facility.
organizacione de revisión colegial Grupo de revisores médicos contrata dos por HCFA para garantizar el control de calidad y la necesidad médica de los servicios ofrecidos por un establecimiento.

pegboard system A method of tracking patient accounts that allows the figures to be proven accurate by using mathematic formulas; also called the "write it once" system.
sistema de tablero perforado Método de controlar las cuentas de los pacientes que permite la demostración de la exactitud de las cifras por medio de fórmulas matemáticas; también conocido como sistema "escríbelo una vez."

perceiving The process by which an individual looks at information and sees it as real.
percibir Proceso en el cual un individuo mira la información y la ve como real.

perception A quick, acute, and intuitive cognition; the capacity for comprehension; an awareness of the elements of the environment.
percepción Conocimiento rápido, agudo e intuitivo; capacidad de comprensión; conocimiento de los elementos del medio ambiente.

pericardium The membranous sac that encloses the heart.
pericardio Saco membranoso que envuelve el corazón.

periosteum The thin, highly innervated, membranous covering of a bone.
periostio Membrana fina y sin nervios que recubre un hueso.

peristalsis The wavelike movement by which the gastrointestinal tract moves food downward.
peristalsis Movimiento ondulatorio por el cual el tracto gastrointestinal mueve la comida hacia abajo.

perjured testimony Testimony involving the voluntary violation of an oath or vow, either by swearing to what is untrue or by failing to do what has been promised under oath; false testimony.

Copyright © 2011, 2007, 2003 by Saunders, an imprint of Elsevier Inc. All rights reserved.

perjuro Testimonio que comprende la violación voluntaria de un juramento o promesa, ya sea jurando algo que es falso o no cumpliendo lo que se ha prometido bajo juramento; falso testimonio.

"perks" Perquisites; extra advantages or benefits from working in a specific job that may or may not be commonplace in that particular profession.
beneficios adicionales Ventajas o beneficios adicionales del trabajar en un puesto de trabajo específico que pueden ser o no comunes a esa profesión en particular.

permeable Allowing a substance to pass or soak through.
permeable Permite el paso o penetración de una sustancia.

persona An individual's social facade or front that reflects the role the individual is playing in life; the personality a person projects in public.
persona Lo que vemos de un individuo, la imagen social que refleja el papel que dicho individuo tiene en la sociedad; la personalidad que una persona proyecta en público.

pertinent Having a clear, decisive relevance to the matter at hand.
pertinente Que tiene una importancia clara y decisiva en el asunto que se está tratando.

petechiae Small, purplish hemorrhagic spots on the skin.
petequia Pequeñas manchas en la piel, hemorrágicas y de color violeta.

phenylalanine An essential amino acid found in milk, eggs, and other foods.
fenilalanina Aminoácido esencial que se encuentra en la leche, los huevos y otros alimentos.

philanthropist An individual who makes an active effort to promote human welfare.
filántropo Individuo que se ocupa activamente de promover el bienestar humano.

philosopher A person who seeks wisdom or enlightenment; an expounder of a theory in a certain area of experience.
filósofo Persona que busca la sabiduría o el esclarecimiento; persona que expone una teoría en cierta área de experiencia.

phlebotomy The invasive procedure used to obtain a blood specimen for testing, experimentation, or diagnosis of disease.
flebotomía Procedimiento invasivo que se usa para obtener un espécimen de sangre para analizar, experimentar o diagnosticar una enfermedad.

phonetic Referring to an alteration of ordinary spelling that better represents the spoken language, that uses only characters of the regular alphabet, and that is used in a context of conventional spelling.
escritura fonética Alteración de la escritura normal que representa mejor el lenguaje hablado, emplea sólo caracteres del alfabeto normal y se usa en un contexto de escritura convencional.

phosphors Fluorescent crystals that give off light when exposed to x-rays.
fósforos Cristales fluorescentes que alumbran cuando se exponen a los rayos x.

photometer An instrument for measuring the intensity of light, specifically to compare the relative intensities of different lights or their relative illuminating power.
fotómetro Instrumento para medir la intensidad de la luz, específicamente para comparar las intensidades relativas de luces diferentes o su poder de iluminación relativo.

photophobia Abnormal visual sensitivity to light.
fotofobia Sensibilidad visual anómala a la luz.

physiologic noise Physiologic interference with the communication process.
ruido fisiológico Interferencia fisiológica con el proceso de comunicación.

pipet A cylindric glass or plastic tube used to deliver fluids.
pipeta Tubo cilíndrico de vidrio o plástico que se usa para distribuir fluidos.

pitch The property of a sound, especially a musical tone, that is determined by the frequency of the waves producing it; the highness or lowness of sound; the relative level, intensity, or extent of some quality or state.
tono Propiedad de un sonido, especialmente de un tono musical, que está determinada por la frecuencia de las ondas que lo producen; cualidad alta o baja de un sonido; nivel, intensidad o extensión relativos de alguna cualidad o estado.

plaque An abnormal accumulation of a fatty substance.
placa Acumulación anómala de una sustancia grasa.

plasma The liquid portion of whole blood that contains active clotting agents.
plasma Parte líquida de la sangre completa que contiene agentes coagulantes activos.

policyholder The person who pays a premium to an insurance company (and in whose name the policy is written) in exchange for the protection provided by a policy of insurance.

Copyright © 2011, 2007, 2003 by Saunders, an imprint of Elsevier Inc. All rights reserved.

titular de la póliza Persona que paga una prima a una compañía aseguradora (y a cuyo nombre se contrata la póliza) a cambio de la cobertura que proporciona una póliza de seguro.

polycythemia vera A condition marked by an abnormally large number of red blood cells in the circulatory system.
policitemia vera Afección que se caracteriza por una cantidad anómalamente elevada de glóbulos rojos en el sistema circulatorio.

polydipsia Excessive thirst.
polidipsia Sed excesiva.

polymorphonuclear white blood cells Leukocytes with a segmented nucleus; also known as *polymorphonuclear neutrophils* (PMNs) or *segmented neutrophils.*
glóbulos blancos polimorfonucleares Leucocitos que tienen un núcleo segmentado; también se conocen como *neutrófilos polimorfonucleares* (PMN) o *neutrófilos segmentados.*

polyphagia Excessive appetite.
polifagia Aumento del apetito.

polyps Tumors on stems; they are frequently found in or on mucous membranes and in the mucosal lining of the colon.
pólipos Tumores en racimos que se encuentran con frecuencia en las membranas mucosas y en el recubrimiento mucoso del colon.

polyuria Excessive urine production; excretion of an unusually large amount of urine.
poliuria Producción y excreción de orina excesivas.

portal hypertension Increased venous pressure in the portal circulation caused by cirrhosis or compression of the hepatic vascular system.
hipertensión portal Aumento de la presión venosa en la circulación portal causado por cirrosis o compresión del sistema vascular hepático.

portfolio A set of pictures, drawings, documents, or photographs either bound in book form or loose in a folder.
portafolio Conjunto de ilustraciones, dibujos, documentos o fotografías, organizadas ya sea archivadas en forma de libro, o sueltas en una carpeta.

posteroanterior (PA) A frontal projection in which the patient is prone or facing the x-ray film or image receptor.
posterioanterior (PA) Proyección frontal en la que el paciente está boca abajo o de frente a la película de rayos x o al receptor de imagen.

post To transfer or carry from a book of original entry to a ledger; to enter figures in an accounting system.
asentar Transferir o traer desde un libro de entradas originales a un libro mayor; entrar cifras en un sistema de contabilidad.

postmortem Done, collected, or occurring after death.
postmortem Hecho, recogido o sucedido después de la muerte.

power of attorney A legal instrument authorizing a person to act as the attorney or agent of the grantor. The authority may be limited to the handling of specific procedures. The person authorized to act as the agent is known as the *attorney in fact.*
potestad legal Instrumento legal que autoriza a una persona a actuar como abogado o agente de la persona que le concede el poder. La autorización puede estar limitada al manejo de procedimientos específicos. La persona autorizada a actuar como agente se conoce como *abogado de hecho.*

precedence Superiority in rank, dignity, or importance; the condition of being, going, or coming ahead or in front of another.
precedencia Superioridad en rango, dignidad o importancia; condición de estar, ir o venir primero o antes.

precedent A person or thing that serves as a model; something done or said that may serve as an example or rule to authorize or justify a subsequent act of the same kind.
precedente Persona o cosa que sirve como modelo; algo hecho o dicho anteriormente y que puede servir como ejemplo o norma para autorizar o justificar un acto subsiguiente del mismo tipo.

pre-existing condition A physical condition of an insured person that existed before the issuance of the insurance policy.
afección preexistente Afección física de una persona asegurada que ya existía antes de la emisión de la póliza de seguro.

premium The consideration paid for a contract of insurance; the periodic (monthly, quarterly, or annual) payment of a specific sum of money to an insurance company that in return agrees to provide certain benefits.
prima Pago por un contrato de seguro; pago periódico (mensual, trimestral o anual) de una suma específica de dinero a una compañía aseguradora, la cual, a cambio, acepta proporcionar ciertos beneficios.

preponderance A superiority or excess in number or quantity; majority.
preponderancia Superioridad o mayor número o cantidad; mayoría.

preponderance of the evidence Evidence that is of greater weight or more convincing than the evidence

Copyright © 2011, 2007, 2003 by Saunders, an imprint of Elsevier Inc. All rights reserved.

offered in opposition to it; evidence that, as a whole, shows that the fact sought to be proven is more probable than not.
preponderancia de evidencia Evidencia que tiene mayor peso o que es más convincente que la evidencia con la que se confronta; evidencia que, en conjunto, muestra que el hecho que se pretende probar es más posible que imposible.

prerequisite Something that is necessary to achieve a result or to carry out a function.
requisito previo Algo que es necesario para obtener un resultado o para desempeñar una función.

present illness The chief complaint, written in chronologic sequence with dates of onset.
enfermedad actual Problema principal, descrito en secuencia cronológica con las fechas de cada acceso.

preservatives Substances added to a specimen to prevent deterioration of cells or chemicals.
preservativos Sustancias añadidas a un espécimen para prevenir el deterioro de células o sustancias químicas.

pressboard A strong, highly glazed composition board resembling vulcanized fiber; heavy card stock.
cartón prensado Cartón de composición resistente y muy satinado que se parece a la fibra vulcanizada; cartulina de gran resistencia.

primary diagnosis The condition or chief complaint for which a patient is treated in outpatient medical care (e.g., the physician's office or a clinic).
diagnóstico primario Afección o problema principal por el cual se trata a un paciente con atención médica externa (en un consultorio médico o una clínica).

principal A capital sum of money due as a debt or used as a fund, for which interest is either charged or paid.
principal Capital o suma de dinero que se debe como deuda o que se usa como fondo, por el cual se cargan o se cobran intereses.

principal diagnosis A condition, established after study, that is chiefly responsible for the admission of a patient to the hospital. It is used in coding inpatient hospital insurance claims.
diagnóstico principal Enfermedad o lesión que, tras su estudio, se determina que es la causa principal por la que un paciente ingresa en el hospital. Es usado en la codificación de reclamaciones de seguros de pacientes hospitalizados.

privately owned laboratories (POLs) Laboratories owned by a private individual or corporation, such as a freestanding laboratory or the laboratory inside a physician's office.
laboratorios privados (POLs) Laboratorios cuyo propietario es un individuo o una corporación privada, como el laboratorio dentro de un consultorio médico o un laboratorio independiente.

processing The way an individual internalizes new information and makes it his or her own.
procesar Forma en la que un individuo interioriza y asimila la información nueva.

procrastination Intentionally putting off doing something that should be done.
procrastinación Dejar a un lado o retrasar, de manera intencional, algo que debe hacerse.

professional behaviors Actions that identify the medical assistant as a member of a healthcare profession, including dependability, respectful patient care, initiative, positive attitude, and teamwork.
comportamientos profesionales Características que identifican al asistente médico como profesional de la atención sanitaria, incluyendo confiabilidad, trato respetuoso a los pacientes, iniciativa, actitud positiva y disposición para trabajar en equipo.

professional courtesy The reduction or omission of a fee for professional associates.
cortesía profesional Reducción o supresión de un cargo para los asociados profesionales.

professionalism Characterizing or conforming to the technical or ethical standards of a profession; exhibiting a courteous, conscientious, and generally businesslike manner in the workplace.
profesionalismo Actitud que se caracteriza por cumplir o actuar de acuerdo con los estándares técnicos y éticos de una profesión; dar muestras de cortesía, meticulosidad y, en general, mostrar un comportamiento adecuado en el lugar de trabajo.

proficiency Competency as a result of training or practice.
pericia Estado de competencia en algo, que se alcanza por medio de entrenamiento o práctica.

profit sharing An offer of part of the company's profits to employees or other designated individuals or groups.
participación en los beneficios Oferta de parte de los beneficios de la compañía a los empleados u otros individuos o grupos designados.

progress notes Notes entered in a patient's chart to track the individual's progress and condition.
notas del progreso Notas escritas en historial médico del paciente para seguir el progreso y estado del mismo.

prokaryote A unicellular organism that lacks a membrane-bound nucleus.
procaryota Organismo unicelular cuyo núcleo no está unido por una membrana.

Copyright © 2011, 2007, 2003 by Saunders, an imprint of Elsevier Inc. All rights reserved.

prolactin (PRL) A hormone secreted by the anterior pituitary gland that stimulates the development of the mammary gland.
prolactina (PRL) Hormona que segrega la glándula pituitaria anterior y que estimula el desarrollo de la glándula mamaria.

proofread To read text and mark corrections.
corregir pruebas Leer un texto y marcar correcciones.

prosthesis An artificial replacement for a body part.
prótesis Pieza artificial para reemplazar una parte del cuerpo.

proteins Organic compounds in plants and animals that contain the major elements carbon, hydrogen, oxygen, and nitrogen and the amino acids essential to maintain life.
proteínas Compuestos orgánicos que existen en plantas y animales y que contienen los elementos principales: carbón, hidrógeno, oxígeno y nitrógeno y los aminoácidos esenciales para el mantenimiento de la vida.

provider An individual or company that provides medical care and services to patients or the public.
proveedor Individuo o compañía que proporciona atenciones y servicios médicos pacientes o al público.

provisional diagnosis A temporary diagnosis made before all test results have been received.
diagnóstico provisional Diagnóstico temporal llevado a cabo antes de recibir todos los resultados de las pruebas.

proxemics The study of the nature, degree, and effect of the spatial separation individuals naturally maintain.
proxemia Estudio de la naturaleza, grado y efecto de la separación espacial que los individuos mantienen de forma natural.

prudent Marked by wisdom or judiciousness; shrewd in the management of practical affairs.
prudente Caracterizado por poseer sabiduría o sensatez; hábil en el manejo de los asuntos prácticos.

psoriasis A usually chronic, recurrent skin disease marked by bright red patches covered with silvery scales.
psoriasis Enfermedad recurrente de la piel, por lo general crónica, caracterizada por manchas de color rojo brillante cubiertas por escamas plateadas.

psychosocial Pertaining to a combination of psychological and social factors.
psicosocial Perteneciente o relativo a una combinación de factores psicológicos y sociales.

public domain The realm embracing property rights that belong to the community at large, are unprotected by copyright or patent, and are subject to appropriation by anyone.
dominio público Campo que abarca los derechos de propiedad que pertenecen a la comunidad en general, que no están protegidos por leyes de derechos de autor ni por patentes y están sujetos a apropiación por parte de cualquiera.

pulmonary consolidation In pneumonia, the process by which the lungs become solidified as they fill with exudates.
solidificación pulmonar Proceso por el cual los pulmones se vuelven rígidos a medida que se llenan con exudados en los casos de pulmonía.

pulse deficit A condition in which the radial pulse is less than the apical pulse. It may indicate a peripheral vascular abnormality.
déficit del pulso Cuando el pulso radial es menor que el apical. Puede indicar una anomalía vascular periférica.

pulse pressure The difference between the systolic and the diastolic blood pressures (less than 30 points or more than 50 points is considered normal).
presión del pulso Diferencia entre las presiones sanguíneas sistólica y diastólica (menos de 30 puntos o más de 50 puede considerarse normal).

pure culture A bacterial or fungal culture that contains a single organism.
cultivo puro Cultivo de bacterias u hongos que contiene un solo organismo.

putrefaction The decomposition of organic matter, which produces a foul smell.
putrefacción Descomposición de materia orgánica que da como resultado un olor fétido.

pyemia The presence of pus-forming organisms in the blood.
piemia Presencia en la sangre de organismos formadores de pus.

quackery The pretense of curing disease.
curanderismo Práctica del que finge curar enfermedades.

quality control An aggregate of activities designed to ensure adequate quality, especially in manufactured products or in the service industries.
control de calidad Conjunto de actividades destinadas a garantizar la calidad adecuada, en especial en productos manufacturados o en las industrias de servicios.

queries Requests for information from a database.
consultas Peticions de información de una base de datos.

Copyright © 2011, 2007, 2003 by Saunders, an imprint of Elsevier Inc. All rights reserved.

rad The conventional unit of absorbed radiation dose.
rad Unidad convencional de dosis de radiación absorbido.

radiograph An x-ray image.
radiografía Imagen obtenida con el uso de rayos-x.

radiographer A person qualified to perform radiographic examinations.
técnico de radiología Persona cualificada para realizar exámenes radiológicos.

radiography Making diagnostic images using x-rays.
radiografía Proceso de diagnosticar imágenes usando rayos x.

radiologist A physician who specializes in medical imaging and/or therapeutic applications of radiation.
médico radiólogo Médico especialista en formación de imágenes o en aplicaciones terapéuticas de la radiación.

radiolucent Referring to a substance that is easily penetrated by x-rays; these substances appear dark on radiographs.
transparente a la radiación Término que se aplica a una substancia que puede ser penetrada con facilidad por los rayos x; estas substancias aparecen oscuras en las radiografías.

radiopaque Referring to a substance that can be easily seen on an x-ray image (i.e., is is not easily penetrated by x-rays); these substances appear light on radiographs.
opaco a la radiación Sustancia que puede visualizarse con facilidad en la imagen de rayos x. Término que se aplica a una substancia que no puede ser penetrada con facilidad por los rayos x; estas substancias aparecen claras en las radiografías.

rales Abnormal or crackling breath sounds during inspiration.
estertores Sonidos respiratorios o crujidos anómalos durante la inspiración.

ramifications Consequences produced by a cause or following from a set of conditions.
ramificaciones Consecuencias producidas por una causa o que siguen a una serie de estados.

rapport A relationship of harmony and accord between the patient and the healthcare professional.
concordia Relación de armonía y acuerdo entre el paciente y el profesional de la atención sanitaria.

Raynaud's phenomenon Intermittent attacks of ischemia in the extremities that result in cyanosis, numbness, tingling, and pain.
fenómeno de Raynaud Ataques intermitentes de isquemia en las extremidades, resultando en cianosis, entumecimiento, picazón y dolor.

RBRVS (resource-based relative value system) A fee schedule designed to provide national uniform payment of Medicare benefits after adjustment to reflect the differences in practice costs across geographic areas.
RBRVS (sistema de valor relativo basado en recursos) Escala de cargos diseñada para proporcionar un pago de beneficios de Medicare uniforme a nivel nacional después de haber sido ajustado para reflejar las diferencias en los costos prácticos a través de áreas geográficas.

ream A quantity of paper consisting of 20 quires or variously 480, 500, or 516 sheets.
resma Una cantidad de papel que consiste de 20 manos o que varía entre 480, 500 o 516 hojas.

reasonable doubt Doubt based on reason and arising from evidence or lack of evidence; not doubt that is imagined or conjured up, but doubt that would cause reasonable persons to hesitate before acting in a manner important to themselves.
duda razonable Duda basada en la razón o que surge de evidencia o falta de evidencia; no es una duda imaginaria ni inventada, sino una duda que puede hacer que una persona razonable vacile antes de dar un paso importante.

receipts Amounts paid on patients' accounts.
recibos Sumas pagadas en las cuentas de los pacientes.

recipient The receiver of something.
receptor El que recibe un artículo u objeto.

rectify To correct by removing errors.
rectificar Corregir eliminando errores.

reduction The return of a structure to its correct anatomic position, as in the reduction of a fracture.
reducción Regreso a la posición anatómica correcta, como en el caso de reducción de una fractura.

referral (reference) laboratory A private or hospital-based laboratory that performs a wide variety of tests, many of them specialized. Physicians often send specimens collected in the office to referral laboratories for testing.
laboratorio de referencia Laboratorio privado o de un hospital que realiza una amplia gama de análisis, muchos de ellos especializados. Con frecuencia los médicos envían especímenes recogidos en la consulta a estos laboratorios para ser analizados.

reflection The process of considering new information and internalizing it to create new ways of examining information.

Copyright © 2011, 2007, 2003 by Saunders, an imprint of Elsevier Inc. All rights reserved.

reflexión Proceso de estudiar información nueva e interiorizarla para crear formas nuevas de examinar información.

refractile Capable of causing light rays to bend, thus altering or distorting an image.
refractante Capaz de provocar la refracción de la luz, desviación alterando o distorcionando una imagen.

registered dietitian (RD) A professionally certified person with a bachelor's degree in food and nutrition who is concerned with the maintenance and promotion of health and the treatment of diseases through proper diet.
dietista registrado (RD) Profesional certificado persona con titulación universitaria en alimentos y nutrición y que se preocupa del mantenimiento y-la promoción de la salud y el tratamiento de las enfermedades a través de la dieta adecuado.

relapse The recurrence of disease symptoms after apparent recovery.
recaída Recurrencia de los síntomas de una enfermedad tras una aparente recuperación.

relevant Having a significant and demonstrable bearing on the matter at hand.
pertinente Que tiene una relación importante y demostrable con el asunto que se está tratando.

rem The dose of ionizing radiation equivalent to 1 roentgen of x-ray exposure.
rem La dosis de radiación ionizante equivalente a un roentgen de exposición a rayos x.

remission A decrease in the severity of a disease or symptoms; the partial or complete disappearance of the clinical and subjective characteristics of a chronic or malignant disease.
remisión Disminución de la gravedad de una enfermedad o sus síntomas; desaparición parcial o total de las características clínicas y subjetivas de una enfermedad crónica o maligna.

remittent fever A fever in which a patient's temperature fluctuates greatly but never falls to the normal level.
fiebre remitente Fiebre en la cual la temperatura fluctúa mucho pero nunca baja al nivel normal.

renal threshold The level above which a substance cannot be reabsorbed by the renal tubules and therefore is excreted in the urine.
umbral renal Nivel por encima del cual una sustancia no puede ser reabsorbida por los túbulos renales y por lo tanto es excretada en la orina.

reparations The act of making amends, offering atonement, or giving satisfaction for a wrong or injury.
reparaciones Acción de enmendar u ofrecer compensaciones por un error o un daño.

reprimands Criticisms for a fault; a severe or formal reproof.
reprimendas Críticas por una falta; reprobación severa o formal.

reproach An expression of rebuke or disapproval; a cause or occasion for blame, discredit, or disgrace.
reproche Expresión de crítica o desaprobación; causa o motivo de culpa, descrédito u oprobio.

requisites Things considered essential or necessary.
requisitos Cosas que se consideran esenciales o necesarias.

resolution The ability of the eye to distinguish two objects that are very close together; the sharpness of an image.
resolución Capacidad del ojo para distinguir dos objetos que están muy cerca uno del otro; nitidez de una imagen.

retention Keeping something in possession or use; to keep someone's pay or service.
retención El hecho de mantener en posesión o en uso; mantener a alguien a su servicio o como empleado.

retention schedule A method or plan for retaining or keeping track of medical records and their movement from active to inactive to closed filing.
plan de retención Método o plan para retener o guardar expedientes médicos, y el paso de los mismos del estado de expediente activo a pasivo y a cerrado.

retribution The giving or receiving of reward or punishment; something given or exacted in recompense.
retribución Acto de dar o recibir una recompensa o castigo; algo que se da o se cobra como recompensa.

rhinitis Inflammation of the mucous membranes of the nose.
rinitis Inflamación de las membranas mucosas de la nariz.

rhonchi Abnormal rumbling sounds during expiration that indicate airway obstruction caused by thick secretions or spasms; a continuous, dry rattling in the throat or bronchial tube resulting from partial obstruction.
ronquido Ruido sordo y anómalo durante la expiración que indica obstrucción de las vías respiratorias debido a secreciones espesas o a espasmos; ruido seco y continuo en la garganta o en el tubo bronquial debido a una obstrucción parcial.

rider A special provision or group of provisions added to an insurance policy to expand or limit the benefits otherwise payable. A rider may increase or decrease benefits, waive a condition or coverage, or in any other way amend the original contract.

Copyright © 2011, 2007, 2003 by Saunders, an imprint of Elsevier Inc. All rights reserved.

cláusula adicional Provisión o conjunto de provisiones especiales añadidas a una póliza de seguro para ampliar o limitar los beneficios que de otro modo se pueden pagar. Puede aumentar o disminuir beneficios, anular una condición o cobertura o puede enmendar el contrato original de otra manera.

robotics Technology dealing with the design, construction, and operation of robots in automation.
robótica Tecnología de la automatización que se ocupa del diseño, construcción y operación de robots.

rods Structures in the retina of the eye that form the light-sensitive elements.
bastoncillos Estructuras que están en la retina del ojo y constituyen los elementos sensibles a la luz.

Roentgen (R) The conventional unit of radiation exposure.
Roentgen (R) Unidad convencional de exposición a radiación.

router A device used to connect any number of LANs that communicate with other routers and determine the best route between any two hosts.
direccionador Dispositivo usado para conectar cualquier cantidad de LAN que se comunican con otros direccionadores para determinar la mejor ruta entre dos computadoras conectadas a una red.

sagittal plane The plane that divides the body into right and left halves.
plano sagital Plano que divide el cuerpo en la mitad derecha y la mitad izquierda.

salutation Words or gestures that express greeting, good will, or courtesy.
saludo Expresión de saludo, buenos deseos o cortesía por medio de palabras o gestos.

sanitization Reduction of the number of potentially harmful microorganisms to a relatively safe level.
saneamiento Reducción del número de microorganismos a un nivel relativamente seguro.

sarcasm A sharp or satiric response or ironic utterance designed to cause pain.
sarcasmo Respuesta aguda y frecuentemente satírica o declaración irónica destinada a burlarse o a lastimar.

scanner A device that reads text or illustrations on a printed page and translates the information into a form the computer can understand.
escáner Dispositivo que lee texto o ilustraciones de una página impresa y traduce esa información a un formato comprensible para la computadora.

sclera The white part of the eye that encloses the eyeball.
esclerótica Parte blanca del ojo que encierra el globo ocular.

scleroderma An autoimmune disorder that affects the blood vessels and connective tissue, causing fibrous degeneration of the major organs.
escleroderma Trastorno autoinmune que afecta a los vasos sanguíneos y los tejidos conectivos provocando degeneración en las fibras de los órganos principales.

sclerotherapy The injection of sclerosing (hardening) solutions to treat hemorrhoids, varicose veins, or esophageal varices.
escleroterapia Inyección de soluciones de esclerosis (endorecedores) para tratar hemorroides, venas varicosas o varices esofágicas.

scoliosis An abnormal lateral curvature of the spine.
escoliosis Curvatura lateral anómala de la columna.

scored tablet A drug tablet manufactured with an indentation that allows the tablet to be broken or cut into equal parts.
tableta con hendidura Tableta que se fabrica con una hendidura que permite dividirla o romperla en partes iguales.

screen Something that shields, protects, or hides; to select or eliminate products or applicants by comparing them with a set of desired criteria.
pantalla Algo que actúa como escudo, que protege u oculta para permitir un proceso de selección.

search engines Computer programs that search documents for keywords and return a list of documents containing those words.
buscadores Programas de computadoras que buscan documentos a partir de palabras clave y proporcionan una lista de los documentos que contienen esas palabras.

seborrhea An excessive discharge of sebum from the sebaceous glands, forming greasy scales on the skin or cheesy plugs in skin pores.
seborrea Descarga excesiva de sebo de las glándulas sebáceas, formando escamas de grasa en la piel o tapones con aspecto de queso en los poros de la piel.

secondary hypertension Elevated blood pressure caused by another medical condition.
hipertensión secundaria Presión sanguínea elevada causada por otra enfermedad o afección médica.

"see" In coding manuals, an instruction to the coder to look in another place; found in volumes 2 and 3 of the Alphabetic Index, this instruction must always be followed.
"ver" Instrucción que se le da a la persona encargada de la codificación para que consulte en

Copyright © 2011, 2007, 2003 by Saunders, an imprint of Elsevier Inc. All rights reserved.

otro lugar. Siempre debe seguirse esta instrucción; la expresión se encuentra en el Índice alfabético, tomos 2 y 3.

"see also" In coding manuals, an instruction to the coder to look elsewhere if the main term or subterm(s) for an entry are not sufficient for coding the information. If a code number follows, "see also" is enclosed in parentheses; if there is no code number, "see also" is preceded by a dash.
"ver también" Instrucción que se le da a la persona encargada de la codificación para que consulte en algún otro lugar si el término o subtérminos principales para una entrada no son suficientes para codificar la información. Si "ver también" va seguido por un número de código, dicho código va entre paréntesis; si no hay número de código, "ver también" va precedido por un guión.

"see category" In coding manuals, an instruction to the coder to refer to a specific category (three-digit code); it must always be followed.
"ver categoría" Instrucción que se le da a la persona encargada de la codificación para que consulte una categoría específica (código de tres dígitos); Siempre debe seguirse.

self-insured plans Insurance plans funded by organizations with a large enough employee base that they can afford to fund their own insurance program.
planes de autoaseguración Planes de seguros implementados por organizaciones con un número de empleados lo suficientemente grande como para permitirles financiar su propio programa de seguros.

sequentially Happening in relation to or by arrangement in a sequence.
secuencial Aquello que ocurre relativo a una secuencia o que es ordenado en secuencia.

serous Pertaining to a thin, watery, serumlike drainage.
seroso Perteneciente o relativo a una materia poco espesa, acuosa, parecida al suero.

serum The portion of whole blood that remains liquid after the blood has clotted.
suero La porción de la sangre que queda líquida después de la coagulación.

service benefit plan A plan that provides benefits in the form of certain surgical and medical services rendered rather than in cash. A service benefit plan is not restricted to a fee schedule.
plan de beneficios de servicio Plan que proporciona beneficios en forma de ciertos servicios médico-quirúrgicos en vez de con dinero en metálico. Un plan de servicio de beneficio no está restringido por una escala de cargos.

sheath The covering surrounding the axon of the nerve cell that acts as an electrical insulator to speed conduction of nerve impulses.
película Recubrimiento que rodea los axones de la célula nerviosa y que se comporta como aislante eléctrico para aumentar la velocidad de conducción del impulso nervioso.

shingling A method of filing whereby each new report is laid on top of the previous report, resembling the shingles of a roof.
laminado Método de archivo en el cual cada informe nuevo se coloca encima del informe anterior, del mismo modo que se colocan las tejas en un techo.

Sievert (Sv) The international unit of radiation dose equivalent.
Sievert (Sv) Unidad internacional de dosis equivalentes de radiación.

sinoatrial (SA) node The pacemaker of the heart, located in the right atrium.
nódulo sinoauricular (SA) Marcapasos del corazón que se halla en la aurícula derecha.

sinus arrhythmia An irregular heartbeat that originates in the sinoatrial (pacemaker) node.
arritmia de seno Ritmo cardiaco irregular que tiene su origen en el nódulo sinoauricular (marcapasos).

socioeconomic Relating to a combination of social and economic factors.
socioeconómico Perteneciente o relativo a una combinación de factores sociales y económicos.

sociologic Oriented or directed toward social needs and problems.
sociologico Que se orienta o dirige hacia las necesidades y problemas sociales.

sonography An imaging modality that uses sound waves to produce images of soft tissues; also called *diagnostic ultrasound.*
sonografía Modalidad de formación de imágenes que usa ondas sonoras para producir imágenes de los tejidos blandos; también se conoce como *ultrasonido de diagnóstico.*

sound card A device that allows a computer to output sound through speakers connected to the main circuitry board (motherboard).
tarjeta de sonido Dispositivo que le permite a una computadora emitir sonido a través de altavoces conectados a la tarjeta principal del circuito.

specimen A sample of body fluid, waste product, or tissue that is collected for analysis and diagnosis.
espécimen Muestra de un fluido corporal, residuo o tejido que se usa para análisis y diagnósticos.

Copyright © 2011, 2007, 2003 by Saunders, an imprint of Elsevier Inc. All rights reserved.

spirometer An instrument that measures the volume of inhaled and exhaled air.
espirómetro Instrumento que sirve para medir el volumen del aire inhalado y exhalado.

spores Thick-walled reproductive cells formed within bacteria and capable of withstanding unfavorable environmental conditions; they are very resistant to disinfection measures.
esporas Células reproductoras de paredes gruesas que se forman dentro de las bacterias y son capaces de resistir condiciones ambientales adversas; tipos de bacterias letárgicas de paredes gruesas que son muy resistentes a las medidas de desinfección.

staff privileges Authorization for a healthcare professional to practice within a specific facility.
privilegios del personal Autorización para un profesional de atención sanitaria, para ejercer la práctica dentro de unas instalaciones específicas.

standards Items or indicators used to measure quality or compliance with a statutory or accrediting body's policies and regulations.
estándares Artículos o indicadores usados para medir la calidad o cumplimiento de las pólizas y-regulaciones de un cuerpo normativo o acreditativo.

stat A medical term meaning "immediately" or "at this moment"; an order found on a laboratory requisition that indicates that the test must be done immediately (from the Latin word *statin,* meaning "at once").
stat Abreviatura usada en medicina que significa inmediatamente o ahora mismo. Orden encontrada en un pedido de laboratorio que indica que el análisis debe llevarse a cabo inmediatamente (de la palabra latina statin, que significa "ahora"); inmediatamente.

stationers Sellers of writing paper.
dependientes de papelería Vendedores de artículos de papelería.

statute A law enacted by the legislative branch of a government.
estatuto Ley sancionada por la rama legislativa de un gobierno.

stereotactic An x-ray procedure to guide the insertion of a needle into a specific area of the breast.
estereotáctico Procedimiento de rayos x para guiar la inserción de una aguja en zonas específicas del pecho.

stereotype Something conforming to a fixed or general pattern; a standardized mental picture that is held in common by many and represents an oversimplified opinion, prejudiced attitude, or uncritical judgment.
estereotipo Algo que se ajusta a un patrón fijado o general; imagen mental estandarizada que tienen en común muchas personas y que representa opiniones simplificadas, actitudes con prejuicios o razonamientos carentes de sentido crítico.

sterilization Complete destruction of all forms of microbial life.
esterilización Destrucción total de toda forma de vida microbiana.

stertorous Referring to a strenuous respiratory effort marked by a snoring sound.
estertóreo Esfuerzo respiratorio penoso que tiene el sonido de un ronquido.

stipulate To specify as a condition or requirement of an agreement or offer; to make an agreement or covenant to do or forbear from doing something.
estipular Especificar como condición o requisito de un acuerdo u oferta; establecer un acuerdo o prometer hacer, o dejar de hacer, algo.

stock option An offer of stocks for purchase to a certain individual or to certain groups, such as employees of a for-profit hospital.
opción sobre acciones Oferta de venta de acciones que se le hace a un ciertos individuos o grupos, como a los empleados de un hospital.

stressors Stimuli that cause stress.
estresantes Dícese de los estímulos que causan estrés.

stridor A shrill, harsh respiratory sound heard during inhalation during laryngeal obstruction.
estridor Sonido respiratorio estridente que se oye durante la inhalación en los casos de obstrucción laríngea.

stroke Sudden paralysis and/or loss of consciousness caused by extreme trauma or injury to an artery in the brain.
apoplejía Súbita pérdida de conocimiento y parálisis causada por una lesión o daño grave de una arteria del cerebro.

stylus A metal probe inserted into or passed through a catheter, needle, or tube to clear the device or to facilitate its passage into a body orifice.
punzón Sonda metálica que se inserta o pasa por medio de un catéter, aguja o tubo y que se usa para limpiar o para facilitar el paso a un orificio del cuerpo.

subjective information Information gained by questioning the patient or taking it from a form.
información subjetiva Información obtienida haciendo preguntas al paciente o tomándola de un formulario.

Copyright © 2011, 2007, 2003 by Saunders, an imprint of Elsevier Inc. All rights reserved.

subluxation Incomplete dislocation of a bone from its normal anatomic location.
subluxación Dislocación incompleta de un hueso desde su posición anatómica normal.

subluxations Slight misalignments of the vertebrae or partial dislocations.
subluxaciones Alineamientos ligeramente defectuosos o dislocaciones parciales de las vértebras.

subordinate Submissive to or controlled by authority; placed in or occupying a lower class, rank, or position.
subordinado Que está sometido a una autoridad o controlado por ella; que ostenta un cargo u ocupa una clase, rango o puesto inferior.

subpoena A writ or document commanding a person to appear in court under penalty for failure to appear.
subpoena Documento escrito ordenando a una persona comparecer en el juzgado bajo penalidad en caso de no comparecencia.

substance number A number based on the weight of a ream of paper containing 500 sheets.
número de sustancia Número basado en el peso de una resma de papel de 500 hojas.

subtle Difficult to understand or perceive; having or marked by keen insight and the ability to penetrate deeply and thoroughly.
sutil Difícil de comprender o percibir; que tiene perspicacia y la capacidad de penetrar a fondo y en toda su extensión en un asunto.

succinct Marked by compact, precise expression without wasted words.
sucinto Caracterizado por una expresión precisa y concisa sin palabras inútiles.

superfluous Exceeding what is sufficient or necessary.
superfluos Que exceden aquello que es suficiente o necesario.

suppurative Forming and/or discharging pus.
supuración Formación o emisión de pus.

surrogate A substitute; something put in place of another.
subrogado Sustituto; puesto en lugar de otro.

switch In networks, a device that filters information between LAN segments, reduces overall network traffic, and increases the speed and efficiency of bandwidth use.
conmutador En las redes de comunicación, dispositivo que filtra información entre segmentos de LAN y disminuye el tráfico global de la red, aumentando la velocidad y la eficacia en el uso del ancho de banda.

syncope Fainting; a brief lapse in consciousness.
síncope Desmayo; lapso breve en estado de consciencia.

syndrome A group of signs and symptoms related to a common cause or presenting a clinical picture of a disease or an inherited abnormality.
síndrome Conjunto de signos y síntomas relacionados con una causa común o que presentan el cuadro clínico de una enfermedad o una anomalía heredada.

synopsis A condensed statement or outline.
sinopsis Declaración resumida; resumen.

synovial fluid Clear fluid found in joint cavities that facilitates smooth movement and nourishes joint structures.
fluido sinovial Fluido claro que se halla en las cavidades de las articulaciones y que facilita los movimientos suaves y nutre las estructuras articulatorias.

tachycardia A rapid but regular heart rate; one that exceeds 100 beats per minute.
taquicardia Ritmo cardiaco rápido pero regular que sobrepasa los 100 latidos por minuto.

tachypnea Respiration that is rapid and shallow; hyperventilation.
taquipnea Respiración rápida y profunda; hiperventilación.

tactful Having a keen sense of what to do or say to maintain good relations with others or avoid offense.
tacto Tener un sentido de lo que se debe hacer o decir para mantener buenas relaciones con los demás y evitar ofenderlos.

target organ The organ affected by a particular hormone.
órgano objetivo Órgano afectado por una hormona específica.

target tissue A group of cells affected by a particular hormone.
tejido objetivo Grupo de células afectadas por una hormona específica.

targeted to Directed toward a specific desire, position, or effect.
dirigido a Dirigido a un fin o meta específico, usado hacia un fin; dirigido hacia un deseo o un puesto específico.

TCP/IP Abbreviation for *transmission control protocol/Internet protocol;* a suite of communications protocols used to connect users or hosts to the Internet.

Copyright © 2011, 2007, 2003 by Saunders, an imprint of Elsevier Inc. All rights reserved.

TCP/IP Abreviatura de *protocolo de control de transmisión/protocolo Internet;* conjunto de protocolos de comunicación que se usa para conectar usuarios o computadoras a Internet.

tedious Tiresome because of length or dullness.
tedioso Que cansa porque es demasiado largo o aburrido.

telecommunications The science and technology of communication by transmission of information from one location to another via telephone, television, telegraph, or satellite.
telecomunicaciones Ciencia y tecnología de la comunicación basada en la transmisión de información de un lugar a otro por teléfono, televisión, telégrafo o satélite.

telemedicine The use of telecommunications in the practice of medicine, allowing great distances between healthcare professionals, colleagues, patients, and students.
telemedicina Uso de las telecomunicaciones en la práctica médica, permitiendo la comunicación entre profesionales de atención sanitaria, colegas, pacientes y estudiantes que se hallan a grandes distancias.

teleradiology The use of telecommunications devices to enhance and improve the results of radiologic procedures.
telerradiología Uso de dispositivos de telecomunicación para mejorar y perfeccionar los resultados de procedimientos radiológicos.

tendon A tough band of connective tissue that connects muscle to bone.
tendón Banda resistente de tejido conectivo que conecta los músculos con los huesos.

teratogen Any substance that interferes with normal prenatal development.
teratógeno Cualquier sustancia que interfiere con el desarrollo prenatal normal.

teratogenic A substance known to cause birth defects.
teratogénico Sustancia que se sabe que provoca defectos de nacimiento.

testimony A solemn declaration usually made orally by a witness under oath in response to interrogation by a lawyer or an authorized public official.
testimonio Declaración solemne, por lo general oral, hecha por un testigo bajo juramento como respuesta a una pregunta (o preguntas) de un abogado o un funcionario público autorizado.

thanatology The description or study of the phenomena of death and of psychological methods of coping with death.
tanatología Descripción o estudio del fenómeno de la muerte y de los métodos psicológicos para hacerle frente.

third-party payer An entity (usually an insurance company) that makes a payment on an obligation or debt but is not a party to the contract that created the debt.
pagador mediador Entidad (por lo general una compañía aseguradora) que hace un pago de una obligación o deuda pero que no es parte del contrato que ha creado dicha deuda.

third-party payer Someone other than the patient, spouse, or parent who is responsible for paying all or part of the patient's medical costs.
pagador mediador Alguien ajeno al paciente, cónyuge, padre o madre que es responsable del pago de todo o parte de los gastos médicos del paciente o de parte de ellos.

thixotropic gel A material that appears to be a solid until subjected to a disturbance, such as centrifugation, when it becomes a liquid.
gel tisotrópico Material que parece ser sólido hasta el momento en que se somete a una alteración como la centrifugación, cuando se convierte en líquido.

thoracic Pertaining to the region between the neck and low back that contains the 12 thoracic vertebrae.
torácica Perteneciente o relativo a región de la espalda entre el cuello y la región lumbar inferior en la que hay 12 vértebras torácicas.

thready pulse A pulse that is scarcely perceptible.
pulso débil Pulso que es apenas perceptible.

thrombus A blood clot.
trombo Cóagulo de sangre.

thyroid-stimulating hormone (TSH) A hormone secreted by the anterior lobe of the pituitary gland that stimulates the secretion of hormones produced by the thyroid gland.
hormona estimulante de la tiroides (TSH) Hormona que segrega el lóbulo anterior de la glándula pituitaria y que estimula la secreción de hormonas producidas por la glándula tiroides.

tickler file A chronologic file used as a reminder that something must be taken care of on a certain date.
archivo cronológico Archivo que se usa para recordar que algo que debe llevarse a cabo en una fecha determinada.

tinea A fungal skin disease that results in scaling, itching, and inflammation.
tinea Enfermedad de la piel causada por hongos y que produce descamación, picazón e inflamación.

Copyright © 2011, 2007, 2003 by Saunders, an imprint of Elsevier Inc. All rights reserved.

tissue culture The technique or process of keeping tissue alive and growing in a culture medium.
cultivo de tejidos Técnica o proceso de mantener un tejido vivo y en fase de crecimiento en un medio de cultivo.

toxemia An abnormal condition of pregnancy characterized by hypertension, edema, and protein in the urine.
toxemia Característica anómala del embarazo, con presencia de hipertensión, edema y proteínas en la orina.

tracer A radioactive substance administered to a patient undergoing a nuclear medicine imaging procedure.
trazador Sustancia radioactiva que se administra al paciente para someterlo a procedimientos de formación de imágenes en medicina nuclear.

tracheostomy A surgical opening through the neck into the trachea that is made to facilitate breathing.
traqueotomía Abertura realizada quirúrgicamente en el cuello a la altura de la tráquea para facilitar la respiración.

transaction An exchange or transfer of goods, services, or funds.
transacción Intercambio o transferencia de bienes, servicios o fondos.

transcription A written copy made either in longhand or by machine.
transcripción Copia escrita de algo, hecha a mano, o con la ayuda de una máquina.

transducer The part of the sonography machine in contact with the patient that sends high-frequency sound waves and receives the sound echoes that return from the patient's body.
transductor Parte de una máquina de sonografía que está en contacto con el paciente envía ondas sonoras de alta frecuencia y recibe los ecos de los sonidos que regresan del cuerpo del paciente.

transection A cross-section; division by cutting across.
sección transversal División cortando a través.

transient ischemic attack A condition of temporary neurologic symptoms caused by gradual or partial occlusion of a cerebral blood vessel.
ataque isquémico transitorio Síntomas neurológicos temporales causados por una oclusión gradual o parcial de un vaso sanguíneo del cerebro.

transillumination Inspection of a cavity or an organ by passing light through its walls.
diafanoscopia Inspección de una cavidad u órgano haciendo pasar luz a través de sus paredes. transport medium A medium used to keep an organism alive during transport to the laboratory. medio para transporte Medio usado para mantener un organismo vivo durante el transporte al laboratorio.

transverse plane The plane that divides the body into superior and inferior parts.
plano transversal Plano que divide el cuerpo en parte superior e inferior.

trauma A physical injury or wound caused by an external force or by violence.
trauma Lesión física o herida causada por una fuerza externa o violencia.

treatises Systematic expositions or arguments in writing, including methodic discussion of the facts and principles involved and the conclusions reached.
tratados Exposiciones sistemáticas o argumentos escritos que incluyen una descripción metódica de los hechos y principios involucrados y las conclusiones a las que se ha llegado.

triage A process of responding to requests for immediate care and treatment after evaluating the urgency of the need and prioritizing the treatment; the sorting and allocation of treatment to patients according to a system of priorities designed to maximize the number of survivors and treat the sickest patients first.
criterio de selección Responder a peticiones de atención y tratamiento inmediato tras evaluar la urgencia de la necesidad y establecer prioridades de tratamiento. Clasificación y asignación de tratamiento a pacientes según un sistema de prioridades destinado a maximizar el número de sobrevivientes y tratar primero a los pacientes más enfermos.

triglycerides Fatty acids and glycerols that are bound to proteins and form high- and low-density lipoproteins.
triglicéridos Ácidos grasos y gliceroles que se unen a las proteínas y forman lipoproteínas de alta y baja densidad.

truss An elastic, canvas, or metallic device for retaining a reduced hernia within the abdominal cavity.
braguero Malla elástica o dispositivo metálico para retener una hernia reducida dentro de la cavidad abdominal.

turgor The resistance of the skin to being grasped between the fingers and released; normal skin tension, which is reduced with dehydration and increased with edema.
turgor Resistencia de la piel a ser pellizcada; tensión normal de la piel que disminuye con la deshidratación y aumenta con el edema.

type and cross-match Tests performed to assess the compatibility of blood intended for transfusion with the person's own blood.

Copyright © 2011, 2007, 2003 by Saunders, an imprint of Elsevier Inc. All rights reserved.

prueba de tipo y RH Análisis que se realizan para evaluar la compatibilidad de la sangre que va a ser usada en una transfusión.

unequal pulses Pulses in which the beats vary in intensity.
pulso desigual Pulso en el cual los latidos varían en intensidad.

Uniform Commercial Code A unified set of rules covering many business transactions; often referred to simply as the UCC, it has been adopted in all 50 states, the District of Columbia, and most U.S. territories.
Código de Comercio Uniforme Conjunto de normas unificadas que cubren muchas transacciones comerciales; se conoce simplemente como UCC y ha sido adoptado en los 50 estados, el Distrito de Columbia y la mayoría de los territorios estadounidenses.

unique identifiers Codes used as part of a method of anonymous HIV testing in which the code is used, instead of a name, to protect the patient's confidentiality.
identificadores únicos Método de prueba de VIH (HIV) anónimo en el cual se usa un código en lugar de nombres, para proteger la confidencialidad del paciente.

unit-dose A method used by a pharmacy to prepare individual doses of medications.
dosis unitaria Método usado por la farmacia para preparar dosis individuales de medicamentos.

universal claim form The form developed by the HCFA (now known as the Centers for Medicare and Medicaid Services [CMS]) and approved by the American Medical Association (AMA) for use in submitting all government-sponsored claims.
formulario de reclamación universal Formulario desarrollado por la Administración financiera de la atención sanitaria (HCFA, ahora conocida como Centros de servicios de Medicare y Medicaid, o CMS) y aprobado por AMA para usarse al someter todas las reclamaciones subvencionadas por el gobierno.

upper GI series Fluoroscopic examination of the esophagus, stomach, and duodenum in which orally administered barium sulfate is used a contrast medium.
serie GI superior Examen fluoroscópico del esófago, estómago y duodeno usando una administración oral de sulfato de bario como medio de contraste.

urea The major nitrogenous end product of protein metabolism and the chief nitrogenous component of the urine.
urea Principal producto final nitrogenado del metabolismo de las proteínas y el principal componente nitrogenado de la orina.

urease An enzyme that catalyzes the hydrolysis of urea to form ammonium carbonate.
ureasa Enzima que cataliza la hidrólisis de la urea para formar carbonato de amonio.

uremia A toxic renal condition characterized by an excess of urea, creatinine, and other nitrogenous end products in the blood.
uremia Enfermedad renal tóxica que se caracteriza por un exceso de urea, creatinina y otros productos finales en la sangre.

urgency A sudden, compelling desire to urinate and the inability to control the release of urine.
urgencia Deseo repentino y apremiante de orinar y la incapacidad de controlarlo.

URL Abbreviation for *uniform resource locator;* the global address of documents or information on the Internet. The URL provides the IP address and the domain name for the Web page, such as "microsoft.com."
URL Abreviatura de *localizador universal de recursos;* la dirección a nivel mundial, de documentos o de información en Internet. El URL proporciona la dirección IP y el nombre del dominio de una página web, como por ejemplo: "microsoft.com."

urticaria A skin eruption marked by inflamed wheals; hives.
urticaria Erupción cutánea que produce ampollas imflamadas.

"use additional code" In coding manuals, this term appears only in volume 1 of the ICD-9-CM in those subdivisions where the user should add further information by means of an additional code to give a more complete picture of the diagnosis. In some cases, "if desired" follows the term. However, "if desired" is not used for coding in military medical treatment facilities; in these cases, when the term "use additional code... if desired" appears, "if desired" is disregarded and the appropriate additional code is assigned.
"usar código adicional" Esta expresión aparece sólo en el tomo 1, en aquellas subdivisiones en las que el usuario debe añadir más información por medio de un código adicional para proporcionar un cuadro más completo del diagnóstico. En algunos casos, se verá "si se desea" tras el término. En la codificación en establecimientos militares de tratamiento médico, no se usará la expresión "si se desea." Por lo tanto, cuando aparezca el término "usar código adicional... si se desea," no se tendrá en cuenta "si se desea" y se asignará el código adicional correspondiente.

utilization review The review of individual cases by a committee to make sure that services are medically necessary and to study how providers use medical care resources.

Copyright © 2011, 2007, 2003 by Saunders, an imprint of Elsevier Inc. All rights reserved.

revisión de utilización Revisión de casos individuales por un comité, para asegurarse de que los servicios son médicamente necesarios y estudiar cómo los proveedores usan los recursos de cuidados de salud.

Valsalva's maneuver A maneuver that occurs when a person strains to defecate and urinate, uses the arms and upper trunk muscles to move up in bed, or strains during laughing, coughing, or vomiting. It causes blood to become trapped in the great veins, preventing it from entering the chest and right atrium, which may cause a heart attack and death.
maniobra de Valsalva Ocurre cuando uno hace fuerza para defecar y orinar, usa los brazos y los músculos de la parte superior del tronco para levantarse de la cama, o hace fuerza al reír, toser o vomitar. Causa una retención de sangre en las venas mayores, impidiendole que entre en el pecho y la aurícula derecha y puede provocar un ataque al corazón y la muerte.

vasodilation An increase in the diameter of a blood vessel.
vasodilatación Aumento en el diámetro de un vaso sanguíneo.

vector An organism, such as an insect or a tick, that transmits the causative organisms of disease.
vector Organismos, tales como un insecto o garrapata, que transmite los organismos que provocan enfermedades.

ventricles The two lower chambers of the heart.
ventrículos Las dos cavidades inferiores del corazón.

veracity Devotion to or conformity with the truth.
veracidad Compromiso o conformidad con la verdad.

verdict The finding or decision of a jury on a matter submitted to it in trial.
veredicto Conclusión o decisión de un jurado en un asunto sometido a juicio.

versatile Embracing a variety of subjects, fields or skills; having a wide range of abilities.
versátil Que abarca diferentes sujetos, campos o destrezas; que tiene una amplia gama de destrezas.

vertigo Dizziness; a sensation of faintness or an inability to maintain normal balance.
vertigo Mareo; sensación de desmayo o de incapacidad de mantener el equilibrio normal.

vested Granted or endowed with a particular authority, right, or property; having a special interest in something.
conferirido Concedido o dotado con una autoridad, derecho o propiedad particular; que tiene un interés especial en algo.

viable Capable of living, developing, or germinating under favorable conditions.
viable Capaz de vivir, desarrollarse o germinar bajo condiciones favorables.

virtual reality An artificial environment experienced by a computer user, often by using special gloves, earphones, and goggles to enhance the experience, that feels as if it were a real environment.
realidad virtual Entorno artificial que experimenta el usuario de una computadora, muchas veces usando guantes especiales, audífonos y lentes para mejorar la experiencia, y que parece ser un ambiente real.

virulent Exceedingly pathogenic, noxious, or deadly.
virulento Excesivamente patógeno, nocivo o mortal.

viscosity The quality of being thick and lacking the capability of easy movement.
viscosidad Cualidad de espeso e incapaz de moverse con facilidad.

vocation The work in which a person is regularly employed.
profesión Trabajo en el que una persona está empleada regularmente.

volatile Referring to a flammable substance's capacity to vaporize at a low temperature; easily aroused; tending to erupt in violence.
volátil Referente a la capacidad de una sustancia flamable para evaporarse a baja temperatura. Que reacciona con facilidad y tiene tendencia a entrar en erupción de forma violenta.

vulva The external female genitalia, which begins at the mons pubis and terminates at the anus.
vulva Zona genital exterior femenina que comienza en el monte púbico y termina en el ano.

watermark A mark in paper resulting from differences in thickness usually produced by pressure from a projecting design in the mold or on a processing roll; it is visible when the paper is held up to the light.
filigrana Marca en un papel que resulta de diferencias de espesor, por lo general se produce presionando un diseño en relieve en el molde o en un rodillo de procesamiento, y es visible por transparencia.

wet mount A slide preparation in which a drop of liquid specimen is protected by a coverslip and observed with a microscope.
montaje húmedo Preparación de una lámina en la que una gota de espécimen líquido por ejemplo, se

Copyright © 2011, 2007, 2003 by Saunders, an imprint of Elsevier Inc. All rights reserved.

protege con una cubierta de vidrio y se observa con un microscopio.

wheal A localized area of edema or a raised lesion.
roncha Área localizada de un edema o una lesión protuberante.

"with" In ICD-9-CM coding, the term "with," "with mention of," or "associated with" in a title dictates that both parts of the title must be present in the statement of the diagnosis to assign the particular code.
"con" En el contexto de la ICD-9-CM, las expresiones "con", "con mención de" y "asociado con" en un título exigen que ambas partes del título estén presentes en la descripción del orden de diagnóstico para asignar el código específico.

workers' compensation Insurance against liability imposed on certain employers to pay benefits and furnish care to injured employees and to pay benefits to dependents of an employee killed in the course of or in a situation arising out of the worker's employment.
compensación laboral Seguro contra la responsabilidad impuesta a ciertos patronos para pagar beneficios y proporcionar atenciones a los trabajadores lesionados, y pagar beneficios a las personas que dependan de trabajadores que mueran en el trabajo o a causa de él.

Zip drive A small, portable disk drive that is used primarily for backing up information and archiving computer files; a 100-megabyte Zip disk holds the equivalent of about 70 floppy disks.
unidad Zip Unidad de un disco pequeño y portátil que se usa principalmente para hacer copias de seguridad de información y para guardar archivos electrónicos. Un disco Zip de 100 megabytes tiene una capacidad equivalente a la de unos 70 disquetes.

Copyright © 2011, 2007, 2003 by Saunders, an imprint of Elsevier Inc. All rights reserved.

NOTES

NOTES

NOTES

NOTES

NOTES

NOTES

NOTES

NOTES

NOTES

NOTES

NOTES

NOTES

NOTES